EMT Skills Supplement 2011 Edition Forward

The UCLA Center for Prehospital Care, *"EMT Skills Supplement"* was prepared using the *"Los Angeles County Skills Guide"* as the main reference. We wish to especially thank those individuals of the Los Angeles County Skills Revision Subcommittee for their unselfish work and devotion in putting together that document. These members include:

Greg Anderson	American Medical Response
Joan Lockwood	LADHS EMS Agency
Matt Goodman	California Institute of EMT
Patti Haley	College of the Canyons
Steve Lockwood	LA Harbor College
Justin McCullough	UCLA/DF Paramedic Education
Lucy Adams	LADHS EMS Agency
Erika Reich	LADHS EMS Agency
David Wells	LADHS EMS Agency

We would also like to recognize the UCLA Center for Prehospital Care Skills Committee for their work in the creation of this text. They include but are not limited to:

Barry Jensen	EMT Program Director
Jeff Pollakoff	EMT Program Educator
Joe Kalilikani	EMT Program Coordinator
Jessica Evans	EMT Program Coordinator
Joseph Herrick	EMT Senior Clinical Instructor
Debra "Case" Kentis	EMT Senior Clinical Instructor

Special Recognition is also given to the Baxter Larmon MICP PhD., and Todd LeGassick MPH, the directors of the Center, for their inspiration and leadership in the creation of this document.

UCLA Skills Guide for EMT-1
Table of Contents 2011 Edition

UCLA Skills Guide for EMT-1
Table of Contents 2011 Edition

UCLA Skills Guide for EMT-1
Table of Contents 2011 Edition

UCLA Skills Guide for EMT-1
Table of Contents 2011 Edition

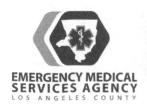

LOS ANGELES COUNTY PREHOSPITAL CODE OF ETHICS

EMERGENCY MEDICAL SERVICES AGENCY
LOS ANGELES COUNTY

Our EMS Community consists of a team of health care professionals including EMT-Is, paramedics, nurses, physicians, and system educators and administrators. This Code defines our ethical responsibilities and can be beneficial in guiding our practice. With regard to the following patient-oriented domains...

We believe that...

Patient Care & Patient Rights

competent medical care must be provided with compassion and regard for human dignity to all persons.

we cannot allow financial considerations to influence professional judgment or quality of care.

patients have the right to determine what shall be done to their body and to receive or refuse medical service, except where the patient is unable (incompetent) to make such determination.

patients (or legal representatives) need to be advised of the consequences of a refusal for treatment or transportation.

Accountability & Confidentiality

we are accountable for providing medical care to the best of our ability and for accurately and completely documenting all patient care.

in all matters pertaining to patient information and medical care, confidentiality and privacy must be respected, except where transmitting such information is necessary to deliver appropriate patient care.

Honesty & Truthfulness

patients and colleagues must be dealt with in an honest and truthful manner.

it is dishonorable to participate in or cover up misconduct of a colleague and it is also wrong to harass anyone who discloses information about situations potentially harmful to the public.

Professionalism

the highest standard of professional conduct must be maintained when providing medical care.

the hallmark of the professional is the willingness to do more than is required.

for the benefit of the patient, members of the health care team must willingly cooperate and respect each other.

colleagues lacking competence should not be misguidedly protected, but offered the opportunity for remedial action.

support of prehospital care research is important to validate our practice and to promote professional growth.

Respect & Equality

regardless of nationality, race, creed, religion, sex, or status, medical services must be delivered with compassion and respect for human dignity.

Ethical Decision Making & Conflicts of Interest

we must refuse to participate in unethical activities or procedures that exceed our scope of practice.

personal interests, such as economic gain, recognition, power, or promotion must not influence our provision of patient care.

Education & Competence

competence in all areas of our certification or licensure is our responsibility and is accomplished through education and training, skill practice and maintenance, and continuing education.

all requirements of educational programs leading to certification or licensure must be followed.

we must refrain from activities which may impair our professional judgment and ability to act competently.

Societal Obligation & Law of Practice

knowledge of prehospital care regulations and policies is necessary for optimal patient care.

we have a responsibility to contribute to an improved community.

Citizenship

our EMS system, organization, supervisors, peers, and subordinates deserve our utmost loyalty.

we must be loyal to the Constitution and the Government, and obey and respect the law.

where conflicts of interest arise, the ultimate obligation is to the public that we serve.

Commitment

we must desire to accomplish our job in a competent manner with dedication to patient care.

commitment stems from the desire to be the best one can possibly be, and the affirmation of all the preceding elements of this code.

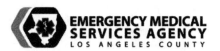

**EMERGENCY MEDICAL
SERVICES AGENCY**
LOS ANGELES COUNTY

AIRWAY EMERGENY / AIRWAY MANAGEMENT
NASOPHARYNGEAL AIRWAY (NPA)
Supplemental Information

INDICATIONS:

- Conscious or unconscious Adults (*with or without a gag reflex*) who are unable to maintain a patent airway or requires positive pressure ventilations

- Conscious or unconscious children greater than 12-months-of –age (*with or without a gag reflex*) who are unable to maintain a patent airway or requires positive pressure ventilations

- Teeth are clenched and oropharyngeal airway cannot be inserted

- Oral trauma when an oropharyngeal airway is contraindicated

CONTRAINDICATIONS:

- Infants less than 12 months due to small diameter of nostril and adenoidal tissue
- Head injury when clear fluid drains from the nose or ears (Basilar skull fracture)
- Head injury with suspected facial fractures

COMPLICATIONS:

- Vomiting
- Laryngospasm
- Injury and pressure necrosis to nasal mucosa
- Laceration of adenoids or tissue lining the nasal cavity
- Severe nosebleed
- Airway obstruction if kinked or clogged

NOTES:

- Every unresponsive patient needs to be evaluated for a patent airway and have an appropriate airway adjunct (NPA or OPA) inserted if they have or do not have a gag reflex.

- Too short of an airway that does not extend past the tongue may obstruct the airway if the tongue falls back into the oropharynx.

- Too long of an airway may pass into the esophagus and cause hypoventilation and gastric distention.

- A nasopharyngeal airway does not protect the lower airway from vomitus or secretions or hold the tongue forward.

- Never force a nasopharyngeal airway into nostril. If an obstruction or deviated septum is encountered, remove the NPA and try the other nostril.

- Use soft, flexible NPAs rather than the rigid, clear plastic NPAs which will less likely cause soft-tissue damage or nose bleeds.

- A second rescuer is needed to maintain in-line axial stabilization if spinal immobilization is required.

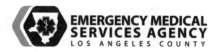

EMERGENCY MEDICAL
SERVICES AGENCY
LOS ANGELES COUNTY

EMS SKILL

AIRWAY EMERGENCY / AIRWAY MANAGEMENT
NASOPHARYNGEAL AIRWAY (NPA)

PERFORMANCE OBJECTIVES

Demonstrate competency in sizing, inserting, and removing a nasopharyngeal airway.

CONDITION

Insert a nasopharyngeal airway in a simulated adult or child who is breathing and has a gag reflex, but has difficulty maintaining a patent airway. Necessary equipment will be adjacent to the manikin or brought to the field setting.

EQUIPMENT

Adult and pediatric airway manikin, various sizes of nasopharyngeal airways, silicone spray, water-soluble lubricant, goggles, masks, gown, gloves.

PERFORMANCE CRITERIA

- Items designated by a diamond (♦) must be performed successfully to demonstrate skill competency.
- Items identified by double asterisks (**) indicate actions that are required if indicated.
- Items identified by (§) are not skill component items, but should be practiced.

INSERTION OF NASOPHARYNGEAL AIRWAY
PREPARATION

Skill Component	Key Concepts
♦ Take body substance isolation precautions	• Mandatory personal protective equipment - gloves • Situational - long sleeves, goggles, masks, gown
♦ Assess for partial or complete airway obstruction ** **Suction - _if indicated_** ** **Administer foreign body airway maneuvers - _if indicated_**	• Noisy upper airway sounds such as grunting, snoring, stridor, etc indicate a partial airway obstruction. • Suction or perform airway maneuvers to assure a patent airway.
♦ Select the largest and least deviated or obstructed nostril	• Usually the right nostril is preferred since it is generally larger than the left.

♦ Select appropriate size nasopharyngeal airway by measuring the:
 	
  • <u>Diameter</u> - size of the patient's nostril or tip of little finger
 	
  • <u>Length</u> – tip of the nose to the tip of the earlobe, tragus, or angle of the lower jaw
	• Contraindicated in patients less than 12 months due to the small diameter of the nostrils and adenoidal tissue.
	
	• Tragus is the small pointed prominence of the external ear, situated in front of the ear canal.
	
	• To ensure correct length:
	  - if the airway has an adjustable flange - use this to mark length.
	  - if no adjustable flange - hold finger at correct mark throughout insertion (depth point).

♦ Lubricate with a water-soluble lubricant	• Use <u>only</u> water soluble lubricants. DO NOT use petroleum based lubricants which may cause damage to the tissue lining of the nasal cavity and the pharynx increasing the risk of infection and bronchial pneumonia. • Lubrication minimizes resistance and decreases irritation to the nasal passage.

PROCEDURE

Skill Component	Key Concepts
♦ Hold the NPA in a "pencil-grip" fashion near the flange or depth point and gently push the tip of the nose upward while maintaining the head in a neutral position	• This provides appropriate alignment for the insertion of the NPA.

Skill Component	Key Concepts
♦ Insert the NPA with the bevel towards nasal septum	• Usually the right nostril is attempted first unless the left nostril is larger than the right or there is a contraindication for using the right. • Insertion of the NPA into the nares should not blanch the nostril. If blanching occurs, the NPA is too large for patient and a smaller diameter must be used to prevent injury to the nostril and turbinates. • If resistance is met, a gentle back-and-forth rotation between the fingers will help guide the NPA into the pharynx. If resistance continues, withdraw the NPA, re-lubricate and attempt to insert into the other nostril.

♦ Advance NPA by directing tip along floor of nasal cavity:
 	
• <u>Right</u> nostril
  - advance 2/3 of the measured length while maintaining chin-lift or jaw-thrust position
  - Continue to advance NPA until flange is seated against outside of nostril or marked area is reached
 	
• <u>Left</u> nostril
  - insert approximately 1" or until resistance is met
  - rotate 180° into position
  - advance 2/3 of the measured length while maintaining chin-lift or jaw-thrust position
  - advance until flange is seated against outside of nostril or marked area is reached
	• Performing either a chin-lift or jaw-thrust maneuver when the NPA has been inserted 2/3 of the measured length moves the mandible anteriorly and elevates the tongue so that the NPA passes beyond the posterior margin of the tongue.
	
	• Rotating the NPA 180° allows for the curvature of the NPA to conform to the natural curve of the nasal cavity.
	
	• When NPA is in position, the tip is in the posterior pharynx and should prevent possible obstruction by the tongue if it falls back into the oropharynx.

♦ Confirm proper position of the NPA: • Patient tolerates airway • Feel at proximal end of airway for airflow on expiration • Check nostril for blanching	• An NPA is usually well tolerated by conscious or semi-conscious patients who are having difficulty maintaining an airway. • If the patient gags in the final stage of insertion, the airway is too long and the NPA needs to be withdrawn slightly. • If nostril shows signs of blanching, the NPA is too large and a smaller diameter needs to be inserted.

♦ Reassess airway patency and breathing:
 	
• Skin color
• Rise and fall of chest
• Upper airway sounds
 	
** **Reposition head, check position of NPA, or suction - *if indicated***
 	
** **Administer oxygen via mask or ventilate with BVM at appropriate rate - *if indicated***
	• Noisy upper airway sounds such as grunting, snoring, stridor, etc indicate a partial airway obstruction.
	
	• Suction or perform airway maneuvers to assure a patent airway, remove NPA if indicated and repeat ABCs and reconfirm size of NPA.
	
	• Ventilate with bag-valve-mask device at appropriate rate:
	  ~ <u>Adult</u> - 10-12/minute (every 5-6 seconds)
	    Intubated adult 8-10/minute (every 6-8 seconds)
	  ~ <u>Infant/Child</u> - 12-20/minute (every 3-5 seconds)
	  ~ <u>Neonate</u> - 30-60/minute (every 1-2 seconds)

REMOVAL OF NASOPHARYNGEAL AIRWAY
PROCEDURE

Skill Component	Key Concepts

♦ Remove airway by grasping the flange and guiding the NPA out while directing the NPA down toward the chin
 	
** **Suction oropharynx - *if indicated***
	• Remove the NPA if the patient is:
	  - not tolerating the NPA
	  - an advanced airway is to be inserted

♦ Administer oxygen via mask, nasal cannula, or use a BVM device	
♦ Reassess airway and breathing	• Assess airway and breathing at least every 5 minutes or if there are changes in airway sounds or respiratory status.
♦ Dispose of contaminated equipment using approved technique	• Place contaminated equipment in plastic bag, seal, and dispose of at designated sites.

REASSESSMENT
(Ongoing Assessment)

Skill Component	Key Concepts

◆ Assess airway and breathing:
   • Continuously or at least every 5 minutes
   • Changes in airway sounds
   • Changes in respiratory status
	• A patient requiring an NPA is considered a priority patient and must be monitored continuously or re-evaluated at least every 5 minutes.

◆ Evaluate response to treatment	• Patients must be re-evaluated at least every 5 minutes if any treatment was initiated, medication administered, or a change in the patient's condition is anticipated.
◆ Evaluate results of on-going assessment and compare to baseline condition and vital signs ****Manage patient condition as indicated.**	• Evaluating and comparing results assists in recognizing if the patient is improving, responding to treatment or condition is deteriorating.

PATIENT REPORT AND DOCUMENTATION

Skill Component	Key Concepts
§ Give patient report to equal or higher level of care personnel	• Report should consist of all pertinent information regarding the assessment finding, treatment rendered and patient response to care provided.

§ Verbalize/Document:
   • Indication for insertion
   • Indication for removal - *if applicable*
   • Patient tolerance
   • Size of NPA used
   • Respiratory assessment:
     - rate
     - effort/quality
     - tidal volume
   • Oxygen administration - *If needed*
     - airway adjunct/ventilatory devices used
     - oxygen liter flow
     - ventilation rate
	• Documentation must be on either the Los Angeles County EMS Report form or departmental Patient Care Record form.

Developed: 9/02   Revised: 6/09

AIRWAY EMERGENCY / AIRWAY MANAGEMENT
OROPHARYNGEAL AIRWAY (OPA)

INDICATIONS:

- Unconscious patient <u>without</u> a gag reflex who has difficulty maintaining a patent airway.
- When a Bag-valve-mask device is used to ventilate an unconscious patient.

CONTRAINDICATIONS:

- Conscious or semi-conscious patient
- Gag reflex
- Clenched teeth
- Oral trauma

COMPLICATIONS:

- Vomiting
- Laryngospasm
- Injury to hard or soft palate or teeth (tearing, bleeding, etc)
- Airway obstruction

NOTES:

- A noisy airway is considered a partially obstructed airway.

- Purpose of an OPA is to prevent obstruction of the upper airway by the tongue and allows for air exchange.

- An oropharyngeal airway does not protect the lower airway from vomitus or secretions.

- Too small of an airway will not adequately hold the tongue forward, and might obstruct the airway.

- Too long of an airway can press the epiglottis against the opening of the trachea and result in an airway obstruction.

- Improper positioning or insertion of the airway can push the tongue against the oropharynx and result in airway obstruction.

- DO NOT secure an OPA with tape. This may result in an airway obstruction or aspiration if the patient vomits and the airway cannot be removed rapidly.

- A second rescuer is needed to maintain in-line axial stabilization if spinal immobilization is required.

- NOTE: An OPA is an "airway adjunct" and does not act alone. Proper positioning of the patient's airway (i.e. "head-tilt, chin-lift") in addition to the insertion / positioning of the OPA is needed to maintain a "patent" (open) airway.

Developed 1/01

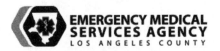

EMERGENCY MEDICAL SERVICES AGENCY
LOS ANGELES COUNTY

EMS SKILL

AIRWAY EMERGENCY / AIRWAY MANAGEMENT
OROPHARYNGEAL AIRWAY (OPA)

PERFORMANCE OBJECTIVES
Demonstrate competency in sizing, inserting and removing an oropharyngeal airway.

CONDITION
Insert an oropharyngeal airway in a simulated unconscious adult, child or infant who is breathing, has no gag reflex, but has difficulty maintaining a patent airway. Necessary equipment will be adjacent to the manikin or brought to the field setting.

EQUIPMENT
Adult, infant or child airway manikin, various sizes of oropharyngeal airways (0-#6), tongue blade or equivalent, pediatric resuscitation tape, goggles, mask, gown, gloves.

PERFORMANCE CRITERIA
- Items designated by a diamond (♦) must be performed successfully to demonstrate skill competency.
- Items identified by double asterisks (**) indicate actions that are required if indicated.
- Items identified by (§) are not skill component items, but should be practiced.

INSERTION OF OROPHARYNGEAL AIRWAY	
PREPARATION	
Skill Component	**Key Concepts**
♦ Take body substance isolation precautions	• Mandatory (minimal) personal protective equipment – gloves
♦ Assess for partial or complete airway obstruction ** **Suction - _if indicated_** ** **Administer foreign body airway maneuvers - _if indicated_**	• Noisy upper airway sounds such as grunting, snoring, strider, etc indicate a partial airway obstruction. • Suction or perform airway maneuvers to assure a patent airway.
♦ Assess for indications for insertion of an airway adjunct	• Any unconscious patient <u>without</u> a gag reflex who has difficulty maintaining a patent airway. • Performing positive pressure ventilations for an unconscious patient.
♦ Select appropriate size by measuring the OPA from : • Corner of the mouth to the tragus or the earlobe **OR** • Center of the mouth to the angle of the lower jaw	• Should take both measurements and choose appropriate size. If the fit is not perfect, choose the smaller one, because if the OPA is too large it may obstruct the airway. • If the size is not located on the OPA, document as infant, small, medium or large. • Too small of an airway will not adequately hold the tongue forward. Too long of an airway can press the epiglottis against the opening of the trachea and result in an airway obstruction.
PROCEDURE	
Skill Component	**Key Concepts**
♦ Open the airway: • <u>Medical</u> - head-tilt/chin-lift maneuver • <u>Trauma</u> - jaw-thrust maneuver	• A second rescuer is needed to maintain in-line axial stabilization if spinal immobilization is required.
♦ Open the mouth by applying pressure on the chin with thumb ** **Remove visible obstruction or suction - _if indicated_**	• Thumb pressure on the chin displaces the jaw. DO NOT use fingers to open the mouth. The "crossed-finger" technique may result in injury to the rescuer and may puncture gloves. (However, the crossed-finger method is a step found on the National Registry Skills Exam.) • DO NOT force teeth open. Insert a nasopharyngeal airway if unable to open the mouth. • Have suction ready at all times and use as indicated.

Skill Component	Key Concepts
◆ Insert the OPA airway into the oropharynx by inserting the tip: • <u>Toward</u> the hard palate and rotate 180° when tip passes the soft palate **OR** • <u>Straight</u> while displacing the tongue anteriorly with a tongue blade or equivalent device **OR** • <u>Sideways</u> while displacing the tongue anteriorly with a tongue blade or equivalent device and rotate OPA 90° when tip passes the soft palate	• Avoid pressure on the palate to prevent injury to the hard and soft palate. • DO NOT push the tongue back into the oropharynx. This will result in an airway obstruction. • Displacing the tongue anteriorly is the recommended method for inserting an OPA in a pediatric patient. _This is the only method that should be used for inserting an OPA in infants._
◆ Advance the airway until the flange rests on lips	• Do not secure the OPA with tape. If the OPA is taped it cannot be removed quickly and aspiration may occur if the patient regains consciousness or a gag reflex and vomits. • The curvature of the OPA follows the contour of the tongue with the flange resting against the lips and the tip of the OPA opening into the pharynx.
◆ Reassess airway patency and breathing: • Skin color • Rise and fall of chest • Upper airway sounds ** **Reposition head, check position of OPA, and suction - _if indicated_** ** **Administer oxygen via mask or ventilate with BVM - _if indicated_**	• Noisy upper airway sounds such as grunting, snoring, stridor, etc indicate a partial airway obstruction. Perform airway maneuvers to ensure a patent airway, remove OPA if indicated and repeat ABCs and reconfirm size of OPA. • Ventilate with bag-valve-mask device at appropriate rate: ~ Adult - 10-12/minute (every 5-6 seconds) Intubated adult 8-10/minute (6-8 seconds) ~ <u>Infant/Child</u> - 12-20/minute (3-5 seconds) ~ <u>Neonate</u> - 30-60/minute (1-2 seconds)

REMOVAL OF OROPHARYNGEAL AIRWAY
PROCEDURE

Skill Component	Key Concepts
◆ Remove airway: • Grasp flange and guide the OPA out by directing airway down toward chin **Suction oropharynx - _if indicated_**	• Remove airway if patient: - is not tolerating the OPA - is vomiting - regains consciousness - regains a gag reflex
◆ Administer oxygen via mask, nasal cannula, or BVM device - _as indicated_	
◆ Reassess airway and breathing	
◆ Dispose of contaminated equipment using approved technique	• Place contaminated equipment in plastic bag, seal, and dispose of at designated site.

REASSESSMENT
(Ongoing Assessment)

Skill Component	Key Concepts
◆ Assess airway and breathing: • Continuously or at least every 5 minutes • Changes in airway sounds • Changes in respiratory status	• A patient requiring an OPA is considered a priority patient and must be monitored continuously or re-evaluated at least every 5 minutes.
◆ Evaluate response to treatment	
◆ Evaluate results of reassessment and compare to baseline condition and vital signs **Manage patient condition as indicated.**	

Skill Component	Key Concepts
§ Give patient report to equal or higher level of care personnel	• Report should consist of all pertinent information regarding the assessment finding, treatment rendered and patient response to care provided.

§ Verbalize/Document
  • Indication for insertion
  • Indication for removal - _if applicable_
  • Patient tolerance/effect
  • Size of OPA used
 	
  • Respiratory assessment:
    - rate
    - effort/quality
    - tidal volume
 	
  Oxygen administration - _If needed_
    - airway adjunct/ventilatory devices used
    - oxygen liter flow
    - ventilation rate
	• Documentation must be on either the Los Angeles County EMS Report or departmental Patient Care Record form.

Developed: 1/01   Revised: 4.02, 10/02, 9/04, 4/09

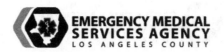
AIRWAY EMERGENCY / AIRWAY MANAGEMENT
SUCTIONING - OROPHARYNGEAL
Supplemental Information

INDICATIONS: To clear the airway in patients who are unable to maintain a patent airway due to oral secretions.

- Excessive oral secretions (noisy respirations)
- Respiratory distress due to oral secretions/vomitus
- Prevent aspiration of secretions/vomitus

COMPLICATIONS:

- Hypoxia
- Bronchospasm
- Cardiac dysrhythmias
- Hypotension
- Oral trauma/broken teeth
- Infection/sepsis
- Vomiting
- Aspiration

CONTRAINDICATION:

- Infants less than 1 year of age – use bulb syringe

NOTES:

- A clean technique must be maintained throughout suctioning procedure to prevent infection.

- Use rigid catheters with caution in conscious or semiconscious patients. Put the tip of the catheter in only as far as can be visualized to prevent activating the gag reflex.

- Rigid catheters are best for suctioning large amount of secretions or large particles.

- Keep suction settings between 80-120 mmHg and adjust lower for pediatric and elderly patients (50-100mmHg). Excessive negative pressures may cause significant hypoxia and damage to tracheal mucosa. Too little suction will be ineffective.

- Hand-powered suction devices may be used as long as they have an adaptor for a flexible catheter.

- Pre-oxygenation may be required depending on patient's condition. This offsets volume and oxygen loss during suctioning.

- Suctioning longer than recommended time will result in hypoxia. Maximum suction time depends on patient's age and tolerance:
  - Adults maximum 10-15 seconds
  - Children maximum of 5-10 seconds
  - Infants - no longer than 5 seconds

- If vagal stimulation occurs, the patient may experience bradycardia, especially pediatric patients.

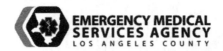

EMERGENCY MEDICAL SERVICES AGENCY
LOS ANGELES COUNTY

EMS SKILL

AIRWAY EMERGENCY / AIRWAY MANAGEMENT
SUCTIONING - OROPHARYNGEAL

PERFORMANCE OBJECTIVES

Demonstrate competency in performing oropharyngeal suctioning using a rigid and flexible suction catheter and a bulb syringe.

CONDITION

Suction a simulated patient who is either conscious or unresponsive and is unable to maintain a patent airway due to copious oral secretions. Necessary equipment will be adjacent to the patient or brought to the field setting.

EQUIPMENT

Simulated adult and pediatric airway management manikin, oxygen tank with connecting tubing, suction device with connecting tubing, or hand-powered suction device with adaptor, hard and flexible suction catheters, bulb syringe, normal saline irrigation solution, container, gloves, goggles, masks, gown, waste receptacle, timing device.

PERFORMANCE CRITERIA

- Items designated by a diamond (♦) must be performed successfully to demonstrate skill competency.
- Items identified by double asterisks (**) indicate actions that are required if indicated.
- Items identified by (§) are not skill component items, but should be practiced.
- A clean technique must be maintained throughout suctioning procedure.

PREPARATION	
Skill Component	**Key Concepts**
♦ Take body substance isolation precautions	• Mandatory personal protective equipment - gloves, goggles • Situational - masks, gown
♦ Assess patient for the need to suction oral secretions	• Indications for suctioning: noisy respirations, coughing up secretions, respiratory distress or patient request.
♦ Open suction kit or individual supplies	• Use the inside of the wrapper to establish a clean field.
♦ Fill container with irrigation solution	• Saline or water is used to flush suction catheter as needed.
♦ Ensure suction device is working ** *Set appropriate suction setting:* • *Adult - between 80-120 mmHg* • *Pediatric and the elderly - between 50-100mmHg*	• Battery operated suction machine or hand-powered suction devices may be used. An adaptor for a flexible catheter is required with hand-powered suction devices. • Excessive negative pressures may cause significant hypoxia, damage to tracheal mucosa or lung collapse.
♦ Measure depth of catheter insertion from corner of mouth to edge of ear lobe	• Never insert catheter past the base of the tongue. This may stimulate the gag reflex and cause vomiting.

RIGID CATHETER (TONSIL TIP, YANKAUER) PROCEDURE	
Skill Component	**Key Concepts**
♦ Remove oxygen source - *if indicated*	• Oxygen should be maintained until ready to suction. • A nasal cannula does not need to be removed for oropharyngeal suctioning.
♦ Connect rigid catheter to suction tubing/device	• Keep catheter in package until ready to use. • Provide a clean field for catheter if reuse is indicated.

Skill Component	Key Concepts
◆ Open patient's mouth by applying pressure on the chin with your thumb	• Thumb pressure on the chin displaces the jaw. DO NOT use fingers to open the mouth. The "crossed-finger" technique may result in injury to the rescuer and may puncture gloves. *Note: The crossed-finger method is a step found on the National Registry Skills Exam.* • DO NOT force teeth open. Use a flexible catheter if unable to open the mouth.
◆ Insert rigid catheter into mouth without applying suction	• The patient is not being oxygenated during this step and applying suction would deplete any oxygen reserve.
◆ Advance catheter gently to depth measured	• Never insert catheter past the base of the tongue. This may stimulate the gag reflex, cause vomiting and bradycardia.
◆ Suction while withdrawing using a circular motion around mouth, pharynx and gum line ** *Maximum suction time of 5-15 seconds:* • *Adults maximum 10-15 seconds* • *Peds maximum of 5-10 seconds*	• Suctioning longer than recommended time will result in hypoxia. Maximum suction time depends on patient's age and tolerance. • Rigid catheters are contraindicated for infants less than 1 year of age.
◆ Replace oxygen source or ventilate patient at approximate rate of: • Adult - 10-20/minute • Peds - 12-20/minute	• Ventilation rates for pediatric patients vary due to a wide age range.
◆ Evaluate airway patency and heart rate - *repeat procedure if needed*	• Observe patient for hypoxemia: dysrhythmias, cyanosis, anxiety, bronchospasms and changes in mental status. • If vagal stimulation occurs, the patient may experience bradycardia, especially pediatric patients. • Allow patient to rest and regain adequate oxygen levels between suction attempts.
◆ Suction remaining water into canister, discard container and change gloves	• Irrigation solution is contaminated and should be treated the same as secretions.
◆ Discard or secure contaminated catheter in a clean area: • Discard into an approved receptacle **OR** • Return used catheter to package and place in clean area for future use	• Provide a clean field for catheter if reuse is indicated.

FLEXIBLE CATHETER (WHISTLE STOP, FRENCH) PROCEDURE

Skill Component	Key Concepts
◆ Remove oxygen source - *if indicated*	• Oxygen should be maintained until ready to suction. • A nasal cannula does not need to be removed for oropharyngeal suctioning.
◆ Connect flexible catheter to suction tubing/device	• Keep catheter in package until ready to use. • Provide a clean field for catheter if reuse is indicated.
◆ Open patient's mouth by applying pressure on the chin with your thumb	• Thumb pressure on the chin displaces the jaw. DO NOT use fingers to open the mouth. The "crossed-finger" technique may result in injury to the rescuer and may puncture gloves. *Note: The crossed-finger method is a step found on the National Registry Skills Exam.* • DO NOT force teeth open. Use a flexible catheter if unable to open the mouth.

Skill Component	Key Concepts
◆ Insert flexible catheter along the roof of the mouth without applying suction	• The patient is not being oxygenated at this time and applying suction would deplete any oxygen reserve that is present.
◆ Advance catheter gently to depth measured	• Never insert catheter past the base for the tongue. This may stimulate the gag reflex, cause vomiting and bradycardia.
◆ Suction while withdrawing moving catheter from side to side around mouth, pharynx and gum line ** *Maximum suction time of 5-15 seconds:* • *Adults maximum 10-15 seconds* • *Children maximum of 5-10 seconds* • *Infants - no longer than 5 seconds*	• Suctioning longer than recommended time will result in hypoxia. Maximum suction time depends on patient's age and tolerance:
◆ Replace oxygen source or ventilate patient at approximate rate of: • Adult - 10-12/minute • Child - 12-20/minute • Infant - 20-30/minute • Neonate - 30-60/minute	• The range for pediatric patients varies due to a wide age range.
◆ Evaluate airway patency and heart rate - *repeat procedure if needed*	• Observe patient for hypoxemia: dysrhythmias, cyanosis, anxiety, bronchospasms and changes in mental status. • If vagal stimulation occurs, the patient may experience bradycardia, especially pediatric patients. • Allow patient to rest and regain adequate oxygen levels between suction attempts.

◆ Discard or secure in a clean area contaminated catheter:
• Discard into an approved receptacle:
  - Coil contaminated catheter around sterile (dominant) hand and pull glove over catheter
  - Pull glove from other hand over packaged catheter and discard in approved waste receptacle
    OR
• Return used catheter to package and place in clean area for future use	

◆ Suction remaining water into canister, discard container and change gloves	• Rinse solution is contaminated and should be treated the same as secretions.

BULB SYRINGE PROCEDURE

Skill Component	Key Concepts
◆ Prime bulb (squeeze out air) and hold in depressed position	• The bulb syringe acts as both the "pump" and collection container for manual suction. • To prime bulb syringe depress (squeeze) it to remove all air and hold.
◆ Open patient's mouth by applying pressure on the chin with your thumb	• Thumb pressure on the chin displaces the jaw. DO NOT use fingers to open the mouth. The "crossed-finger" technique may result in injury to the rescuer and may puncture gloves. *Note: The crossed-finger method is a step found on the National Registry Skills Exam.*
◆ Insert tip of primed syringe into mouth and advance gently to back of mouth	• DO NOT insert tip past the base of the tongue. This may stimulate the gag reflex, cause vomiting and bradycardia.
◆ Slowly release pressure on bulb to draw secretions into syringe	• The bulb syringe acts as both the "pump" and collection container for manual suction.

Skill Component	Key Concepts
◆ Remove syringe from mouth	
◆ Empty secretions into designated container by squeezing bulb several times	• All secretions are to be treated as contaminated waste.

◆ Replace oxygen source or ventilate patient at approximate rate of:
  • Adult - 10-12/minute
  • Child - 12-20/minute
  • Infant - 20-30/minute
  • Neonate - 30-60/minute
	• The rate for ventilating pediatric patients varies due to a large age range.

◆ Evaluate airway patency and heart rate - _repeat procedure if needed_	• Observe patient for hypoxemia: dysrhythmias, cyanosis, anxiety, bronchospasms and changes in mental status. • If vagal stimulation occurs, the patient may experience bradycardia, especially pediatric patients. • Allow patient to rest and regain adequate oxygen levels between suction attempts.
◆ Rinse bulb syringe with irrigation solution	• Rinsing bulb syringe removes secretions for future use.
◆ Return used bulb syringe to package/container and place in clean area for future use	
◆ Discard irrigation solution into designated container and change gloves	• Irrigation solution is contaminated and should be treated the same as secretions.

REASSESSMENT
(Ongoing Assessment

Skill Component	Key Concepts nts

§ Assess airway, breathing and heart rate:
  • Continuously or at least every 5 minutes
  • Changes in airway sounds
  • Changes in respiratory status
	• If vagal stimulation occurs, the patient may experience bradycardia, especially pediatric patients.

◆ Evaluate response to treatment	• Patients must be re-evaluated at least every 5 minutes if any treatment was initiated or medication administered.

PATIENT REPORT AND DOCUMENTATION

Skill Component	Key Concepts

§ Verbalize/Document
  • Indication for suctioning
  • Oxygen liter flow
  • Patient's tolerance of procedure
  • Problems encountered
  • Type of secretions:
    - color
    - consistency
    - quantity
    - odor
  • Respiratory assessment and heart rate:
    - respiratory rate
    - effort/quality
    - tidal volume
    - lung sounds
	• Documentation must be on either the Los Angeles County EMS Report form or departmental Patient Care Record form.

Developed: 12/02   Revised: 1/05, 1/10

	• Allow patient to rest and regain adequate oxygen levels between suction attempts.
♦ Rinse bulb syringe with irrigation solution	• Rinsing bulb syringe removes secretions for future use.
♦ Return used bulb syringe to package/container and place in clean area for future use	
♦ Discard irrigation solution into designated container and change gloves	• Irrigation solution is contaminated and should be treated the same as secretions.

ONGOING ASSESSMENT

Skill Component	Teaching Points
§ Assess airway, breathing and heart rate • Continuously or at least every 5 minutes • Changes in airway sounds • Changes in respiratory status	• If vagal stimulation occurs, the patient may experience bradycardia, especially pediatric patients.

DOCUMENTATION

Skill Component	Teaching Points

§ Verbalize/Document
 	
• Indication for suctioning
• Oxygen liter flow
• Patient's tolerance of procedure
• Problems encountered
 	
• Type of secretions:
  - color
  - consistency
  - quantity
  - odor
 	
• Respiratory assessment and heart rate:
  - respiratory rate
  - effort/quality
  - tidal volume
  - lung sounds
	• Documentation must be on either the Los Angeles County EMS Report form or departmental Patient Care Record form.

Developed: 12/02
Revised: 1/05

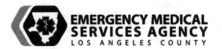

AIRWAY EMERGENCY / AIRWAY MANAGEMENT
SUCTIONING - TRACHEOSTOMY TUBE AND STOMA
Supplemental Information

DEFINITIONS:

- <u>Inner cannula</u> - a "sleeve" which fits inside the tracheostomy tube and may be removed for cleaning

- <u>Pre-oxygenation</u> - increasing oxygen liter flow for a brief period of time or ventilating the patient 3-4 times with a bag-valve device to increase the blood oxygen level

- <u>Tracheotomy</u> - a surgical incision into the trachea to establish an airway that may be temporary or permanent

- <u>Tracheostomy (trach)</u> - a tracheal stoma (opening) that results from a tracheotomy

- <u>Tracheostomy</u> (trach) tube - a plastic or metal tube inserted below the 2nd or 3rd tracheal ring bypassing the epiglottis

INDICATIONS: To maintain a patent airway in patients with a tracheostomy tube or stoma.

- Rattling mucus sound from tracheostomy (noisy respirations)
- Bubbles of mucus in trach
- Coughing up secretions
- Patient requests to be suctioned
- Respiratory distress due to airway obstruction.

COMPLICATIONS:

• Hypoxia	• Tracheal trauma
• Bronchospasm	• Infection/sepsis
• Cardiac dysrhythmias	• Cardiac arrest
• Hypotension	

NOTES:

- Aseptic technique must be maintained throughout suctioning procedure to prevent infection.

- Excessive suctioning should be avoided to decrease potential for tracheal damage and increase in mucus production.

- Catheter size should not exceed ½ the inner diameter of the airway. Larger catheters may cause suction-induced hypoxia, lung collapse and damage to tracheal tissues.

- Establish and maintain a sterile field. Use the inside of the wrapper to establish field for equipment.

- Hand-operated vacuum suction devices may be used as long as they have an adaptor for a flexible catheter.

- Keep suction setting between 80-120 mmHg and adjust setting lower for pediatric and elderly patients (50-100 mmHg). Excessive negative pressures may cause significant hypoxia, damage to tracheal mucosa or lung collapse. Too little suction is ineffective.

- Pre-oxygenation may be required depending on patient's condition. This offsets volume and oxygen loss during suctioning.

- Patient may or may not be on oxygen and have either a T-bar or tracheal mask for humidification.

- Oxygen should be maintained until ready to suction. Flow rate may need to be adjusted to prepare patient for suctioning.

- Rotating the catheter prevents the direct suctioning of the tracheal mucosa. Roll the catheter between thumb and forefinger for rotating motion.

- Suctioning longer than recommended time will result in hypoxia. Maximum suction time depends on patient's age and tolerance and is timed from the **insertion to withdrawal of the catheter:**

  - Adults maximum 10-15 seconds

  - Children maximum of 5-10 seconds

  - Infants - no longer than 5 seconds

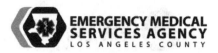

EMERGENCY MEDICAL SERVICES AGENCY
LOS ANGELES COUNTY

EMS SKILL

AIRWAY EMERGENCY / AIRWAY MANAGEMENT
SUCTIONING - TRACHEOSTOMY TUBE AND STOMA

PERFORMANCE OBJECTIVES

Demonstrate competency in suctioning a patient with a tracheostomy tube while maintaining aseptic technique.

CONDITION

Suction a simulated patient that who has a tracheostomy tube/stoma and has copious secretions and difficulty breathing. Necessary equipment will be adjacent to the manikin or brought to the field setting.

EQUIPMENT

Simulated adult and pediatric tracheostomy manikin, tracheostomy tube (metal/plastic) with an inner cannula, oxygen tank with connecting tubing, T-bar or tracheal mask, suction device with connecting tubing or hand-powered suction device with adaptor, sterile flexible suction catheter, sterile normal saline irrigation solution, sterile container, plastic saline irrigation vial/ampule, vial of normal saline, 5cc syringe, removable needle, sterile and unsterile gloves, goggles, masks, gown, waste receptacle, timing device.

PERFORMANCE CRITERIA

- Items designated by a diamond (♦) must be performed successfully to demonstrate skill competency.
- Items identified by double asterisks (**) indicate actions that are required if indicated.
- Items identified by (§) should be practiced.
- Ventilations must be at least at the minimum rate required.
- Must maintain aseptic technique.

PREPARATION	
Skill Component	**Key Concepts**
♦ Take body substance isolation precautions	• Mandatory personal protective equipment – gloves
♦ Assess patient for the need to suction tracheal secretions	• Indications for suctioning: noisy respirations, coughing up secretions, respiratory distress or patient request.
♦ Open suction kit or individual supplies	• Establish and maintain a sterile field. Use the inside of the wrapper to establish field. • Catheter size should not exceed ½ the inner diameter of the airway.
♦ Open/unfold sterile container and fill with irrigation solution	• Sterile saline is used to flush suction catheter as needed. • Depending on kit, container may be under gloves and catheter; this should be removed without contaminating gloves and catheter. Not a problem to put on sterile gloves if an assistant is present.
♦ Ensure suction device is working ** *Set appropriate suction setting:* • *Adult - between 80-120 mmHg* • *Pediatric and the elderly - between 50-100mmHg*	• Hand-powered suction devices may be used as long as they have an adaptor for a flexible catheter. • Excessive negative pressures may cause significant hypoxia, damage to tracheal mucosa or lung collapse.

PROCEDURE	
Skill Component	**Key Concepts**
♦ Pre-oxygenate patient - *if indicated*: • Increase Oxygen liter flow **OR** • Ventilate with Bag-valve device 4-5 times	• Hyper-oxygenation may be required in patient's dependent on O_2 source or if ventilator dependant to offset volume or oxygen loss during suctioning.
♦ Remove oxygen source - *if indicated*	• Patient may or may not be on oxygen and have either a T-bar or tracheal mask for humidification. • Oxygen should be maintained until ready to suction. Flow rate may need to be adjusted to prepare patient for suctioning.

Skill Component	Key Concepts
◆ Unlock and remove inner cannula - *if indicated*	• Not all trach tubes have inner cannulas. • The inner cannula does not need to be removed for routine suctioning. However, if the patient is in respiratory distress the inner cannula must be removed in order to avoid pushing thick secretions back down the trachea. • Sometimes just removing the inner cannula corrects the problem. The cannula may only need to be cleaned and replaced.
◆ Put on sterile gloves	• Sterile gloves are pulled over existing clean gloves.
◆ Connect sterile catheter to suction tubing/device ** ***Keep one (dominant) hand sterile***	• The suction catheter should only be handled using sterile glove. • Keep catheter in sterile package until ready to use. • Catheter size should be ½ the inner diameter of the trach tube to allow for ease of insertion and air to enter during suctioning.
◆ Suction small amount of irrigation solution to: • Ensure suction device is working • Lubricate tip of catheter	• Lubricating the tip of the catheter with irrigation solution prevents the catheter from adhering to the sides of the trach tube or tracheal mucosa.
◆ Insert catheter into tracheostomy tube/stoma without applying suction	• The patient is not being oxygenated at this time and applying suction would deplete any oxygen reserve. • If patient has a stoma, suctioning during insertion may damage the lining of the tracheal mucosa.

◆ Advance catheter gently to appropriate level:
• Shallow suctioning - opening of trach tube/stoma
   OR
• Measured suctioning - length of trach tube
   OR
• Deep suctioning - past trach tube to carina
	• Shallow/measured suctioning may be all that is needed. Deep suctioning is usually not necessary unless cough is ineffective and airway is not cleared.
	
	• Deep suctioning is at the level of the carina which is determined by the catheter meeting resistance during insertion.
	
	• The patient may cough when the tip of catheter touches the carina or develop bronchospasms.
	
	• Catheter insertion should be accomplished as rapidly as possible since the patient is not oxygenated during this step.

◆ Withdraw catheter slightly before applying suction - *if beyond trach tube*	• Withdrawing the catheter slightly before applying suction prevents damage to the mucosa of the carina.
◆ Suction while withdrawing catheter using a rotating motion and observe patient's response: ** ***Maximum suction time of 5-15 seconds from insertion to withdrawal of catheter.*** • ***Adults maximum 10-15 seconds*** • ***Children maximum of 5-10 seconds*** • ***Infants - no longer than 5 seconds***	• Rotating the catheter prevents the direct suctioning of the tracheal mucosa and suctions secretions from side of the tube. • Roll the catheter between thumb and forefinger for rotating motion. • Suctioning longer than recommended time will result in hypoxia. Maximum suction time depends on patient's age and tolerance: • Patient's response by coughing or grimacing may indicate the catheter is too deep and irritating the tracheal mucosa or carina.
◆ Place patient on oxygen or replace oxygen source - *if indicated*	• Patients may need supplemental oxygen after suctioning. • If the patient is ventilator dependent, ventilate the patient with a bag-valve device in between suctioning
◆ Evaluate airway patency and heart rate - *repeat procedure if needed* ** ***If secretions are thick and unable to clear tracheostomy tube, instill sterile saline and repeat previous steps***	• Observe patient for hypoxemia, dysrhythmias, cyanosis, anxiety, bronchospasms and changes in mental status. • If vagal stimulation occurs, the patient may experience bradycardia, especially pediatric patients. • EMTs & paramedics may instill normal saline into the trach tube if needed to loosen secretions. However, this procedure poses a great risk for pneumonia and ***should only be done if absolutely necessary***. • Allow patient to rest and regain adequate oxygen levels between suctioning attempts.

Skill Component	Key Concepts
♦ Suction remaining irrigation solution into collection canister and discard appropriately	• Irrigation solution is contaminated and should be treated the same as secretions.

♦ Discard contaminated catheter:
  • Coil contaminated catheter around sterile (dominant) hand and pull glove over catheter
  • Pull glove from other hand over packaged catheter and discard in approved waste receptacle	

REPLACE INNER CANNULA

Skill Component	Key Concepts

♦ Check for spare or clean the inner cannula - *if needed*	• Some patients have a spare inner cannula at the bedside.
	• If the inner cannula needs to be cleaned, this can be done by the rescuer, caregiver or partner.
	• Procedure for cleaning the inner cannula:
	  - rinse the inner cannula with saline/tap water
	  - suction or use a pipe cleaner to remove secretions
	  - gently tap the cannula to remove excess solution before reinsertion

♦ Remove oxygen source	
♦ Replace clean inner cannula and lock	• The inner cannula must be replaced in order to connect to a T-bar, ventilator or bag-valve device.
♦ Replace oxygen source	

REASSESSMENT
(Ongoing Assessment)

Skill Component	Key Concepts

§ Assess airway, breathing and heart rate:
  • Continuously or at least every 5 minutes
  • Changes in airway sounds
  • Changes in respiratory status
	• If vagal stimulation occurs, the patient may experience bradycardia, especially pediatric patients.

PATIENT REPORT AND DOCUMENTATION

Skill Component	Key Concepts

§ Verbalize/Document
  • Indication for suctioning
  • Oxygen liter flow
  • Patient's tolerance of procedure
  • Problems encountered
  • Type of secretions:
    - color
    - consistency
    - quantity
    - odor
  • Respiratory assessment and heart rate:
    - respiratory rate
    - effort/quality
    - tidal volume
    - lung sounds
	• Documentation must be on either the Los Angeles County EMS Report form or departmental Patient Care Record form.

NSTILLATION OF NORMAL SALINE
Normal Saline is only instilled if absolutely necessary

Skill Component	Key Concepts

§ Prepare saline irrigation solution - _if indicated_
 	
  • Check saline for:
    - drug name
    - integrity of container/medication
    - concentration/dose
    - clarity
    - expiration date
  • Twist off top of saline irrigation vial /ampule
          OR
  • Prepare a syringe with 5cc normal saline and remove needle - _if within scope of practice_
	• EMTs & paramedics may instill normal saline into the trach tube if needed to loosen secretions. However, this procedure poses a great risk for pneumonia and **should only be done if absolutely necessary**.
	
	• Each patient must be evaluated early to determine the need for irrigation to loosen secretions.
	
	• EMTs & paramedics may use prepared saline irrigation vial /ampule. _Caution - the rescuer must ensure that the vial/ampule contains normal saline and not a medication such as albuterol._
	
	• Paramedics may use a syringe to draw up saline and after removing needle instill into the trach tube.

§ Instill 1-5ml of sterile saline down tracheostomy tube
  • 3-5ml for adults
  • 1-2 ml for pediatric patients
	• Amount of saline instilled depends on patient's age and tolerance.
	
	• Pediatric patients falling into any color zone on the Broselow tape should have only 1-2 ml of solution instilled and those bigger than the Broselow tape may tolerate 3-5 ml of solution.

§ Repeat suction procedure	

Developed: 10/02   Revised: 1/05, 1/10

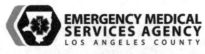

EMERGENCY MEDICAL SERVICES AGENCY
LOS ANGELES COUNTY

EMS SKILL

AIRWAY EMERGENCY: AIRWAY OBSTRUCTION
ADULT

PERFORMANCE OBJECTIVES
Demonstrate competency in recognizing and managing a foreign body airway obstruction in an adult who is choking

CONDITION
Recognize and manage an airway obstruction in an adult who is found choking. Necessary equipment will be adjacent to the manikin or brought to the field setting.

EQUIPMENT
Adult CPR manikin, adult bag-valve-mask or barrier device, O_2 connecting tubing, oxygen source with flow regulator, goggles, various masks, gown, gloves, timing device.

PERFORMANCE CRITERIA
- Items designated by a diamond (♦) must be performed successfully to demonstrate skill competency.
- Items identified by double asterisks (**) indicate actions that are required, if indicated.
- Items identified by (§) should be practiced.
- Ventilations and compressions must be performed at the minimum rate required.

PREPARATION	
Skill Component	**Key Concepts**
♦ Take body substance isolation precautions	• Mandatory (minimal) personal protective equipment – gloves
♦ Assess scene safety/scene size-up ** *Consider spinal immobilization - if indicated*	• If unknown as to possible trauma, manage as trauma (determined by environment and information obtained from bystanders).
♦ Evaluate need for additional BSI precautions	• Situational - goggles, mask, gown
♦ Approach the patient and introduce yourself to the patient/caregivers	

RESPONSIVE ADULT PROCEDURE	
Skill Component	**Key Concepts**
♦ Establish that the person is choking: ** *Call for additional resources – if needed*	• <u>Mild Obstruction:</u> - adequate air exchange - coughing - gagging - wheezing • <u>Severe Obstruction:</u> - poor or no air exchange - increased respiratory distress - weak, ineffective cough or no cough - high-pitched noise while inhaling (stridor) or no noise - unable to speak - clutching the neck (universal sign of choking) - cyanosis - decreasing level of consciousness
♦ Attempt to remove foreign body obstruction: • <u>Mild obstruction</u> - Encourage patient to cough • <u>Severe obstruction</u> - Perform abdominal thrusts (Heimlich maneuver)	• DO NOT interfere if the patient has an effective cough. • If the patient is sitting or standing, place the patient in a position that allows for balance and supports the patient when performing abdominal thrusts.
Continued	**Continued**

Skill Component	Key Concepts
<ul><li>- Stand or kneel behind the victim and place thumb side of fist between the patient's xiphoid and umbilicus</li><li>- Grasp fist with other hand and give quick inward and upward thrusts - *as many times as needed*</li></ul>	<ul><li>If the patient is found supine, straddle the patient and perform abdominal thrusts.</li><li>Deliver as many abdominal thrusts as needed until the object is expelled, the patient starts to breathe or becomes unresponsive.</li></ul>
♦ Continue abdominal thrusts until obstruction is relieved or the patient becomes unresponsive. ** **If unresponsive – start sequence for airway obstruction for unresponsive adult.**	

♦ Manage ventilations after removal of obstruction:
 	
• If breathing is restored and adequate:
  - medical - place in recovery position if patient is altered or unresponsive
  - trauma - initiate spinal immobilization – *if indicated*
 	
• If breathing is absent or inadequate:
  - perform rescue breathing of 10-12 per minute (1 breath every 5-6 seconds) with BVM or barrier device
	<ul><li>Patients who are responsive and <u>not</u> altered should be placed in a position of comfort, unless spinal immobilization is indicated.</li><li>Patients who are altered or unresponsive should be placed in the recovery position to reduce the chance of the airway being occluded by the tongue and the aspiration of mucus or vomitus.</li><li>Some signs of inadequate breathing are: respiratory distress, fast/slow respirations, cyanosis, poor perfusion, and altered LOC.</li><li>Supplemental oxygen should always be used after spontaneous breathing has resumed.</li><li>Use <u>*only*</u> enough force when providing positive pressure ventilation to allow for adequate chest rise. Over-inflation results in gastric distention and decreases tidal volume by elevating the diaphragm.</li><li>Use of a BVM by a single rescuer can result in an inadequate seal on the face and may not be as effective as a barrier device.</li><li>If the airway is open and it is difficult to compress the bag and/or air leaks around the seal, an airway obstruction may <u>still</u> be present.</li></ul>

UNRESPONSIVE ADULT

PROCEDURE

(Patients who were previously responsive may have the obstruction relieved when muscles relax)

Skill Component	Key Concepts
♦ Establish unresponsiveness ** ***Call for additional resources – if needed***	

♦ Open airway:
• <u>Medical</u>
  - head-tilt/chin-lift
 	
• <u>Trauma</u>
  - jaw-thrust
  - neutral position (tragus of ear should be level with top of shoulder)
 	
** ***Clear/suction airway - if indicated***
	<ul><li>The tongue is the most common cause of airway obstruction due to decreased muscle tone.</li><li>The tongue and epiglottis may obstruct the entrance of the trachea due to inspiratory efforts creating negative pressure in the airway.</li><li>Move the patient no more than necessary to maintain an open airway. A second rescuer is needed to maintain in-line axial stabilization if spinal immobilization is required.</li><li>If the patient is found in a prone position with suspected trauma, the patient should be turned using the log-roll method to avoid flexion or twisting of the neck and back.</li></ul>

♦ Assess for adequate breathing 5-10 seconds: • Look • Listen • Feel	<ul><li>Look at chest for adequate tidal volume and rate.</li><li>Check breathing for at least 5 seconds and no more than 10 seconds.</li></ul>

Skill Component	Key Concepts

◆ Manage ventilations:
  • If breathing is adequate:
    - medical - place in recovery position – *if altered or unresponsive*
    - trauma - maintain spinal immobilization - *if indicated*
  • If breathing is absent or inadequate:
    - attempt 2 breaths with BVM or barrier device – (1 second/breath)
** *If 1ˢᵗ breath is unsuccessful, reposition the head, attempt 2ⁿᵈ ventilation and initiate obstructed airway procedures.*
	• Patients who are altered or unresponsive should be placed in the recovery position to reduce the chance of the airway being occluded by the tongue and aspiration of mucus or vomitus.
	• DO NOT hyperventilate. Hyperventilation reduces the success of survival due to:
	  - cerebral vasoconstriction resulting in decreased cerebral perfusion
	  - increase in intrathoracic pressure and decrease in venous return to the heart resulting in decreased cardiac output. ***Rescuers have a tendency to ventilate too rapidly.***
	• Ventilate using *only* enough force to cause the chest to rise. Over-inflation causes gastric distention decreasing tidal volume by elevating the diaphragm.
	• Using a BVM by a single rescuer can result in an inadequate seal on the face, and may not be as effective as a barrier device.
	• Remove dentures *only* if they cannot be kept in place. Dentures maintain facial form for a good seal.

◆ Look in mouth for foreign body:
  • If object is visible – remove foreign body
  • If object is not visible – begin CPR, starting with compressions
** *Clear/suction airway - if indicated*
	• DO NOT perform a blind finger sweep, this may force object further down the trachea. Perform finger sweep *only* if object is visible.
	• To remove foreign body:
	  - Insert the index finger inside the cheek and into the throat to the base of the tongue.
	  - Use a hook like motion to grasp the foreign body and maneuver it into the mouth so it can be removed.

◆ Perform chest compressions - *if indicated*:
  • Center of chest (lower half of sternum) between the nipples
  • Heel of one hand on the sternum and other hand on top of the 1ˢᵗ
  • Depth: 1½ - 2 inches
  • Rate: approximately 100/minute
  • Ratio cycle: 30 compressions to 2 ventilations
** ***Always look in mouth for foreign body prior to giving breaths:***
  - Remove object - *if visible*
  - Clear/suction airway - *if indicated*
** ***DO NOT compress on or near the xiphoid process.***
** ***Compressions must be deep, hard, fast, and allow for full chest recoil***
	• Chest compressions must be performed on a hard surface, place a board under the patient or move the patient to the floor.
	• **Compression landmark**: Place the heel of 1 hand on the center of chest (lower half of sternum) between the nipples.
	• **Compression method**: push hard and fast
	  - place the heel of one hand on top of the 1ˢᵗ hand
	  - fingers may be extended or interlaced, but must be kept off chest
	  - shoulders directly over hands
	  - arms straight and elbows locked - delivers force of compression straight down in order to be more effective
	  - allow chest to recoil (return to normal position) after down stroke to allow blood to flow into the chest and heart (50% of time for down stroke and 50% for chest relaxation)
	• Compressions need to be hard and fast to be effective.
	• **Compression rate**: 100/minute (speed of compressions) delivers fewer than 100/minute due to interruption of providing ventilations. The actual number is determined by the accuracy and consistency of the compression cycle (30 compressions should be delivered within 23 seconds). Five (5) cycles of 30:2 should take approximately 2 minutes.

◆ Continue compressions until foreign body obstruction is relieved
** ***Call for additional resources - If not called for previously***
	• *Always look in mouth for foreign body prior to giving breaths:*
	  - *Remove object - if visible*
	  - *Clear/suction airway - if indicated*

◆ Reassess patient after obstruction is relieved
  • Check for:
  - Responsiveness to stimuli
  - Breathing
  - Pulse
** ***Provide rescue breathing - 10-12/minute (every 5-6 seconds) - if indicated***
	• If a pulse is present and the patient is not breathing adequately, start BVM ventilations.
	• Patients <u>not</u> altered should be placed in a position of comfort.
	• Patients who are altered should be placed in the recovery position to reduce the chance of the airway being occluded by the tongue, and aspiration of mucus or vomit.

REASSESSMENT
(Ongoing Assessment)

Skill Component	Key Concepts

◆ Reassess a patient at least every **5 minutes once the obstruction is relieved once the patient has return of spontaneous respirations and circulation (ROSC):**
  • Primary assessment
  • Relevant portion of the secondary assessment
  • Vital signs
	• This is a priority patient and must be re-evaluated at least every 5 minutes or sooner, if any treatment is initiated, medication administered, or condition changes.

◆ Evaluate response to treatment	• The patient must be re-evaluated at least every 5 minutes if any treatment was initiated or medication administered.
◆ Evaluate results of reassessment and compare to baseline condition and vital signs ****Manage patient condition as indicated.**	• Evaluating and comparing results assists in recognizing if the patient is improving, responding to treatment or condition is deteriorating.
§ Explain the care being delivered and transport destination to the patient/caregiver	• Communication is important when dealing with the patient, family or caregiver. This is a very critical and frightening time for all involved and providing information helps in decreasing the stress they are experiencing.

PATIENT REPORT AND DOCUMENTATION

Skill Component	Key Concepts
§ Give patient report to equal or higher level of care personnel	• Report should consist of all pertinent information regarding the assessment findings, treatment rendered and patient response to care provided.

§ Verbalize/Document:
 	
  • Cause of obstruction - identify foreign body
  • Observed or reported signs of obstruction:
    - skin signs
    - absent or inadequate respirations
  • Response to obstruction maneuver
    Reassessment of airway
  • Additional treatment provided
	• Reassessment of airway includes:
	  - chest rise and fall
	  - skin color
	  - airway patency
	
	• Documentation must be on either the Los Angeles County EMS Report or departmental Patient Care Record form.

Developed: 10/01   Revised: 1/05, 6/06, 10/07, 9/08, 3/09

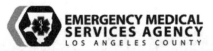

EMERGENCY MEDICAL SERVICES AGENCY
LOS ANGELES COUNTY

AIRWAY EMERGENCY: AIRWAY OBSTRUCTION
CHILD
Supplemental Information

INDICATIONS:
- Children who are choking with signs of mild or severe airway obstruction (1 year of age to puberty)

CAUSES:
- Intrinsic cause - tongue (most common), infection and swollen air passages
- Extrinsic cause - foreign body, facial injuries, vomitus, etc

CONTRAINDICATIONS:
- None when above condition applies.

COMPLICATIONS:
- Gastric distention
- Rib fractures
- Sternal fractures
- Separation of ribs from sternum
- Laceration of liver or spleen
- Pneumothorax
- Hemothorax
- Lung and heart contusion
- Fat emboli
- Other internal injuries

Recognizing Choking in the Responsive Child	
Mild Airway Obstruction Signs	**Severe Airway Obstruction Signs**
• Adequate air exchange • Responsive and able to cough forcefully • May wheeze between coughs	• Poor or no air exchange • Weak, ineffective cough or no cough • Stridor (high-pitched noise while inhaling) or no noise • Increased respiratory difficulty • Possible cyanosis • Unable to speak • Clutching the neck (universal choking sign) • Decreasing level of consciousness

Rescuer Actions	
Mild Airway Obstruction	**Severe Airway Obstruction**
• Encourage victim to continue coughing and attempt to breathe as long as there is adequate air exchange. • DO NOT interfere with the child's attempts to expel the foreign body. Monitor his/her condition. • Activate ALS response if mild obstruction persists.	• Activate ALS response • If responsive, perform abdominal thrusts • If unresponsive, start chest compressions • Activate ALS

NOTES:
- Child Obstructed Airway technique is indicated for children 1 year of age to puberty. A child reaches puberty when the child displays secondary sexual characteristics.

- Some signs of inadequate breathing are: respiratory distress, fast/slow respirations, bradycardia, stridor, cyanosis, poor perfusion, and altered LOC.

- Obstruction may have been relieved prior to EMS arrival. The child should be transported for medical evaluation.

- An additional rescuer is needed to maintain in-line axial stabilization if spinal immobilization is required.

- If the child is in a prone position with suspected trauma, the child should be turned using log-roll method to avoid flexion or twisting of the neck or back.

- *There is no universal recovery position for children.* A child who is altered should be placed in a position to protect the airway and reduce the chances of the airway being occluded by the tongue and from aspiration of mucus or vomit.

- DO NOT perform a blind finger sweep. This may force object further down trachea. Perform finger sweep _only_ if object is visible.

- Supplemental oxygen should always be used after spontaneous breathing has resumed.

- The tongue is the most common cause of airway obstruction due to decreased muscle tone. Intrinsic causes of an obstruction include infection and swollen air passages. Extrinsic causes include foreign body, facial injuries, vomitus, etc.

- The tongue and epiglottis may obstruct the entrance of the trachea due to inspiratory efforts creating negative pressure in the airway

- Any child who received abdominal thrusts must be evaluated medically to ensure there are no complications, injuries or retained foreign body fragments.

- DO NOT hyperventilate. Hyperventilation reduces the success of survival due to cerebral vasoconstriction resulting in decreased cerebral perfusion. In addition, hyperventilation increases intrathoracic pressure and decreases venous return to the heart resulting in diminished cardiac output. *Rescuers have a tendency to ventilate too rapidly.*

- Priority patients are patients who have abnormal vital signs, signs/symptoms of poor perfusion, or if there is a suspicion that the patient's condition may deteriorate.

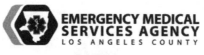

SKILL

AIRWAY EMERGENCY: AIRWAY OBSTRUCTION
CHILD

PERFORMANCE OBJECTIVES
Demonstrate competency in recognizing and managing an airway obstruction in a child (1-year-old to puberty) who is choking.

CONDITION
Recognize and manage an airway obstruction in a child who is found choking. Necessary equipment will be adjacent to the manikin or brought to the field setting.

EQUIPMENT
Child manikin, child bag-valve-mask device, O₂ connecting tubing, oxygen source with flow regulator, pediatric resuscitation tape, goggles, various masks, gown, gloves, timing device.

PERFORMANCE CRITERIA
* Items designated by a diamond (♦) must be performed successfully to demonstrate skill competency.
* Items identified by double asterisks (**) indicate actions required, if indicated.
* Items identified by the symbol (§) should be practiced.
* Ventilations and compressions must be performed at the minimum rate required.

PREPARATION	
Skill Component	**Key Concepts**
♦ Take body substance isolation precautions	• Mandatory (minimal) personal protective equipment – gloves
♦ Assess scene safety/scene size-up ** ***Consider spinal immobilization - if indicated***	• If unknown as to possible trauma, manage as trauma (determined by environment and information obtained from bystanders). • Depending on the size of the child and if spinal immobilization is required, an additional rescuer is needed to maintain in-line axial stabilization.
♦ Evaluate need for additional BSI precautions	• Situational - goggles, mask, gown
♦ Approach the patient and introduce yourself to the child and caregiver	• Use age appropriate techniques to introduce yourself to the child • The caregiver should hold the young child during the assessment if the child is in distress and responsive.

RESPONSIVE CHILD	
PROCEDURE	
Skill Component	**Key Concepts**

♦ Establish that the child is choking:
 	
** ***Call for additional resources – if needed***
	• Mild Obstruction:
	  - adequate air exchange
	  - coughing
	  - gagging
	  - stridor/wheezing
	• Severe Obstruction:
	  - poor or no air exchange
	  - increased respiratory distress
	  - weak, ineffective cough or no cough
	  - stridor (high-pitched noise while inhaling) or no noise
	  - unable to speak
	  - clutching the neck (universal sign of choking)
	  - cyanosis
	  - decreasing level of consciousness

	Continued

Skill Component	Key Concepts
	• Signs and symptoms of airway obstruction may be caused by a foreign body or infection of the upper airway such as epiglottitis and croup. • Infection should be suspected if the child has a fever and is congested, hoarse, drooling, lethargic, or is limp.

♦ Attempt to remove foreign body obstruction:
 	
  • <u>Mild obstruction</u> - Encourage child to cough
 	
  • <u>Severe obstruction</u> - Perform abdominal thrusts (Heimlich maneuver)
    - Stand or kneel behind the victim and place thumb side of fist above child's umbilicus
    - Grab fist with other hand and give quick inward and upward thrusts - *as many times as needed*
	• DO NOT interfere if child has an effective cough.
	• <u>ONLY</u> attempt to remove an obstruction caused by a foreign body. An obstruction caused by an infection will not clear with obstruction maneuvers and the child must be transported immediately to the closest emergency department approved for pediatrics (EDAP).
	
	• Straddle responsive child and perform Heimlich maneuver if found lying down.
	
	• Deliver as many abdominal thrusts as needed until the object is expelled, the child starts to breathe, or becomes unresponsive.

♦ Continue abdominal thrusts until obstruction is relieved or the child becomes unresponsive. ** *If unresponsive – start sequence for airway obstruction for unresponsive child.*	

♦ Manage ventilations after removal of obstruction:
 	
  • <u>If breathing is restored and adequate:</u>
-    - medical - place in position to protect airway – *if child is altered or unresponsive*
    - trauma - initiate spinal immobilization – *if indicated*
 	
  • <u>If breathing is absent or inadequate:</u>
    - perform rescue breathing of 12-20 per minute (1 breath every 3-5 seconds) with BVM or barrier device
	• *There is no universal recovery position for children.* A child who is altered should be placed in a position to protect the airway and reduce the chances of the airway being occluded by the tongue and from aspiration of mucus or vomit.
	
	• Signs of inadequate breathing are: respiratory distress, fast/slow respirations, bradycardia, stridor, cyanosis, poor perfusion, and altered LOC.
	
	• Supplemental oxygen should always be used after spontaneous breathing has resumed.
	
	• When ventilating use *only* enough force when providing positive pressure ventilation to allow for adequate chest rise. Over-inflation causes gastric distention that will affect tidal volume by elevating the diaphragm.
	
	• Use of a BVM by a single rescuer can result in an inadequate seal on the face and may not be as effective as a barrier device.
	
	• If the airway is open and it is difficult to compress the bag and air leaks around the seal, an airway obstruction may still be present.

UNRESPONSIVE CHILD

PROCEDURE
(Children who were previously responsive may have obstruction relieved when muscles relax)

Skill Component	Key Concepts
♦ Establish unresponsiveness ** *Call for additional resources – if needed*	

♦ Open airway:
  • <u>Medical</u>
    - head-tilt/chin-lift
 	
  • <u>Trauma</u>
    - jaw-thrust
    - neutral position (tragus of ear should be level with top of shoulder)
 	
** *Clear/suction airway - if indicated*
	• Use the jaw thrust maneuver when a head, neck or spine injury is suspected.
	
	• If the jaw thrust maneuver does not open the airway to allow for adequate ventilation, use the head tilt-chin lift technique.
	
	• Use shoulder padding to maintain airway and spinal alignment.
	
	• The tongue and epiglottis may obstruct the entrance of the trachea due to inspiratory efforts creating negative pressure in the airway.
	
	• The child's airway is more compliant and may collapse during their respiratory effort. The airway is easily obstructed by mucus, blood, pus, edema, external compression and hyperextension.

Skill Component	Key Concepts
♦ Assess for adequate breathing for 5-10 seconds: • Look • Listen • Feel	• Look at chest for adequate tidal volume and rate. • Check breathing for at least 5 seconds but no more than 10 seconds.

♦ Manage ventilations:
• If breathing is adequate:
  - medical - place in position to protect airway
  - trauma - maintain spinal immobilization - *if indicated*
• If breathing is absent or inadequate:
  - give 2 breaths with BVM or barrier device –
   (1 second/breath)
** *If 1st breath is unsuccessful, reposition the head, attempt 2nd ventilation and initiate obstructed airway procedures.*
	• *There is no universal recovery position for children.* A child who is altered should be placed in a position to protect the airway and reduce the chances of the airway being occluded by the tongue and from aspiration of mucus or vomit.
	• Rescue breathing for a child is 1 breath every 3-5 seconds (12-20 breaths/minute).
	• DO NOT hyperventilate. Hyperventilation reduces the success of survival due to:
	  - cerebral vasoconstriction resulting in decreased cerebral perfusion
	  - an increase in intrathoracic pressure and decrease in venous return to the heart resulting in decreased cardiac output. **Rescuers have a tendency to ventilate too rapidly.**
	• Ventilate using *only* enough force to cause the chest to rise. Over-inflation causes gastric distention which decreases tidal volume by elevating the diaphragm.
	• Use of a BVM by a single rescuer can result in an inadequate seal on the face and may not be as effective as a barrier device.
	• If the airway is open and it is difficult to compress the bag and air leaks around the seal, an airway obstruction is present.

♦ Look in mouth for foreign body:
• If object is visible – remove foreign body
• If object is not visible – begin CPR, starting with compressions
** *Clear/suction airway - if indicated*
	• In children, the most common cause of cardiac arrest is an inadequate airway.
	• DO NOT perform a blind finger sweep, this may force object further down the trachea. Perform finger sweep only if object is visible.
	• To remove foreign body:
	  - insert the index finger inside the cheek and into the throat to the base of the tongue.
	  - use a hook like motion to grasp the foreign body and maneuver it into the mouth so it can be removed.

♦ Perform chest compressions - *if indicated*:
• Center of chest
• Use 1 or 2 hands:
  - 1 hand - heel of hand on sternum
  - 2 hands – heel of one hand on sternum with the other hand on top of the 1st hand
• Depth: ⅓ to ½ of anterior-posterior chest size
• Rate: approximately 100/minute (hard and fast)
• Ratio cycle: 30 compressions to 2 ventilations (2 Rescuer CPR ratio is 15:2)
** *Always look in mouth for foreign body prior to giving breaths:*
  - *Remove object - if visible*
  - *Clear/suction airway - if indicated*
** *DO NOT compress on or near the xiphoid process.*
** *Compressions must be deep, hard, fast, and allow for full chest recoil*
	• Chest compressions must be performed on a hard surface. Place a board under the child or move the child to a table or the floor.
	• **Compression landmark:** center of the chest on the lower ½ of the sternum
	• **Compression method:** push hard and fast
	Use 1 or 2 hands:
	  - 1 hand - heel of hand on sternum
	  - 2 hands – heel of one hand on the sternum with other hand on top of the 1st hand.
	  - fingers may be extended/interlaced, but must be kept off chest
	  - shoulders directly over hands
	  - arms straight and elbows locked - delivers force of compression straight down in order to be more effective
	  - allow chest to recoil (return to normal position) after down stroke to allow blood to flow into the chest and heart (50% of time for down stroke and 50% for chest relaxation)
	• Compressions need to be hard and fast to be effective.
	• **Compression rate:** 100/minute (speed of compressions) delivers fewer than 100/minute due to interruption of providing ventilations. The actual number is determined by the accuracy and consistency of the compression cycle.

Skill Component	Key Concepts
◆ Complete 5 compression cycles of 30:2 ** ***Call for additional resources - If not called for previously*** **[end with ventilations]**	• Five (5) compression cycles should take approximately 2 minutes.

◆ Continue compressions until foreign body obstruction is relieved	• *Always look in mouth for foreign body prior to giving breaths:*
	  - *Remove object - if visible*
	  - *Clear/suction airway - if indicated*

◆ Reassess child after obstruction is relieved
  • Check for:
  - Unresponsiveness
  - Breathing
  - Pulse
	• If a pulse is present and the child is not breathing adequately, start BVM ventilations.
	• A child who is awake and alert should be placed in a position of comfort.
	• *There is no universal recovery position for children.* A child who is altered should be placed in a position to protect the airway and reduce the chances of the airway being occluded by the tongue and from aspiration of mucus or vomit.

REASSESSMENT
(Ongoing Assessment)

Skill Component	Key Concepts

◆ Reassess the child at least every **5 minutes once the child has return of spontaneous respirations and circulation (ROSC):**
  • Primary assessment
  • Relevant portion of the secondary assessment
  • Vital signs
	• This is a priority patient and must be re-evaluated at least every 5 minutes or sooner, if any treatment is initiated, medication administered, or condition changes.

◆ Evaluate response to treatment	• The child must be re-evaluated at least every 5 minutes if any treatment was initiated or medication administered.
◆ Evaluate results of reassessment and compare to baseline condition and vital signs ****Manage the child's condition as indicated.**	• Evaluating and comparing results assists in recognizing if the child is improving, responding to treatment or condition is deteriorating.
§ Explain the care being delivered and the transport destination to the child/caregivers	• Communication is important when dealing with the child, family or caregiver. This is a very critical and frightening time for all involved and providing information helps in decreasing the stress they are experiencing.

PATIENT REPORT AND DOCUMENTATION

Skill Component	Key Concepts
§ Give patient report to equal or higher level of care personnel	• Report should consist of all pertinent information regarding the assessment finding, treatment rendered and patient response to care provided.

§ Verbalize/Document:
  • Cause of obstruction - identify foreign body
  • Observed or reported signs of obstruction:
    - skin signs
    - absent or inadequate respirations
  • Response to obstruction maneuver
  • Reassessment of airway
  • Additional treatment provided
	• Reassessment of airway includes:
	  - chest rise and fall
	  - skin color
	  - airway patency
	• Documentation must be on either the Los Angeles County EMS Report or departmental Patient Care Record form.

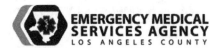

AIRWAY EMERGENCY: AIRWAY OBSTRUCTION
INFANT
Supplemental Information

INDICATIONS:

• Infants who are choking with signs of mild or severe airway obstruction

CAUSES:

• Intrinsic cause - tongue (most common), infection and swollen air passages
• Extrinsic cause - foreign body, facial injuries, vomitus, etc

CONTRAINDICATIONS:

• None when above conditions apply.

COMPLICATIONS:

• Gastric distention	• Pneumothorax
• Rib fractures	• Hemothorax
• Sternal fractures	• Lung and heart contusion
• Separation of ribs from sternum	• Fat emboli
• Laceration of liver or spleen	• Other internal injuries

Recognizing Choking in the Responsive Infant	
Mild Airway Obstruction **Signs**	**Severe Airway Obstruction** **Signs**
• Adequate air exchange • Responsive and able to cough forcefully • May wheeze between coughs	• Poor or no air exchange • Weak, ineffective cough or no cough • Stridor (high-pitched noise while inhaling) or no noise • Increased respiratory difficulty • Possible cyanosis • Unable to make noise(cry) • Decreasing level of consciousness
Rescuer Actions	
Mild Airway Obstruction	**Severe Airway Obstruction**
• Encourage infant to continue coughing and attempt to breathe as long as there is adequate air exchange. • DO NOT interfere with the infant's attempts to expel the foreign body. Monitor his/her condition. • Activate ALS response if mild obstruction persists.	• Activate EMS response • If responsive, perform chest thrusts • If unresponsive, to stimuli start chest compressions • Activate ALS

NOTES:

• Infant is defined as a neonate to 1 year of age (12 months).

• Some signs of inadequate breathing are: respiratory distress, fast/slow respirations, bradycardia, stridor, cyanosis, poor perfusion, and altered LOC.

• Obstruction may have been relieved prior to EMS arrival. Patient should be transported for medical evaluation.

• DO NOT perform a blind finger sweep. This may force object further down trachea. Perform finger sweep *only* if object is visible.

• Supplemental oxygen should always be used after spontaneous breathing has resumed.

• An infant who is altered should be placed in a position to protect the airway to reduce the chance of the airway being occluded by the tongue and protected from aspiration of mucus or vomit.

• The tongue is the most common cause of airway obstruction due to decreased muscle tone. Intrinsic causes of an obstruction include infection and swollen air passages. Extrinsic causes include foreign body, facial injuries, vomitus, etc.

• The tongue and epiglottis may obstruct the entrance of the trachea due to inspiratory efforts creating negative pressure in the airway.

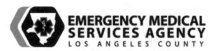

EMERGENCY MEDICAL SERVICES AGENCY
LOS ANGELES COUNTY

EMS SKILL

AIRWAY EMERGENCY: AIRWAY OBSTRUCTION
INFANT

PERFORMANCE OBJECTIVES
Demonstrate competency in recognizing and managing an airway obstruction in an infant who is choking.

CONDITION
Recognize and manage an airway obstruction in an infant who is found choking. Necessary equipment will be adjacent to the manikin or brought to the field setting.

EQUIPMENT
Infant manikin, infant bag-valve-mask device, O_2 connecting tubing, oxygen source with flow regulator, pediatric resuscitation tape, goggles, various masks, gown, gloves, timing device.

PERFORMANCE CRITERIA
- Items designated by a diamond (♦) must be performed successfully to demonstrate skill competency.
- Items identified by double asterisks (**) indicate actions required, if indicated.
- Items identified by the symbol (§) should be practiced.
- Ventilations and compressions must be performed at the minimum rate required.

PREPARATION	
Skill Component	**Key Concepts**
♦ Take body substance isolation precautions	• Mandatory (minimal) personal protective equipment – gloves
♦ Assess scene safety/scene size-up ** *Consider spinal immobilization - if indicated*	• If unknown as to possible trauma, manage as trauma (determined by environment and information obtained from bystanders). • If spinal immobilization is required, an additional rescuer is needed to maintain in-line axial stabilization.
♦ Evaluate need for additional BSI precautions	• Situational - goggles, mask, gown
♦ Approach the patient and introduce yourself to the infant, family or caregiver – *if circumstance, time and resources allow*	• Use age appropriate techniques to introduce yourself to infant. • The caregiver should hold the infant during the assessment if the infant is in distress and responsive.

RESPONSIVE INFANT PROCEDURE	
Skill Component	**Key Concepts**

♦ Establish that the infant is choking:
 	
** *Call for additional resources – if needed*
	• <u>Mild Obstruction:</u>
	  - adequate air exchange
	  - coughing
	  - gagging
	  - stridor/wheezing
	
	• <u>Severe Obstruction:</u>
	  - poor or no air exchange
	  - increased respiratory distress
	  - weak, ineffective cough or no cough
	  - stridor (high-pitched noise while inhaling) or no noise
	  - unable to make noise (cry)
	  - cyanosis
	  - decreasing level of consciousness
	
	• Signs and symptoms of airway obstruction may be caused by a foreign body or infection of the upper airway such as epiglottitis and croup.
	• Infection should be suspected if the infant has a fever and is congested, hoarse, or drooling.

Skill Component	Key Concepts

◆ Attempt to remove foreign body obstruction:
 	
  • <u>Mild obstruction</u> – Do not interfere with infant's attempt to relieve the obstruction
 	
  • <u>Severe obstruction</u> – Perform up to 5 back slaps
    - Place infant prone on forearm
    - Keep head lower than the body
    - Support jaw and face
    - Use heel of hand
    - Deliver slaps, using the heel of the hand, between the shoulder blades
	• DO NOT interfere if infant has an effective cough.
	
	• <u>Only</u> attempt to remove an obstruction caused by a foreign body.
	
	• An obstruction caused by an infection will not clear with obstruction maneuvers and the infant must be transported immediately to an Emergency Department Approved for Pediatrics (EDAP).
	
	• DO NOT perform a blind finger sweep. This may force object further down the distal airway structures. <u>Only</u> perform finger sweep if object is visible.
	
	• Place infant on forearm with head lower than the chest while supporting the head. Hold the jaw and face with fingers extended. *DO NOT cover mouth or compress the soft tissue of the neck.*
	
	• Use the heel of the hand to deliver slaps to the back between the shoulder blades.
	
	• Each slap should be of sufficient force to dislodge the object.

◆ Place infant supine:
  • Turn infant onto the opposite arm
  • Maintain support of the head and neck (keep head lower than the body)
	• Turn the infant by:
	  - placing the free hand on the occiput and back, cradling the infant between both hands and arms
	  - turning the body as one unit
	  - maintain control of head and neck at all times
	  - keep the head slightly lower than the body throughout the procedure

◆ Perform up to 5 chest thrusts:
  • Find lower 1/2 of sternum (1 finger width below nipple line)
  • Use 2 finger pads
  • Compress at a depth of 1/3 - 1/2 of chest diameter
  • Rate of 1 second per thrust
	• Technique for chest thrusts is the same as for chest compressions when performing CPR. *DO NOT use upward compressions.*
	  - Lower half of sternum
	  - 2 finger pads of either index & middle finger or middle & ring finger of one hand
	  - Depth 1/3 - 1/2 the anterior/posterior diameter of the infant
	  - Rate of 1 second per thrust to simulate an "artificial cough"

◆ Call for ALS - *if obstruction is not relieved after 2 minutes or infant becomes unresponsive* ** *If responsive but still obstructed – continue series of back slaps and chest trusts until obstruction is relieved or the infant becomes unresponsive.*	• In children, the most common cause of cardiac arrest is an inadequate airway. Attempt removal of obstruction for 2 minutes before leaving the infant to call for other resources.

◆ Manage ventilations after removal of obstruction:
 	
  • <u>If breathing is restored and adequate</u>:
    - trauma - initiate spinal immobilization
 	
  • <u>If breathing is absent or inadequate</u>:
    - perform rescue breathing of 12-20 per minute (1 breath every 3-5 seconds) with BVM or barrier device
	• Signs of inadequate breathing include: respiratory distress, fast/slow respirations, bradycardia, stridor, cyanosis, poor perfusion, and altered LOC (agitation, irritable cry, non-responsive to caregivers, etc.).
	
	• Supplemental oxygen should always be used after spontaneous breathing has resumed.
	
	• When ventilating <u>only</u> use enough force to allow for adequate chest rise. Over-inflation causes gastric distention that will affect tidal volume by elevating the diaphragm.
	
	• Use of a BVM by a single rescuer can result in an inadequate seal on the face and may not be as effective as a barrier device.
	
	• When using an infant BVM device, occlude the pop-off-valve if unable to achieve adequate chest rise since higher pressures may be necessary.
	
	• If the airway is open and it is difficult to compress the bag and air leaks around the seal, an airway obstruction may still be present.

PROCEDURE

(Infants who were previously responsive may have the obstruction relieved when muscles relax)

Skill Component	Key Concepts
◆ Establish unresponsiveness ** Activate the emergency response system or call for additional EMS personnel - *if not called for previously*	• Tap bottom of feet or gently shake and shout.
◆ Open airway: 　• <u>Medical</u> 　　- head-tilt/chin-lift 　• <u>Trauma</u> 　　- jaw-thrust 　　- neutral position (tragus of ear level with top of shoulder) ** *Clear/suction airway - if indicated* <u>Caution</u>:　**Hyperextension of the neck will cause airway obstruction**	• Use the jaw thrust maneuver when a head, neck or spine injury is suspected • If the jaw thrust maneuver does not open the airway to allow for adequate ventilation, use the head tilt-chin lift technique. • Use shoulder padding to maintain proper airway and spinal alignment. • The tongue and epiglottis may obstruct the entrance of the trachea due to inspiratory efforts creating negative pressure in the airway. • The infant's airway is more compliant and may collapse during hyperextension and can be compromised with respiratory effort.
◆ Look for foreign body: 　• If object is visible – remove foreign body 　• If object is not visible – begin CPR, starting with compressions ** *Clear/suction airway - if indicated*	• In infants, the most common cause of cardiac arrest is an inadequate airway. • DO NOT perform a blind finger sweep, this may force object further down the trachea. Perform finger sweep <u>only</u> if object is visible. The airway is easily obstructed by mucus, blood, pus, edema, external compression and hyperextension. • To remove a foreign body: 　- Insert index finger inside the cheek and into the throat to the base of the tongue. 　- Use a hook like motion to grasp the foreign body so it can be removed.
◆ Perform chest compressions - *if indicated*: 　• Lower 1/2 of sternum (1 finger width below nipple line) 　• Depth: 1/3 to 1/2 of chest diameter 　• Rate: at least 100/minute 　• Ratio cycle: 　　- <u>2 finger technique</u> – 30:2 (1 rescuer) 　　- <u>2 thumb-encircling technique</u> – 15:2 (2 rescuers) ** *Always look in mouth for foreign body prior to giving breaths:* 　- *Remove object - if visible* 　- *Clear/suction airway - if indicated*	• Chest compressions must be performed on a hard surface. Place a board under the infant or move the infant to a table, counter, etc. • Technique for chest compressions when performing CPR : 　*2 finger technique* – Use 2 finger pads (either index & middle finger or middle & ring finger) of one hand 　- **Compression landmark**: center of the chest on the lower 1/2 of the sternum 　- **Compression method**: push hard and fast 　- **Compression rate**: 100/minute (speed of compressions) delivers fewer than 100/minute due to interruption of providing ventilations. The actual number is determined by the accuracy and consistency of the compression cycle. 　*2 thumb-encircling technique* (2 rescuers)– Use both thumbs side by side 　- <u>Compression landmark</u> - center of the chest just below nipple line 　- <u>Compression method</u>: push hard and fast 　- <u>Compression rate</u> of 100/minute (speed of compressions) delivers fewer than 100/minute due to interruption of providing ventilations. The actual number is determined by the accuracy and consistency of the compression cycle.
◆ Complete 5 compression cycles ** *Attempt removal of obstruction for 2 minutes before leaving the infant to call for ALS – if not called for previously* 　　　*[end with ventilations]*	• Five (5) compression cycles should take approximately 2 minutes.

Skill Component	Key Concepts

♦ Continue compressions until foreign body obstruction is relieved	• *Always look in mouth for foreign body prior to giving breaths:*
	    - *Remove object - if visible*
	    - *Clear/suction airway - if indicated*

♦ Reassess infant after obstruction is relieved • Look for: - Responsiveness to stimulus - Breathing - Pulse - Vital signs ** *Start compressions - if heart rate is less than 60/minute with signs of poor perfusion* *[begin with compressions]*	• If a pulse is present and the infant is not breathing adequately, start BVM ventilations. • An infant who is <u>not</u> altered should be placed in a position of comfort. • An infant who is altered should be placed in a position to protect the airway, reduce the chances of the airway being occluded by the tongue, and protected from aspiration of mucus or vomit.

REASSESSMENT
(Ongoing Assessment)

Skill Component	Key Concepts
♦ Reassess the infant at least every **60 seconds once the infant has return of spontaneous respirations and circulation (ROSC):** • Respirations and circulation continuously • Initial assessment • Relevant portion of the secondary assessment • Vital signs	• This is a priority patient and infants must be re-evaluated every 60 seconds or sooner.
♦ Evaluate response to treatment	• Infants must be re-evaluated at least every 5 minutes if any treatment was initiated or medication administered.
♦ Evaluate results of reassessment and compare to baseline condition and vital signs **Manage the infant's condition as indicated.**	• Evaluating and comparing results assists in recognizing if the child is improving, responding to treatment or condition is deteriorating.
§ Explain the care being delivered and the transport destination to the child/caregivers	• Communication is important when dealing with the child, family or caregiver. This is a very critical and frightening time for all involved and providing information helps in decreasing the stress they are experiencing.

PATIENT REPORT AND DOCUMENTATION

Skill Component	Key Concepts
§ Give patient report to equal or higher level of care personnel	• Report should consist of all pertinent information regarding the assessment finding, treatment rendered and patient response to care provided.

§ Verbalize/Document:
 	
 • Event leading up to the obstruction
 • Cause of obstruction – type of obstruction/foreign body
 • Observed or reported signs of obstruction:
   - skin signs
   - absent or inadequate respirations
 • Response to obstruction maneuver
 • Reassessment of airway
 • Additional treatment provided
	• Reassessment of airway includes:
	   - chest rise and fall
	   - skin color
	   - airway patency
	
	 • Documentation must be on either the Los Angeles County EMS Report or departmental Patient Care Record form.

Developed: 10/01   Revises: 6/06, 11/07, 1/08, 4/09

ASSISTING ADVANCED LIFE SUPPORT PERSONNEL
ADVANCED AIRWAY SET-UP

INDICATIONS:

- As directed by ALS personnel on scene

CONTRAINDICATIONS:

- As directed / indicated by ALS personnel on scene

COMPLICATIONS:

- Equipment malfunction might delay intubation of patient, resulting in hypoxia

- Moving of the patient at any time may lead to dislodgement of the Endotracheal Tube (ETT). Any time that the patient is moved, auscultation of the upper-epigastrium, and bi-lateral breath sounds need to be   evaluated again

- Auscultation that reveals: positive upper - epigastric sounds and / or unequal bi-lateral lung sounds could indicate that the ETT is not properly placed by the ALS Personnel

NOTES:
- Be sure to practice all procedures of ETT set-up prior to having perform them on a 911 call

- Proper set-up of the ETT and all it accompanying parts / procedures will be evaluated

- Proper BSI, on-going assessment, and disposal of all materials following the ETT set-up will be evaluated

- Be familiar with the ETCO2 "Colormetric" device, how it adapts to the BVM, and what the proper color changes indicate

- Look for condensation in the actual ETT after proper placement of the ETT, and ventilatory efforts have been started. If there isn't any condensation or condensation disappears, notify the ALS Personnel

Developed 7/07

ASSISTING ADVANCED LIFE SUPPORT PERSONNEL
ADVANCED AIRWAY SET-UP

PERFORMANCE OBJECTIVES
The examinee will demonstrate proficiency in assisting Advanced Life Support Personnel (ALS) with the use of an advanced airway.

CONDITION
The examinee will be requested to, under the direction of ALS personnel, to prepare and set-up for the use of an endotracheal tube (ETT), in the event that an advanced airway device is needed.

EQUIPMENT
Gloves, goggles, (1) packaged E TT, stylette, (1) 10cc syringe, (1) packaged CO2 detector device, (1) ET tube holder, laryngoscope handle with assortment of blades, (1) BVM with oxygen tubing, (1) oxygen cylinder

PERFORMANCE CRITERIA
- 100% accuracy required on all items designated by a diamond (♦) for skills testing and must manage successfully all items indicated by double asterisks (**).
- Documentation, identified by the symbol (§), must be practiced, but is not a required test item.
- Appropriate body substance isolation precautions must be instituted.

ADVANCED AIRWAY SET-UP PREPARATION	
Skill Component	**Teaching Points**
♦ Take body substance isolation precautions	• Mandatory personal protective equipment – gloves, goggles • Situational: masks, gown
♦ Assess scene safety / scene size-up	
** Consider spinal injury precautions – **If Indicated**	• If unknown as to possible trauma, treat as trauma (determined by environment and / or information obtained from bystanders).
PROCEDURE	
Skill Component	**Teaching Points**
♦ Attach "blade" to the laryngoscope handle	• Ensure the light is working properly ("tight, white and bright")
♦ Remove ET tube from packaging	• Place on top of packaging, making sure to keep it clean.
♦ Remove 10cc syringe from packaging	• Pull "plunger" back to the 10cc (or ml) mark
♦ Attach 10cc syringe to the "pilot" balloon attachment on the ET tube	• Depress plunger all the way, (until it stops), then remove it from the "pilot" balloon attachment • Check the "distal" cuff balloon, and the "pilot" balloon to see that they are fully-inflated, and are not leaking
♦ Remove 10cc syringe from the "pilot" balloon, after full-inflation has occurred	• Removal of the 10cc syringe so it will not leak air back into it
♦ Attach 10cc syringe to the "pilot" balloon attachment on the ET tube, and pull back the plunger to the 10 cc mark fully-deflating the "distal" cuff and "pilot" balloon	

♦ Place the ET tube (with 10cc syringe attached to the "pilot" balloon site) on top of the ET tube package, ready for A.L.S. Personnel	• This will help keep the equipment clean and ready for use
♦ Turn on portable suction unit	• This is done to ensure it is working properly

Developed 7/07

BLOOD SAMPLE FROM CAPILLARY FINGER STICK

INDICATIONS:

- As directed by ALS personnel on scene.

CONTRAINDICATIONS

- None.

COMPLICATIONS:

- Equipment malfunction might delay the collection / evaluation of a blood sample from a patient

- If patient's blood glucose level is too high, the glucometer has not been correctly calibrated, or there is not enough blood collected on the reagent strip, the glucometer will give an "error" reading in the display window

NOTES:

- Be sure to practice all of these procedures prior to having to actually perform them on an actual 911 call
- Proper use of the glucometer and all of its procedures will be evaluated
- Proper BSI and disposal of all materials following the collection of a blood sample will also be evaluated

Developed 7/07

ASSISTING ADVANCED LIFE SUPPORT PERSONNEL
BLOOD SAMPLE FROM CAPILLARY FINGER STICK

PERFORMANCE OBJECTIVES
The examinee will demonstrate proficiency in assisting advanced life support personnel (ALS) with correctly setting up and check blood glucose levels utilizing a capillary finger stick.

CONDITION
The examinee will be requested to, under the direction of an advanced life support personnel, to prepare / set-up for the use of a glucometer

EQUIPMENT
Gloves, goggles, alcohol prep pad, 4x4 gauze, Band-Aid, one glucometer with a reagent test strip.

PERFORMANCE CRITERIA
- 100% accuracy required on all items designated by a diamond (♦) for skills testing and must manage successfully all items indicated by double asterisks (**).
- Documentation, identified by the symbol (§), must be practiced, but is not a required test item.
- Appropriate body substance isolation precautions must be instituted.

BLOOD SAMPLE FROM CAPILLARY FINGER STICK PREPARATION	
Skill Component	**Teaching Points**
♦ Take body substance isolation precautions	• Mandatory personal protective equipment – gloves, , goggles • Situational - long sleeves, masks, gown
♦ Open glucometer and place a reagent test strip into the opening of the glucometer	• Be sure to place the correct end of the reagent strip into the glucometer, usually marked with a metal tab on the end • After properly inserting the reagent strip into the glucometer, it will turn "on" • Glucometer will be "ready" for blood sample when indicated on the screen (usually within five seconds after the reagent test strip is placed into the opening of the glucometer
♦ Assist Advanced Life Support Personnel by having an alcohol prep pad, 4x4 gauze, and a Band-Aid ready	• Alcohol prep pad is used for cleansing the site on the patient's finger, prior to ALS personnel puncturing the skin with a "lancet" • 4x4 gauze is used for cleanup around the puncture site • Band-Aid is used in the last step, after the blood sample has been collected, to help stop minimal bleeding, and to keep the puncture-site clean
PROCEDURE	
Skill Component	**Teaching Points**
♦ After the ALS personnel has punctured the selected site with the "lancet", help assist by taking glucometer (with reagent strip in-place) and placing reagent strip on the site, where blood can be seen exiting the punctured area on the patient's finger	• Wait for the ALS personnel's direction to collect blood sample from site. • When collecting a blood sample from the site, make sure that the strip has a sufficient amount of blood. The glucometer will start a countdown (visually, in seconds), usually not lasting longer than ten seconds.
♦ Once the glucometer has calculated the dextrose amount in the patient's blood, it will display a numerical value.	• When the glucometer displays a numeric value, tell the ALS personnel that value. • With gloved-hands, pull the reagent strip from the glucometer opening and properly discard in a biohazard container • Properly discard of gloves and all other materials used in this procedure

ASSISTING ADVANCED LIFE SUPPORT PERSONNEL
INTRAVENOUS (IV) LINE PREPARATION

INDICATIONS:

- As directed by ALS personnel on scene

CONTRAINDICATIONS

- None

COMPLICATIONS:

- None

NOTES:

- *Be sure to practice all of these procedures prior to having to actually perform them on a 911 call*

Developed 7/07

ASSISTING ADVANCED LIFE SUPPORT PERSONNEL
INTRAVENOUS (IV) LINE PREPARATION

PERFORMANCE OBJECTIVES

The examinee will demonstrate proficiency in assisting (Advanced Life Support) A.L.S. with preparing an I.V. solution prior to I.V. therapy

CONDITION

The examinee will be requested to, under the direction of an advanced life support personnel, to prepare / set-up for the use of a glucometer

EQUIPMENT

Gloves, goggles, appropriate size bag of "normal saline" I.V. solution and tubing

PERFORMANCE CRITERIA

- 100% accuracy required on all items designated by a diamond (♦) for skills testing and must manage successfully all items indicated by double asterisks (**).
- Documentation, identified by the symbol (§), must be practiced, but is not a required test item.
- Appropriate body substance isolation precautions must be instituted.

INTRAVENOUS (IV) LINE PREPARATION PREPARATION	
Skill Component	**Teaching Points**
♦ Take body substance isolation precautions	• Mandatory personal protective equipment - gloves, goggles • Situational - long sleeves, masks, gown
♦ Select properly sized bag of normal saline I.V. solution and tubing, as requested by ALS Personnel	

PROCEDURE	
Skill Component	**Teaching Points**
♦ Tear-open packaging (vertically, from top to bottom) that contains the I.V. solution	
♦ Open the appropriate-sized IV tubing	
♦ "DICE" the bag of normal saline	• D - Appropriate drug and dosage • I - Integrity • I - Indication • C - Clarity of the drug • C - Contraindications • E - Expiration of the drug • If you find that any of the above are not met, discard the bag and choose another until it meets the above-criteria
♦ Pull the protective plastic covering from the IV solution port	

Skill Component	Teaching Points
♦ Remove plastic sheath from the end of the IV tubing ♦ "Spike" the bag by inserting the pointed-end of the IV tubing into the solution port	• Be sure to push the sharp end of the IV tubing all the way into the solution port until it stops. Otherwise, it will not properly pierce the opening so that the solution will flow form the port.
♦ Squeeze the "drip chamber" until the IV solution fills to half-way in the chamber	
♦ Allow for the IV solution to flow-through the tubing, until all air bubbles have been removed from the tubing	
♦ Slide the down valve-control tab until the dripping stops	• Located on the IV tubing at the top of the tubing – usually blue in color with a white slide-tab
♦ Loosen the bottom cap of the IV tubing	• Where the tubing ends, there will a end-cap (usually blue in color). • Unscrew counter-clockwise to slightly loosen.
♦ Hang the (now-ready) IV solution from a hanger at the roof line, ready for the ALS personnel	
♦ When the ALS personnel is ready for the IV line, hold the end-cap so that the ALS personnel can easily take the IV tubing for attachment to the catheter in the patient' arm	

Developed 7/07

ASSISTING ADVANCED LIFE SUPPORT PERSONNEL
MONITORING INTRAVENOUS LINES

INDICATIONS:

- Patient with intravenous (IV) isotonic salt solutions of (e.g., Normal Saline (NaCl 0.9%), Lactated Ringers) or glucose solutions

CONTRAINDICATIONS

- Patient with IV solution, piggybacked with medications or medications added to the IV solution directly. (see notes for specific exceptions)
- Central IV Lines
- AV Shunts
- Arterial lines

COMPLICATIONS:

- Infiltration
- Infection
- Inflammation
- Inaccurate Dose

NOTES:

- The following additives are permitted in Los Angeles County if adjusted to a TKO rate by hospital personnel.
  o Folic acid – max 1mg/1000ml
  o Multi-vitamins - max 1 vial/1000ml
  o Thiamine – max 100mg/1000ml

- The following additives are permitted in Los Angeles County for IV solution if administered through an infusion pump at a preset rate.
  o KCL – max 20 mEq/1000ml
  o Total Parenteral Nutrition (TPN)
  o Chemotherapeutic agents with required precautions

Developed 7/07

ASSISTING ADVANCED LIFE SUPPORT PERSONNEL
MONITORING INTRAVENOUS (IV) LINE

PERFORMANCE OBJECTIVES
The examinee will demonstrate proficiency in monitoring a peripheral intravenous line.

CONDITION
The examinee will be requested to properly monitor an intravenous line on a simulated patient receiving fluids. The examinee should also be able to identify signs and symptoms of IV infiltration.

EQUIPMENT
Adult CPR/trauma manikin or live model, IV bag with isotonic solution or D5W, drip chamber with administration line, mask, gown, gloves, goggles'.

PERFORMANCE CRITERIA
*   100% accuracy required on all items designated by a diamond (♦) for skills testing and must manage successfully all items indicated by double asterisks (**).
*   Documentation, identified by the symbol (§), must be practiced, but is not a required test item.
*   Appropriate body substance isolation precautions must be instituted.

SPECIFIC SKILL PREPARATION

Skill Component	Teaching Points
♦ Take body substance isolation precautions	• Mandatory personal protective equipment - gloves • Situational - long sleeves, goggles, masks, gown
♦ Explain Procedure to patient	• Maintain patient rapport

PROCEDURE

Skill Component	Teaching Points
Monitoring IV Flow Rate (rate preset):	
♦ Determine IV flow rate by counting drips/minute	
♦ Adjust flow rate to ordered rate as needed	
♦ Confirm IV flow rate by counting drips/minute	
Discontinuing IV:	
♦ Implement universal precautions	
♦ Explain procedure to patient	The EMT candidate should be able to provide the signs and symptoms indicating IV infiltration.
♦ Turn off flow rate regulator	
♦ Leave tubing attached to IV catheter	The EMT should not remove the IV catheter.

ONGOING ASSESSMENT

Skill Component	Teaching Points
§ Continue to reassess patient	

Skill Component	Teaching Points
§ Verbalize/Document: • Reason for intervention • Description of infiltration • Treatment provided	

Developed 7/07

ASSISTING ADVANCED LIFE SUPPORT PERSONNEL
3 LEAD ECG ELECTRODE PLACEMENT

INDICATIONS:

- As directed by ALS personnel on scene

CONTRAINDICATIONS

- None

COMPLICATIONS:

- A patient exhibiting diaphoresis on the chest area, or who has an excessive amount of chest hair, it will be difficult to achieve adherence of the ECG patches.

- Once the ECG monitor is turned to the "on" position and does not "read" a ECG rhythm, check all electrode connections to ensure that they are properly attached to the patches, and that the patches are properly adhered to the patient's body.

NOTES:
- Be sure to practice all of these procedures prior to having to actually perform them on an actual 911 call.

- There are metal "snaps" on top of the ECG patch. Each different colored electrode wire has an attachment point at the end of the wire where the patch attaches.

- Properly attach the ECG patches to the end of the electrode wires prior to removal of the plastic backing. After the removal of the plastic backing, adhere the ECG patches on the patient's body.

- The ECG patches have a plastic backing on them. This plastic backing needs to be removed prior to the application of the patch to the patient's skin.

- There are three distinct colored "lead" wires:
    - White – to be placed on the patient's (anatomical right-side) right clavicle
    - Black – to be placed on the patient's (anatomical left-side) left clavicle
    - Red – to be placed on the patient's (anatomical left-side) left-upper abdominal quadrant

- If ECG patches are difficult to adhere to the chest and upper abdominal area, the EMT (under the direction of an ALS personnel) may be directed to:
    - Diaphoresis - dry the area before the application of the ECG patches, so that they will properly adhere
    - Excessive body hair – properly use a razor (supplied by ALS personnel) to remove body hair, for the application of the ECG patches, if needed.

Developed 7/07

EMS SKILL

ASSISTING ADVANCED LIFE SUPPORT PERSONNEL
3 - LEAD ECG ELECTRODE PLACEMENT

PERFORMANCE OBJECTIVES
The examinee will demonstrate proficiency in assisting advanced life support personnel (ALS) with correctly setting-up, and successfully placing the ECG electrodes on a patient for advanced life support personnel evaluation of a cardiac rhythm.

CONDITION
The examinee will be requested to, under the direction of an advanced life support personnel, to prepare / set-up and properly place the ecg electrodes on a patient

EQUIPMENT
Gloves, goggles, ECG patches, ECG monitor with 3 electrode leads, 1 patient

PERFORMANCE CRITERIA
- 100% accuracy required on all items designated by a diamond (♦) for skills testing and must manage successfully all items indicated by double asterisks (**).
- Documentation, identified by the symbol (§), must be practiced, but is not a required test item.
- Appropriate body substance isolation precautions must be instituted.

3-LEAD ECG ELECTRODE PLACEMENT PREPARATION	
Skill Component	**Teaching Points**
♦ Take body substance isolation precautions	• Mandatory personal protective equipment – gloves, , goggles • Situational - long sleeves, masks, gown

PROCEDURE	
Skill Component	**Teaching Points**
♦ Open the pouch on the ECG monitor and take out the 3 lead electrodes and ECG patches	• The electrode wires might be tangled. Untangle prior to attaching the ECG patches
♦ Attach an ECG patch to each one of the leads	• The ECG patch will make a "snap" noise when pushed-onto the end of the electrode
♦ Peel-off the plastic backing, one at a time, before placing on the patient	
♦ Place each of the ECG patches, with the electrodes attached to the appropriate location on the patient's body	
♦ Once all of the ECG patches are placed, turn the ECG monitor to the "on" position. Notify the ALS Personnel that the monitor is ready to read the cardiac rhythm	

Developed 7/07

ASSISTING WITH ESOPHAGEAL TRACHEAL COMBITUBE (ETC) INTUBATION

INDICATIONS:

- Respiratory failure
- Respiratory arrest

CONTRAINDICATIONS

- Gag reflex
- Children under 16 years of age
- Adults shorter than 5'
- Patients who have ingested caustic substances
- Patients with known esophageal disease

COMPLICATIONS:

- Hypoxia if inserted improperly
- Soft tissue injury

NOTES:

- When inserted, the device will enter the esophagus 90% of the time and the trachea 10% of the time. If used correctly the patient can be ventilated regardless of entry.

Developed 7/07

BREATHING EMERGENCY / AIRWAY MANAGEMENT
ASSISTING WITH ESOPHAGEAL TRACHEAL COMBITUBE (ETC) INTUBATION

PERFORMANCE OBJECTIVES
The examinee will demonstrate proficiency in assisting ventilating a patient with a Flow Restricted Oxygen Powered Breathing Device

CONDITION
The examinee will be requested assist in securing an airway maintaining an airway manikin utilizing an Esophageal Tracheal Combitube

EQUIPMENT
Adult CPR/Airway manikin, all necessary airways oral pharyngeal and nasal pharyngeal airways, suction, gloves, goggles, and gown

PERFORMANCE CRITERIA
- 100% accuracy required on all items designated by a diamond (♦) for skills testing and must manage successfully all items indicated by double asterisks (**).
- Documentation, identified by the symbol (§), must be practiced, but is not a required test item.
- Appropriate body substance isolation precautions must be instituted.

SPECIFIC SKILL PREPARATION	
Skill Component	**Teaching Points**
♦ Take body substance isolation precautions	• Mandatory personal protective equipment - gloves • Situational - long sleeves, goggles, masks, gown

PROCEDURE	
Skill Component	**Teaching Points**
♦ Check and assemble components when instructed.	• Inflate cuff #1 (blue) with 100ml or 85 ml of air and remove syringe • Check for integrity of cuff then remove air but leave syringe attached with 100ml of air • Inflate cuff #2 (clear) with 15ml or 12 ml of air and remove syringe • Check for integrity of cuff then remove air but leave syringe attached with 15ml of air
♦ Upon instruction pre-oxygenate patient (5-6 breaths). Prepare for 30 second time count.	
♦ Position patient's head	• No trauma - neutral or slightly extended position • Trauma - neutral position with in-line axial spinal stabilization.
♦ Connect BVM to tube #1 (blue) and ventilate.	
♦ If breath sounds are present bilaterally, chest rises with ventilation and epigastric sounds are absent – ventilate through tube #1 (blue).	• Head-tilt or modified jaw thrust may or may not be required to obtain patency.
♦ If breath sounds are absent, there is no chest rise, and epigastric sounds are auscultated - immediately remove deflector and ventilate through tube #2 (clear).	• Secure tube with tape if patent airway

Skill Component	Teaching Points
◆ If breath sounds are absent, there is no chest rise, and epigastric sounds are not auscultated - deflate both cuffs, recess tube 3cm, re-inflate both cuffs, ventilate tube #1 and reassess breath sounds.	
◆ If unable to verify placement, there is no chest rise, and breath sounds are absent – deflate both cuffs, remove tube and resume BVM ventilation with NP or OP airway.	• Patient should be hyperventilated a minimum of 60 seconds between intubation attempts.
◆ Ventilate patient specific to patient's condition.	• 1 breath every 6-8 secs or 8-10 breaths/min
◆ Dispose of equipment using approved technique.	

ONGOING ASSESSMENT

Skill Component	Teaching Points
§ Reassess patient's condition and effectiveness of ventilations	• Return of normal skin color, decrease in pulse (adult), and good rise and fall of chest indicate adequate clinical response

DOCUMENTATION

Skill Component	Teaching Points
§ Verbalize/Document: • Reason for intervention • Criteria used for assuring correct placement • Signs indicating effectiveness of treatment • Treatment provided	

Developed 8/07

Breathing Emergency – Assisting with Combitube Intubation

© 2007

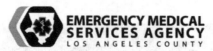
BREATHING EMERGENCY / AIRWAY MANAGEMENT
BAG-VALVE-MASK VENTILATION
UNPROTECTED AIRWAY
Supplemental Information

INDICATIONS:

- Respiratory arrest
- Respiratory compromise (hypoxia)

COMPLICATIONS:

- Gastric distention
- Vomiting

NOTES:

- A second rescuer is needed to maintain in-line axial stabilization if spinal immobilization is required, but may initially be performed by one rescuer by stabilizing the head between the rescuer's legs and anterior thighs.

- BVM device should have either no pressure-relief (pop-off) valve or a valve with an override feature to permit use of high pressures which may be necessary to achieve visible chest rise and effective ventilation.

- Squeezing the bag too forcefully will result in gastric distension and vomiting. Use only the force and tidal volume needed to achieve visible chest rise.

- In cases of gastric distension, continue ventilations using appropriate airway maneuvers.

- Using a bag-valve-mask device with an oxygen reservoir attached to an oxygen source that delivers 15L/minute can provide a 90% or greater concentration of inspired oxygen. However, the effectiveness of the BVM device depends on the volume of gas that is squeezed out of the bag and if a proper seal is maintained.

- In pediatric patients, hypoxia results in bradycardia which may lead to asystole. Reassess heart rate in neonates every 30-60 seconds and in infants and children every 1-2 minutes.

- It is important to maintain a neutral position in <u>pediatric</u> patients to prevent hyperflexion of the neck which may inhibit ventilations or occlude the airway (head is relatively large for size of the body). Appropriate airway alignment is achieved by placing approx. 2" of padding under the shoulders or entire torso if necessary.

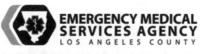

EMERGENCY MEDICAL SERVICES AGENCY
LOS ANGELES COUNTY

EMS SKILL

BREATHING EMERGENCY / AIRWAY MANAGEMENT
BAG-VALVE-MASK VENTILATION
UNPROTECTED AIRWAY

PERFORMANCE OBJECTIVES
The examinee will demonstrate proficiency in ventilating a simulated patient utilizing a bag-valve-mask device.

CONDITION
The examinee will be requested to ventilate a simulated adult, child, or infant in a non-traumatic respiratory arrest with an unprotected airway. The examinee will be required to ventilate for a minimum of 1 minute. The adult or child manikin will be placed supine on the floor. The infant may be placed on a table. Necessary equipment will be adjacent to the manikin.

EQUIPMENT
Adult, child, and infant manikin, adult and pediatric bag-valve-mask device, O_2 connecting tubing, oxygen source with flow regulator, oropharyngeal and nasopharyngeal airways appropriate for manikin, silicone spray, water-soluble lubricant, 10cc syringe, pediatric resuscitation tape, goggles, masks, gown, gloves, timing device.

PERFORMANCE CRITERIA
- 100% accuracy required on all items designated by a diamond (♦) for skills testing and must manage successfully all items indicated by double asterisks (**).
- Documentation, identified by the symbol (§), must be practiced, but is not a required test item.
- Appropriate body substance isolation precautions must be instituted.
- Ventilation must be at least at the minimum rate required for the situation given.

PREPARATION	
Skill Component	**Key Concepts**
♦ Take body substance isolation precautions	• Mandatory personal protective equipment - gloves • Situational - long sleeves, goggles, masks, gown
♦ Select appropriate size mask and bag	• Ideally rescuers should use the appropriate size bag and mask. However, the size of the bag is not as important as the size of the mask. *If an adult bag is used on a pediatric patient, the tidal volume delivered should not exceed the chest rise of normal inspiration.*
♦ Assemble bag-valve-mask device	
♦ Connect bag-valve-mask device to oxygen source	• Immediate ventilation should not be delayed to connect the BVM device to an oxygen source. This may be done once ventilations have started.
♦ Turn oxygen on to deliver 15L/min	

PROCEDURE	
Skill Component	**Key Concepts**
♦ Open the airway: • <u>Medical</u> - head-tilt/chin-lift • <u>Trauma</u> - jaw-thrust	• Move the patient no more than necessary to ensure an open airway. A second rescuer is needed to maintain in-line axial stabilization if spinal immobilization is required. *If only one rescuer is available to maintain spinal immobilization and ventilate with a BVM, the EMT may use his/her knees to stabilize the head between the rescuer's lower legs and thighs.* • It is important to maintain a neutral position in <u>pediatric</u> patients to prevent hyperflexion of the neck which may inhibit ventilations or occlude the airway (head is relatively large for size of the body). Appropriate airway alignment is achieved by placing approx. 2" of padding under the shoulders or entire torso if necessary.

Skill Component	Key Concepts
◆ Insert oropharyngeal/nasopharyngeal airway ** **Remove visible obstruction or suction - *if indicated***	• Nasopharyngeal airway contraindicated in infant that is less than 12 months due to the small diameter of the nostril and adenoidal tissue. • Some NPA airways may extend past the nostrils. This results in inability to maintain a tight seal and inhibits the function of the NPA when the mask is in place.
◆ Place mask over mouth and nose, maintaining a tight seal and patent airway: • Place thumb on apex of mask and index finger on mask over chin area - forming letter "C" • Place remaining 3 fingers on mandible and bring the jaw up toward the mask - forming letter "E"	• Avoid pushing mask down on the face. This results in vagal stimulation if pressure is put on the eyeballs, - especially in pediatric patients. The top of the mask is over the bridge of the nose and the bottom is in the groove between the lower lip and the chin. • Avoid pressure on soft tissue under the chin which may result in airway obstruction.
◆ Ventilate patient with appropriate tidal volume: • Observe for effective rise and fall of chest • Allow for adequate exhalation between ventilations	• Use <u>only</u> enough force to allow for good chest rise. Over-inflation causes gastric distention which will decrease tidal volume by elevating the diaphragm. • To allow for adequate exhalation, say "squeeze-release-release". (Exhalation requires more time than inspiration) • To maintain an adequate seal and provide adequate tidal volume, the EMT may squeeze the bag by using one hand or squeezing the bag against the forearm or anterior thigh. When the patient is on a gurney the bag may be squeezed with one hand and against the rescuers rib cage. • The bag is refilled with oxygen during its expansion when the patient exhales.
◆ Ventilate patient at approximate rate of: • Adult - 10-12/minute • Child - 12-20/minute • Infant - 20-30/minute • Neonate - 30-60/minute	• The range for pediatric patients varies due to a large age range. The range from toddler to 8 years-of-age, rate is 20/minute while a 14 year-old may be ventilated at the adult rate.
◆ Reassess: • Lung compliance • Airway patency • Skin color • Heart rate **Suction - *if indicated***	• Continually assess respiratory status with each ventilation. • Lung compliance provides information of successful inspiration or if there is interference with air delivery due to inadequate mask seal and airway or thoracic problems. • In pediatric patients the resistance felt will generally be greater than in an adult due to the smaller size of the bronchi and bronchioles. • In pediatric patients, hypoxia results in bradycardia which may lead to asystole. Reassess heart rate in neonates every 30-60 seconds and in infants and children every 1-2 minutes.

◆ Clean or dispose of contaminated equipment using approved technique.	• <u>Non-disposable</u>:
	  - Must insure that there is no chance of contamination from one patient to another. Use approved method for disassembling, cleaning and disinfecting all parts of the device.
	
	  <u>Disposable</u>:
	  - Place contaminated equipment in plastic bag, seal, and dispose at designated sites.

ONGOING ASSESSMENT

Skill Component	Key Concepts
§ Repeat an ongoing assessment every **5 minutes**: • Initial assessment • Relevant portion of the focused assessment • Evaluate response to treatment • Compare results to baseline condition and vital signs	• The initial and focused examination is repeated every 15 minutes for stable patients and every 5 minutes for priority patients. • Every patient must be re-evaluated at least every 5 minutes, if any treatment was initiated or medication administered, unless changes in the patient's condition are anticipated sooner. • Priority patients are patients who have abnormal vital signs, signs/symptoms of poor perfusion or if there is a suspicion that the patient's condition may deteriorate.

DOCUMENTATION

Skill Component	Key Concepts

§ Verbalize/Document:
• Percent of oxygen/Liter flow
• Ventilation rate
• Size of nasopharyngeal or oropharyngeal adjunct
• Resistance encountered (lung compliance)
• Gastric distention - *if developed*
• Dentures and location - *if removed*
• Response to ventilation
  - chest rise and fall
  - color
  - level of consciousness
	• Documentation must be on either the Los Angeles County EMS Report or departmental Patient Care Record form.

Developed 11/00   Revised 12/01, 1/03, 6/06

[Handwritten notes:]
15L/min
use adjunct

adult   10-12 /min (every 5-6 sec)
child   12-20 /min (every 3-5 sec)
Infant   20-30/min (every 2-3 sec)
Neonate   36-60 min (every sec)

INDICATIONS:

- Respiratory Failure
- Respiratory Arrest

CONTRAINDICATIONS

- Chest injury
- Suspected cervical spinal injury
- Pediatric patients
- Should be used with caution in patients with COPD

COMPLICATIONS:

- Gastric distention
- Pneumothorax

NOTES:

- If the chest does not adequately rise and you are sure there is no airway obstruction, use an alternative device.

Developed 7/07

Breathing Emergency – Flow Restricted Oxygen Powered Ventilatory Device
© 2007
UCLA Skills Guide for EMT -1
Page 1 of 1
Page 54

BREATHING EMERGENCY / AIRWAY MANAGEMENT
FLOW RESTRICTED OXYGEN POWERED VENTILATORY DEVICE

PERFORMANCE OBJECTIVES
The examinee will demonstrate proficiency in ventilating a patient with a Flow Restricted Oxygen Powered Ventilatory Device (FROPVD)

CONDITION
The examinee will be requested to secure an airway and ventilate an airway manikin utilizing a FROPVD

EQUIPMENT
Adult CPR/Airway manikin, all necessary airways oral pharyngeal and nasal pharyngeal airways, suction, gloves, goggles, and gown

PERFORMANCE CRITERIA
- 100% accuracy required on all items designated by a diamond (♦) for skills testing and must manage successfully all items indicated by double asterisks (**).
- Documentation, identified by the symbol (§), must be practiced, but is not a required test item.
- Appropriate body substance isolation precautions must be instituted.

FLOW RESTRICTED OXYGEN POWERED VENTILATORY DEVICE PREPARATION	
Skill Component	**Teaching Points**
♦ Take body substance isolation precautions	• Mandatory personal protective equipment - gloves • Situational - long sleeves, goggles, masks, gown
♦ Open the airway using appropriate technique	
♦ Insert an airway adjunct if possible	• Insertion of airway adjunct should be done only if patient lacks gag reflex. Insertion is not necessary to accomplish skill.
♦ Attach proper size mask to the manually-triggered oxygen powered ventilating device	
♦ Open oxygen source and ensure pressure is adequate	• Oxygen tank regulator should be set at 15 liters/min

PROCEDURE	
Skill Component	**Teaching Points**
♦ Secure mask to face maintaining a tight seal and patent airway	• Place mask over mouth and nose • Using one hand, place thumb on mask at apex and index finger on the mask at the chin level • With the remaining three fingers, pull mandible forward to maintain patent airway
♦ Ventilate by pressing trigger on manually-triggered oxygen powered ventilating device once every 3- 5 seconds as appropriate for patients condition and age observing for chest rise	• Crycoid pressure is highly recommended to reduce gastric distention.
♦ Observe lung compliance when pressing trigger of demand valve	

Skill Component	Teaching Points
§ Reassess patient's condition and effectiveness of ventilations	• Return of normal skin color, decrease in pulse (adult), and good rise and fall of chest indicate adequate clinical response

DOCUMENTATION

Skill Component	Teaching Points
§ Verbalize/Document: • Reason for intervention • Signs indicating effectiveness of treatment • Treatment provided	

Developed 8/07

BREATHING EMERGENCY / AIRWAY MANAGEMENT
MOUTH-MASK VENTILATION WITH SUPPLEMENTAL OXYGEN

INDICATIONS:

- •Patients who are unresponsive, apneic, or have depressed respirations

CONTRAINDICATIONS:

- None when above conditions apply.

COMPLICATIONS:

- Gastric distention

NOTES:

- Do not start resuscitation if the patient meets the criteria in Ref. No. 814 - Determination / Pronouncement of Death in the Field or Ref. No. 815 - Honoring Prehospital Do-Not Resuscitate (DNR) Orders.

- The tongue is the most common cause of airway obstruction due to decreased muscle tone.

- The tongue and epiglottis may obstruct the entrance of the trachea due to inspiratory efforts creating negative pressure in the airway.

- Move the patient no more than necessary to maintain an open airway. A second rescuer is needed to maintain in-line axial stabilization if spinal immobilization is required.

- Adequate ventilation is indicated by good chest rise and hearing and feeling air escape doing exhalation.

- Improper positioning of head and chin is the most common cause of inadequate ventilations.

- If the patient is in a prone position with suspected trauma, the patient should be turned using log-roll method to avoid flexion or twisting of the neck or back.

- Only remove dentures if they cannot be kept in place to prevent airway obstruction. Fitted dentures maintain form for a good seal.

- Improper positioning of head and chin is the most common cause of inadequate ventilations.

- Adequate ventilation is indicated by good chest rise and hearing and feeling air escape doing exhalation.

- Mouth-mask rescue breathing provides the same tidal volume as mouth-to-mouth rescue breathing, and is easier to use and produces a larger tidal volume than the bag-valve-mask device since the rescuer uses both hands to maintain a seal.

- Using a mouth-to-mask device <u>without</u> supplemental oxygen, breaths should be delivered at 10ml/kg or average of 700-1000ml over a 2 second period.

- Using a mouth-to-mask device <u>with</u> supplemental oxygen, breaths should be delivered at 8-7ml/kg or average 400-600ml over a 1-2 second period which reduces the chance of gastric inflation.

- In pediatric patients, breaths should be delivered a 6-7ml/kg (no average available since weight range varies significantly).

REFERENCES:

- Reference No. 814 - Determination/Pronouncement of Death in the Field
- Reference No. 815 - Honoring Prehospital Do-Not-Resuscitate (DNR) Orders
- Reference No. 818 - Honoring Advance Health Care Directive (AHCD)

Developed: 4/04

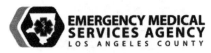

EMERGENCY MEDICAL SERVICES AGENCY
LOS ANGELES COUNTY

EMS SKILL

BREATHING EMERGENCY / AIRWAY MANAGEMENT
MOUTH – MASK OR BARRIER DEVICE VENTILATION
WITH SUPPLEMENTAL OXYGEN

PERFORMANCE OBJECTIVES
Demonstrate proficiency in ventilating a patient using a pocket face mask or barrier device with supplemental oxygen.

CONDITION
The examinee will be requested to assess and ventilate a patient that requires pulmonary resuscitation and/or rescue breathing by using a pocket face mask or barrier device and providing supplemental oxygen. The manikin will be placed supine on the floor. Necessary equipment will be adjacent to the manikin or brought to the field setting.

EQUIPMENT
Adult CPR manikin, pocket face mask or barrier device with an O_2 outlet and a one-way valve, O_2 connecting tubing, oxygen source with flow regulator, oropharyngeal airway, nasopharyngeal airway, goggles, gown, gloves, timing device.

PERFORMANCE CRITERIA
- Items designated by a diamond (♦) must be performed successfully to demonstrate skill competency.
- Items identified by double asterisks (**) indicate actions that are required if indicated.
- Items identified by (§) are not skill component items, but should be practiced.
- Ventilation must be at least at the minimum rate required for the situation given.

PREPARATION	
Skill Component	**Key Concepts**
♦ Take body substance isolation precautions	• Mandatory personal protective equipment – gloves • Situational - long sleeves, goggles, mask, gown
♦ Assess scene safety/scene size-up ** ***Consider spinal injury precautions - if indicated***	• If unknown as to possible trauma, treat as trauma (determined by environment and information obtained from bystanders).
♦ Assess breathing	
♦ Connect one-way valve to pocket mask or barrier device opening	• Test equipment by blowing through it once thus eliminating potential faulty equipment.
♦ Connect oxygen tubing to mask or barrier device and oxygen source	• DO NOT delay <u>initial</u> ventilations to connect O_2 tubing to oxygen source.
♦ Turn oxygen on to deliver 15L/min	

PROCEDURE	
Skill Component	**Key Concepts**
♦ Position self at the head or side of the patient	
♦ Open the airway using head tilt-chin lift or jaw-thrust maneuver	• The jaw-thrust maneuver is used when spinal injuries are suspected
♦ Place the mask or barrier device securely over the patient's nose and mouth:	• If the mask or barrier device is not seated properly it will result in inadequate ventilations.

Skill Component	Key Concepts
♦ Seal the mask or barrier device on the patient's face	• To seal the mask (most common technique): - Place both thumbs and forefingers around the anterior circumference of the mask - Place the ring and middle fingers under the angle of the mandible - Press the mask firmly onto the face
♦ Maintain an open airway using head-tilt/jaw-thrust maneuver	• Head-tilt/Jaw-thrust maneuver - Grasp the mandible with the ring and middle fingers of both hands - Pull mandible upward while compressing the mask onto the patient's face with thumbs and forefingers to maintain a tight seal

♦ Place mouth around the one-way valve and deliver appropriate number of slow breaths:
  • Adult - each breath over 2 seconds
  • Infant and child – each breath 1-1.5 seconds
	• DO NOT over inflate. Provide enough volume for good chest expansion, but prevent gastric distention.
	• Rescuer should take a breath after each ventilation.

♦ Watch for rise and fall of the chest ** *Reposition head if unable to ventilate* ** *Start obstructed airway maneuvers - If still unable to ventilate* ** *Consider an oropharyngeal or nasopharyngeal airway - if indicated*	• View the chest for sufficient chest rise using peripheral vision. • Adequate ventilation is indicated by good chest rise and hearing and feeling air escape during exhalation. • Improper positioning of head and chin is the most common cause of inadequate ventilations. • If force of air is too great and/or rate is too fast, gastric distention will occur when the pharyngeal pressures exceeds esophageal opening pressure allowing air to enter the stomach. • Allow for adequate exhalation between ventilations.

♦ Continue to ventilate at the approximate rate of:
  • Adult - 10-12/minute
  • Child - 12-20/minute
  • Infant - 20-30/minute
  • Neonate - 30-60/minute
 	
** *After 30 seconds attach oxygen to face mask or barrier device – if not already done*
 	
** *Consider Sellick's maneuver (cricoid pressure) to prevent gastric distention*
	• The range of ventilations for pediatric patients varies due to a large age range and emphasis should be placed on signs of adequate perfusion.
	• Performing a Sellick's maneuver requires a second rescuer.

REASSESSMENT
(Ongoing Assessment)

Skill Component	Key Concepts

§ Repeat an ongoing assessment every **5 minutes**:
  • Initial assessment
  • Relevant portion of the focused assessment
  • Evaluate response to treatment
  • Compare results to baseline condition and vital signs
	• Patients must be evaluated every 5 minutes and should be evaluated more often if any treatment was initiated, medication administered, or changes in the patient's condition are anticipated.

PATIENT REPORT AND DOCUMENTATION

Skill Component	Key Concepts

§ Verbalize/Document:
  • Percent of oxygen/Liter flow
  • Ventilation rate
  • Dentures and location - *if removed*
  • Response to ventilation
   - chest rise and fall
   - color
   - level of consciousness
	• Documentation must be on either the Los Angeles County EMS Report or departmental Patient Care Record form.

Breathing Emergency - Mouth-Mask Ventilation © 2004, 2006, 2007, 2010 UCLA Skills Guide for EMT -1   Page Page 59

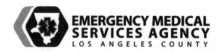
BREATHING EMERGENCY: OXYGEN ADMINISTRATION
Supplemental Information

Definitions:

- Hypoxia – insufficient oxygen delivery to body cells which may lead to organ ischemia and eventually death. Signs/symptoms of hypoxia include: increased respiratory rate, increased heart rate, changes in level of consciousness, restlessness, irritability and cyanosis.

- Inadequate respirations –

- Minute volume – total volume inhaled in a minute calculated by multiplying tidal volume and the number of respirations for one minute.

- Respiratory distress – acute condition in which the patient needs to work harder to breath. Signs/symptoms include: increased respiratory rate, accessory muscle use, nasal flaring, and difficulty speaking in complete sentences. The patient may assume an upright or a tripod position to aid respiratory muscles.

- Respiratory failure – acute condition in which there is inadequate ventilation to support life and requires immediate positive-pressure ventilations. Signs and symptoms of respiratory failure include: altered mental status, loss of muscle tone that progresses to inadequate minute volume. This condition develops when there is respiratory muscle fatigue after prolonged respiratory distress or obstruction of the upper or lower airway.

- Respiratory arrest – agonal or complete cessation of breathing.

- Tidal volume – amount of air inhaled and exhaled during a normal breath.

- Vital capacity (lung capacity) – is compose of the maximum inspiratory reserve volume (IRV), maximum expiratory reserve volume (ERV) and the tidal volume (TV) of a single breath.

Indications for supplemental oxygen administration:

- Goal of providing supplemental oxygen is to treat patients in respiratory distress and prevent respiratory failure and respiratory arrest.

- Consider when respiratory rates do not allow for adequate gas exchange:
  - Adults   < 12 and > 20 breaths per minute
  - Children   < 15 and > 30 breaths per minute
  - Infants   < 25 and > 50 breaths per minute

- Patients that exhibit signs/symptoms of:

- Respiratory problems	- Seizure	- Fever
- Altered level of consciousness	- Abdominal pain	- Overdose
- Shock	- Back pain	- Vomiting
- Trauma	- Chest pain	- Diarrhea

- Exposure to toxins e.g. smoke, carbon monoxide and cyanide

Indications for assisted ventilations:

- Patients with inadequate respirations and tidal volume, respiratory failure and respiratory arrest need positive pressure ventilations. They should not be placed on supplemental oxygen using a nasal cannula or mask.

Contraindications:

- None in prehospital care with the above conditions.

Hazards of Oxygen Administration:

Equipment
- Increased chance of fire if a spark or flame is introduced into an oxygen-rich environment

- Cylinder becomes a missile if punctured or if a valve breaks off

- Explosion may occur if any device attached to the cylinder or outlet valve, or is used for oxygen delivery comes in contact with a petroleum product e.g. lubricant or cleaner; fat-based soap; or adhesive tape

Physiological (depends on patient's condition and rarely occurs in prehospital due to short ETA.)
- Oxygen toxicity – rare in prehospital care

- Damage to the retina in newborns

- Respiratory depression or arrest in patients with COPD

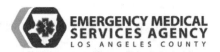

EMS SKILL

BREATHING EMERGENCY: OXYGEN ADMINISTRATION

PERFORMANCE OBJECTIVES
Demonstrate proficiency in the administration of oxygen by utilizing an oxygen tank and regulator, oxygen masks, nasal cannula, and providing oxygen by blow-by method.

CONDITION
Administer oxygen to a patient whose condition requires supplemental oxygenation by a mask, cannula, or blow-by method. Necessary equipment will be adjacent to the manikin or brought to the field setting.

EQUIPMENT
Adult CPR manikin, O_2 connecting tubing, simple O_2 mask, non-re-breather mask, nasal cannula, oxygen source with flow regulator, oropharyngeal and nasopharyngeal airways appropriate for manikin, silicone spray, water-soluble lubricant, goggles, masks, gown, gloves, timing device.

PERFORMANCE CRITERIA
- Items designated by a diamond (♦) must be performed successfully to demonstrate skill competency.
- Items identified by double asterisks (**) indicate actions that are required, if indicated.
- Items identified by (§) should be practiced.

PREPARATION	
Skill Component	**Key Concepts**
♦ Take body substance isolation precautions	• Mandatory (minimal) personal protective equipment – gloves
♦ Assess scene safety/scene size-up ** ***Consider spinal immobilization - if indicated***	• If unknown as to possible trauma, manage as trauma (determined by environment and information obtained from bystanders).
♦ Evaluate need for additional BSI precautions	• Situational - goggles, mask, gown
♦ Approach the patient and introduce yourself to the patient/caregivers	

SETTING UP OXYGEN CYLINDER AND REGULATOR PROCEDURE	
Skill Component	**Key Concepts**
♦ Confirm that it is a "medical grade" oxygen cylinder	• To confirm cylinder contains medical grade oxygen: - check color of cylinder - green and white, solid green, or unpainted aluminum with a green ring around top of cylinder - pin index groupings line up with oxygen regulator
♦ Clear dust or debris from the opening	• To clear dust or debris from the opening, open the main valve slowly until gas flow is heard and then immediately close valve. • The valve stem should not be covered with adhesive tape or petroleum based substances. Both of these may contaminate the oxygen or result in spontaneous combustion due to the presence of pressurized oxygen.
♦ Place a new O-ring (flexible gasket) over the large opening on either the cylinder or regulator	• The O-ring can be placed over the large opening on either the cylinder or regulator opening. • O-rings are manufactured for single-use only and must be replaced every time a regulator is attached.
♦ Secure the regulator to the valve stem: • Align the pin index from the regulator with the holes in the cylinder • Insert the pins of the regulator with the holes in the cylinder • Tighten screw bolt with firm hand pressure to ensure an adequate seal	• Gas regulators have a different pin index and the cylinder valves have specific configurations of holes to prevent accidental administration of the wrong gas. • DO NOT tighten the screw bolt with a wrench or other device as this may cause a break in the seal and damage to the regulator.

Skill Component	Key Concepts
♦ Open valve two (2) full turns *(handwritten: open valve)* ** **If cylinder leaks, turn off valve and check connections**	• A leaking cylinder may be the result of an O-ring this is improperly seated, poor connection between the regulator pins and the cylinder, or debris that does not allow for a proper seal.
♦ Read the pressure gauge to determine the oxygen pressure (psi) in the cylinder *(handwritten: should be 2000 psi)* ** **If cylinder is not in use and is near 500 psi – Do Not put in service** ** **If cylinder is in use and reaches 200 psi – change cylinder immediately**	• Amount of oxygen pressure in cylinder is read as pounds per square inch (psi). • Gauge should read approximately 2000 psi. The volume of oxygen varies in the different size cylinders, but when full are at the same pressure of 2000 psi. • Portable cylinders ideally should be changed if between 1000 and 500 psi. • Cylinders should not be put into service if near 500 psi. • If the cylinder is in use, it should never be allowed to go below 200 psi. Oxygen pressure below 200 psi does not deliver appropriate liter flow and will empty within minutes depending on liter flow.
♦ Attach oxygen tubing or delivery device to regulator and adjust to desired liter flow	
♦ Place oxygen delivery device on patient	

DISCONTINUING OXYGEN ADMINISTRATION AND DISCONNECTING CYLINDER AND REGULATOR PROCEDURE

Skill Component	Key Concepts
♦ Remove oxygen delivery device from patient and regulator	
♦ Check pressure gauge for psi remaining in cylinder	
♦ Close regulator valve	
♦ Remove oxygen tubing from regulator stem	
♦ Close valve at top of cylinder	
♦ Bleed oxygen out of system • Open regulator valve • Listen for oxygen flow to stop • Close regulator • Check that gauge reads zero with the cylinder valve closed.	
♦ Detach regulator by loosening the screw bolt	
♦ Log or label cylinder with psi reading per department or agency protocol	• Cylinder should be labeled as "EMPTY" if near 500 psi. • Various departments and agencies may use a log or use commercial tags. **Never use adhesive tape to label readings.**
♦ Store oxygen cylinder appropriately	• Never leave cylinders standing in an upright position unless properly secured. If cylinder is dropped and the valve breaks off, the cylinder will act as a missile projectile.

NASAL CANNULA (NC)
PROCEDURE

Skill Component	Key Concepts
◆ Attach oxygen supply tubing to oxygen source	• Patients who are mouth breathers receive minimal benefit from nasal cannula oxygen administration.
◆ Set oxygen to appropriate liter flow (2-6 Liters/minute)	• NC is a low-flow, low-oxygen concentration delivery device that delivers 24%-44% of oxygen with flow rates of 2-6 Liters/minute. • DO NOT deliver more than 6 Liters/minute by nasal cannula. This will dry out the mucosa or cause oxygen burns to nostrils, but will not increase oxygen delivery.
◆ Check for oxygen flow through NC	
◆ Place the nasal cannula prongs into the nostrils (nares)	• Curvature of the prongs should be oriented so that the tips will curve down and are slightly posterior once inserted.
◆ Secure tubing by: • Hold loop of tubing anterior to face and neck and slip tubing around the patient's ears and under the chin	• Never place the tubing behind the head since this may decrease the flow of oxygen or the patient may strangle if the cannula slips around the neck.
◆ Adjust fit of the NC under the chin	• Tubing must be secure, but not so tight that it causes discomfort.
◆ Evaluate patient comfort	

MEDIUM CONCENTRATION OXYGEN MASK (SIMPLE FACE MASK)
PROCEDURE

Skill Component	Key Concepts
◆ Attach oxygen supply tubing to oxygen source	
◆ Set oxygen to appropriate liter flow (8-10 Liters/minute)	• Simple face mask delivers up to 60% of oxygen with flow rates of 8-10 Liters/minute. • Flow rates greater than 10 Liters/minute does not increase oxygen delivery and may result in patient discomfort and drying of mucus membranes.
◆ Check for oxygen flow through mask NOTE: **Never apply an oxygen mask without oxygen flowing**	☠ **Never apply an oxygen mask without oxygen flowing, this will result in hypoxia and possible death.**
◆ Place mask on patient's face covering both nose and mouth with narrow end over the bridge of the nose	
◆ Slip elastic strap over patient's head and either above or below ears	• Elastic strap placed above the ears may result in patient discomfort, but is more secure for prehospital transport.
◆ Adjust elastic strap until mask is secure	• Mask must be secure, but not so tight that it causes discomfort.
◆ Form the metal strip over the bridge of the nose for a secure fit	• Leakage around the mask decreases the delivery of oxygen.
◆ Evaluate patient comfort	

HIGH CONCENTRATION OXYGEN MASK (NON-REBREATHER RESERVOIR MASK)
PROCEDURE

Skill Component	Key Concepts
♦ Unroll oxygen reservoir bag and attach to mask - *if not already attached*	• Use a pediatric non-rebreather mask that has a smaller reservoir since infants and children inhale smaller volumes.
♦ Ensure oxygen tubing is attached to oxygen source and reservoir bag	
♦ Set oxygen to appropriate liter flow (12-15 Liters/minute)	• A non-rebreather mask is a low-flow, high-oxygen concentration device that delivers approximately 80-90% with flow rates of 12-15 Liters/minute.
♦ Inflate reservoir bag completely by holding finger over valve located inside the mask above the reservoir bag insertion	• Inflate the bag completely before placing the mask on the patient.
♦ Check for oxygen flow through mask	• Ensure that there is adequate and uninterrupted oxygen flow or the patient may not be able to inhale an adequate volume.
♦ Place mask on patient's face covering both nose and mouth with the narrow end over the bridge of the nose	
♦ Slip elastic strap over patient's head and either above or below ears and just below the occiput	• Elastic strap placed above the ears may result in patient discomfort. However, the mask is more secure in prehospital care if it is applied above the ears.
♦ Adjust elastic strap until the mask is secure	• Mask must be secure, but not so tight that it causes discomfort.
♦ Form the metal strip over the bridge of the nose for a secure fit	• Leakage around the mask decreases the delivery of oxygen.
♦ Adjust the liter flow as needed to keep the bag partially inflated after several breathing cycles	• The correct liter flow has been reached when the bag remains partially inflated at the peak of inspiration. • The liter flow is too high if the bag exceeds its capacity and oxygen flows from the valves on the sides of the mask.
♦ Evaluate patient comfort and that the reservoir bag does not deflate completely ** *If reservoir bag deflates completely, increase oxygen by 2 Liter increments until bag remains partially inflated at end of inspiration.* ** *If the oxygen reservoir bag dislodges, replace the oxygen mask.*	• High flow rates are needed to keep oxygen reservoir bag inflated. • Monitor the bag continually to make sure it does not deflate completely at the end of inspiration. • <u>During inspiration</u> -- exhalation valves located at the sides of the mask close, valve above the reservoir bag opens, and reservoir bag deflates slightly. ☠ *If the reservoir bag collapses completely, the patient is unable to inhale and hypoxia and/or death will occur.* <u>Increase oxygen by 2 Liter increments until the bag remains partially inflated at the end of each inspiration.</u> • <u>During exhalation</u> – exhalation valves at the sides of the mask open, valve above the reservoir bag closes, and reservoir bag expands completely.

BLOW-BY OXYGEN ADMINISTRATION
PROCEDURE

Skill Component	Key Concepts
◆ Attach oxygen supply tubing to oxygen source	• The blow-by technique does not provide a high level of oxygen. But if unable to use other oxygen delivery systems, it is better than not being able to deliver oxygen at all.

◆ Set oxygen to appropriate liter flow:
  • Adult – 10-15 Liters/minute
  • Infant/Child – 6-10 Liters/minute
  • Neonate – 5 Liters/minute
	• Provides 30% - 40% of oxygen concentration with a 10 Liters/minute flow rate.
	• For infant/child the liter flow depends on the flow rate and proximity to the face.

◆ Check for oxygen flow through tubing	

◆ Administer oxygen by appropriate method:
  • Adult –
    - Use face mask and hold approximately 1"-2" from face
  • Infant/Child –
    - Use face mask and hold approximately 1"-2" from face
    - Hold tubing 1"-2" from nose and mouth
    - Place oxygen tubing through small hole in the bottom of a 6-8 oz paper or Styrofoam cup and hold cup approximately 1"-2" from child's nose and mouth
  • Neonate – hold tubing 1"-2" from nose and mouth
	• Can be delivered by mask, corrugated tubing, O2 tubing or through bottom of a paper cup (not Styrofoam cup) or in a toy.
	• Adults who are unable to use a nasal cannula and are too claustrophobic to use a mask may benefit by the blow-by method.
	• Nasal cannulas and masks may frighten young children. By using a cup the child may feel more comfortable and allow the administration of oxygen.
	• The cup also acts as an oxygen reservoir allowing for better oxygen delivery than if only using the tubing.
	• Hold tubing for neonates with opening of oxygen tubing facing the nose and mouth.
	• If there is no improvement and hypoxia is suspected another form of oxygen delivery device should be considered.

REASSESSMENT
(Ongoing Assessment)

Skill Component	Key Concepts

◆ Reassess patient at least every **5 minutes for priority** patients and every **15 minutes for stable** patients.
  • Primary assessment
  • Relevant portion of the secondary assessment
  • Vital signs
	Priority patients are patients who have abnormal vital signs, S/S of poor perfusion, if there is a suspicion that the patient's condition may deteriorate, or when the patient's condition changes.
	• Continue to monitor oxygen level of tank.

◆ Evaluate response to treatment	• Patients must be re-evaluated at least every 5 minutes if any treatment was initiated, medication administered or unless a change in the patient's condition is anticipated.
◆ Evaluate results of on-going assessment and compare to baseline condition and vital signs ****Manage patient condition as indicated.**	• Evaluating and comparing results assists in recognizing if the patient is improving, responding to treatment or condition is deteriorating.

PATIENT REPORT AND DOCUMENTATION

Skill Component	Key Concepts
§ Gives appropriate report to equal or higher level of care personnel **EXCEPTION** – ALS to BLS downgrade	• Report should consist of all pertinent information regarding the assessment finding, treatment rendered and patient response to care provided. • Report may be given to a lower level of care provider when an ALS to BLS downgrade has occurred

§   Document:
  • Oxygen administration device used
  • Percent of oxygen/Liter flow
  • Dentures and location - _if removed_
  • Respiratory rate and tidal volume
  • Skin color
  • Level of consciousness
  • Response to oxygen administration
	• Documentation must be on either the Los Angeles County EMS Report or departmental Patient Care Record form.

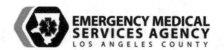
CARDIAC EMERGENCY: AUTOMATED EXTERNAL DEFIBRILLATION (AED)
Supplemental Information

INDICATIONS:

* Patient unresponsive to stimuli, non-breathing, and pulseless. (The AED will shock patients with a pulse if they are in ventricular tachycardia).

CONTRAINDICATIONS:

* Patients who are awake, have a pulse, or are breathing
* Patients who meet conditions outlined in Reference No. 814, 815 and 818.

COMPLICATIONS:

* Burns to chest
* Inappropriate shocks or failure to shock

NOTES:

* EMS personnel are defined as EMTs and Paramedics.

* A **witnessed arrest** is when EMS personnel actually see the patient collapse.

* An **unwitnessed arrest** is when EMS personnel DID NOT witness the arrest even though it was witnessed by a citizen.

* The initial priority in an **unwitnessed** arrest is to start CPR immediately. The initial priority in a **witnessed** arrest is to use the AED as soon as it is available because the "pump" is still primed.

* Never use the AED to triage or monitor patients who complain of chest pain and are awake, breathing or have a pulse.

* CPR for 2 minutes prior to defibrillation results in improved survival rates.

* The only shockable rhythms are ventricular fibrillation and ventricular tachycardia.

* Defibrillation stops all chaotic electrical impulses in the heart and allows for the normal pacemaker to re-establish a viable heart beat.

  The AED operator is responsible to ensure that no one touches the patient when the AED is analyzing or when shocks are given.

* The arcing of electricity results in burns to the chest and/or the myocardium not receiving an appropriate electrical charge.

* Electrical devices may create wave forms that can be misinterpreted by the AED as a shockable rhythm (electric blanket, TV, radio, wireless phones, pagers, etc.). These devices should be turned off or removed.

* DO NOT apply pads over medication patches. Remove medication patches with gloves and clean area before applying pads. Medication patches can block energy delivery to the heart and cause minor burns due to arcing. Gloves should be worn to protect the EMS provider from exposure to medications which may be absorbed through the skin.

* DO NOT place pads over pacemaker or implanted cardiac defibrillator. Place pads inferior to the medical device or to the side of the device. Pacemakers and implantable cardioverter defibrillators (ICDs) may reduce energy delivery to the heart, if pads are placed over them.

* Metal surfaces do not pose a hazard to either the patient or to EMS providers.

* DO NOT defibrillate in free standing water. Remove patient from water and dry chest thoroughly before applying pads. Water conducts electricity and may provide a pathway for energy from the AED to the provider or bystanders or from one electrode pad to another.

* Excessive chest hair may interfere with electrode pad placement. Use safety razor or if no razor is available apply initial pads then remove them quickly to remove hair then apply a second set of pads.

* Body piercing jewelry, such as nipple rings, may cause arcing and skin burns. However, jewelry should not be removed since a special technique is required for removal. If no other option is available, place the pads directly over the jewelry.

* Some manufacturers recommend that pads are placed on specific sides. Follow the manufacturer's guidelines.

* A child, for the purpose of using an AED, is defined as an infant up to 8 years of age. Use pediatric paddles or self-adhering electrodes for infants less than 1 year of age, if available.

* For children, use a defibrillator with a child key/switch, pediatric pads, or adult pads with a pediatric dose-attenuator. If an attenuator system is not available, use adult pads and the adult electrical dose. *Not treating a shockable rhythm in children has the potential for greater harm than using an adult dose if that is all that is available.*

* If a child is older than 8 years-of-age or more than 55 pounds, use adult defibrillation pads and AED.

Cardiac Emergency: Automated External Defibrillation (AED) [© 2001, 2004, 2006, 2008, 2009]

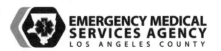

EMS SKILL

CARDIAC EMERGENCY: AUTOMATED EXTERNAL DEFIBRILLATION (AED)

PERFORMANCE OBJECTIVE
Demonstrate competency in assessing for signs of cardiopulmonary arrest and performing defibrillation using a semi-automated external defibrillator.

CONDITION
Manage an adult or pediatric patient who is found unresponsive with no signs of trauma. CPR may or may not be in progress. Necessary equipment will be adjacent to the manikin or brought to the field setting.

EQUIPMENT
Adult , pediatric and infant CPR manikin, AED trainer, adult and pediatric defibrillator pads and attenuator (if available), cables, towel, safety razor, bag-valve-mask device, O₂ connecting tubing, oxygen source with flow regulator, oropharyngeal and nasopharyngeal airways (various sizes), silicone spray (for manikin use), pediatric resuscitation tape, 1-2 assistants (optional), goggles, various masks, gown, gloves, timing device.

PERFORMANCE CRITERIA
- Items designated by a diamond (♦) must be performed successfully to demonstrate skill competency.
- Items identified by double asterisks (**) indicate actions required if indicated.
- Items identified by the symbol (§) should be practiced.
- Ventilations and compressions must be performed at the minimum rate required.

PREPARATION	
Skill Component	**Key Concepts**
♦ Take body substance isolation precautions (BSI)	• Mandatory personal protective equipment – gloves at all times • Situational - long sleeves, goggles, masks, gown as needed
♦ Assess scene safety/scene size-up ** *Consider spinal immobilization – if indicated*	• If unknown as to possible trauma, manage as trauma (determined by environment and information obtained from bystanders).
♦ Evaluate need for additional BSI precautions	• Situational - goggles, mask, gown
♦ Approach the patient and introduce yourself to the caregivers	

PROCEDURE	
Skill Component	**Key Concepts**

♦ Assess patient and initiate BLS procedures:
 	
• **EMS Witnessed Arrest:**
- establish unresponsiveness
- open the airway (head/tilt or jaw/thrust)
- assess for adequate breathing 5-10 seconds
  ** *give 2 breaths if indicated*
- assess pulse 5-10 seconds
 	
  If no pulse in a witnessed arrest:
- perform CPR @ 30:2 until AED is attached
- activate ALS
 	
• **Unwitnessed Arrest** (unwitnessed by EMS)**:**
- activate appropriate resource – ALS and call for AED
- stop CPR - if in progress
- establish unresponsiveness
- open the airway (head/tilt or jaw/thrust)
- assess for adequate breathing 5-10 seconds –
  ** *give 2 breaths if indicated*
- assess pulse 5-10 seconds   *Continued*
	• The AED should NOT be applied to any patient who is conscious, has a pulse, is breathing, or meets Reference No. 814, 815, 818, or 821.
	
	• A <u>witnessed arrest</u> is when EMS personnel actually see the patient collapse.
	
	• An <u>unwitnessed arrest</u> is when EMS personnel DID NOT witness the arrest even though it was witnessed by a citizen.
	
	• The AED will *only* shock ventricular fibrillation and ventricular tachycardia.
	
	• Early defibrillation is critical in improving the survival of patients in ventricular fibrillation and pulseless ventricular tachycardia.
	
	• Defibrillation stops all chaotic electrical impulses in the heart and allows for the pacemaker to re-establish a viable heart beat.
	
	• CPR for 2 minutes prior to defibrillation, in an unwitnessed arrest, results in improved survival rates. The brief period of CPR helps to correct acidosis by providing oxygen and perfusion to the heart.
	
	    Continued

Cardiac Emergency: Automated External Defibrillation (AED) © 2001, 2004, 2006, 2008, 2009

Skill Component	Key Concepts
If no pulse in an unwitnessed arrest: - perform CPR @ 30:2 for 5 cycles (2 minutes) - attach AED as soon as available **NOTE: *If an airway obstruction is present, the rescuer should perform obstructive airway maneuvers.***	• Moving the patient may interfere with rhythm analysis and the resulting artifact may be interpreted by the AED as ventricular fibrillation. • For the purpose of using an AED, a child is defined as starting with an infant and up to 8 years of age. Use self-adhering electrodes for infants < 1 year of age, if available. • For children, use a defibrillator with a child key/switch, pediatric pads, or adult pads with a pediatric dose-attenuator. • If an attenuator system is not available, use adult pads and the adult electrical dose. *Not treating a shockable rhythm in children has the potential for greater harm than using an adult dose if that is all that is available.*
♦ Position the AED near the patient and the operator	• The AED should be placed near the operator to prevent reaching across the patient to press the "analyze" and "shock" buttons.
♦ Turn on the AED	• Some devices have an ON/OFF button; some turn on when the lid is opened. Once the AED is turned on, <u>DO NOT</u> turn off until the patient has been transferred to a higher medical care provider.
♦ Expose the chest and prepare pad sites for secure pad contact	• Metal surfaces do not pose a hazard to either patients or EMS providers. • Water conducts electricity and may provide a pathway for energy from the AED to the provider or bystanders or from one electrode pad to another. • Medication patches can block energy delivery to the heart and cause minor burns due to arcing. Gloves should be worn to protect provider from exposure to medications that may be absorbed through the skin. • Excessive chest hair may prevent pads from adhering to the chest. Use safety razor or apply initial pads then remove them quickly to remove hair and then apply a second set of pads (ensure that unit has multiple sets of pads). • Body piercing jewelry to the torso may cause arcing and skin burns. Attempts should not be made to remove jewelry since a special technique is required for removal. If no other option is available, place the pads directly over the jewelry. • DO NOT place pads over pacemakers or implantable cardioverter defibrillators (ICDs) since this may reduce the energy delivery to the heart and damage these devices.

♦ Apply AED pads (must not touch or overlap):
• **Adult**
  - <u>Upper</u> - right sternal border directly below the clavicle
  - <u>Lower</u> - left midaxillary line, 5th - 6th intercostal space with top margin below the axilla
• **Children**
  - <u>Anterior-Posterior</u>
    1st pad anterior over sternum between nipples
    2nd pad posterior between shoulder blades
  - <u>Anterior-Anterior</u>
    Right pad – wrap over a small child's shoulder
    Left pad – left anterior to cover midclavicular and midaxillary lines
	• Some manufacturers recommend that pads are placed on specific sites/sides – follow the manufacturer's guidelines.
	
	• Ensure that pads NEVER TOUCH in either an adult or child. If the pads touch, this may cause arcing and result in skin burns. If pads overlap, the AED is unable to read the rhythm and will result in <u>no shock</u> being delivered.
	
	• If a child is older than 8 years-of-age or more than 55 pounds, use adult defibrillation pads

Cardiac Emergency: Automated External Defibrillation (AED) [© 2001, 2004, 2006, 2008, 2009]

Skill Component	Key Concepts

◆ Verbalize stand clear:
  • Stop CPR
  • Verbalize "clear" and ensure no one is touching the patient or gurney
	• The AED is unable to analyze the rhythm when there is artifact derived from touching the patient, chest compressions, poor pad contact or other communication devices. This may result in the prompt to defibrillate when the patient is not in ventricular fibrillation or ventricular tachycardia.

◆ Analyze the rhythm:	

◆ Follow AED voice prompt:
  • **If shock advised**
    - administer shock
    - resume CPR
  ** ***Ensure no one is touching the patient***
  • **If no shock advised**
    - resume CPR immediately
	• If there is no pulse and the AED indicates "shock", stand clear and follow voice prompt.
	• DO NOT administer a single shock then turn the AED off and restart it again. This prevents the administration of the higher defibrillation dose needed for successful conversion. *(If an AED has not been reprogrammed to the 2005 ECC Guidelines and still recommends 3 stacked shocks, follow the voice prompt.)*
	• Once the AED is turned on, DO NOT turn off until the patient has been transferred to a higher medical care provider.

◆ Continue CPR for 5 cycles (2 minutes) beginning with chest compressions	• DO NOT check the pulse immediately after defibrillation since checking the pulse delays compressions and the resumption of circulation. • CPR for 2 minutes after delivering a shock helps to correct acidosis by providing oxygen and perfusion to the myocardium. This increases the heart's ability to pump blood more effectively after the shock. • There is no evidence that chest compressions immediately after defibrillation will provoke recurrent ventricular fibrillation.

◆ Analyze rhythm and follow AED voice prompt:
  • **If shock advised**
    - administer shock
    - resume CPR
  ** ***Ensure no one is touching the patient***
  • **If no shock advised**
    - resume CPR immediately
	• Continue shock sequence until patient regains a pulse and has signs of adequate circulation or patient is transferred to a higher medical care provider.
	• Shock Sequence:
	  - 1. CPR for 5 cycles (2 minutes)
	  - 2. analyze
	  - 3. shock if indicated
	  - 4. CPR for 5 cycles (2 minutes)
	• **Resuscitation efforts need to be continued until ALS arrives.** Transport should be considered only after 20 minutes of continuous BLS efforts and ALS is unavailable
	• **Discontinue resuscitation efforts only if**:
	  - EMS providers are unable to continue due to exhaustion
	  - a dangerous environment exists.
	  - immediate family members request resuscitation be discontinued with agreement of others present
	    * if under 18 years of age, parent or legal guardian must be present
	  - collapsed and no CPR provided within10 minutes

◆ Reassess patient every 60 seconds after return of spontaneous circulation (ROSC):
  • Check for:
    - unresponsiveness
    - breathing
    - pulse
  ** ***Provide rescue breathing- if indicated***
  ** ***Obtain baseline vital signs***
  ** ***Place in position to protect airway - if patient has adequate respirations***
	• The 3 main considerations post-resuscitation are:
	  - Perform pulse check every 60 seconds
	  - Perform an initial and focused assessment every 5 minutes.
	  - Keep AED turned on and attached to patient enroute unless switched to a manual monitor/defibrillator mode or unit.
	• If a pulse is present and the patient is not breathing adequately, start BVM ventilations.
	• If a pulse is present and the patient is breathing adequately, place adults in recovery position and children in a position to protect the airway and reduce the chances of the airway being occluded by the tongue and from aspiration of mucus or vomit.

Cardiac Emergency: Automated External Defibrillation (AED) © 2001, 2004, 2006, 2008, 2009

REASSESSMENT
(Ongoing Assessment)

Skill Component	Key Concepts
♦ Perform pulse check every 60 seconds	
♦ Reassess the patient at least every **5 minutes or sooner:** 　• Primary assessment 　• Relevant portion of the secondary assessment 　• Vital signs	• This is a priority patient and must be re-evaluated at least every 5 minutes or sooner, if any treatment is initiated, medication administered, or condition changes.
♦ Evaluate response to treatment	• Patients must be re-evaluated at least every 5 minutes if any treatment was initiated or medication administered.
♦ Evaluate results of reassessment and compare to baseline condition and vital signs ****Manage patient condition as indicated.**	• Evaluating and comparing results assists in recognizing if the patient is improving, responding to treatment or condition is deteriorating.
§ Explain the care being delivered and the transport destination to the patient/caregivers	• Communication is important when dealing with the patient, family or caregiver. This is a very critical and frightening time for all involved and providing information helps in decreasing the stress they are experiencing.

PATIENT REPORT AND DOCUMENTATION

Skill Component	Key Concepts
§ Give patient report to equal or higher level of care personnel	• Report should consist of all pertinent information regarding the assessment finding, treatment rendered and the patient response to care provided.
§ Document: 　• Patient assessment 　• CPR performed 　• Analysis result - shock vs. no shock advised 　• Time and number of shocks - _if applicable_ 　• Patient response to shocks - _if applicable_	• Documentation must be on either the Los Angeles County EMS Report or departmental Patient Care Record form. • Documentation element on EMS Report form asks for "Witnessed by: ☐ Citizen or ☐ EMS. _(This does not change the definition of "Witnessed Arrest" in regards to the use of an AED.)_

Developed 1/01,　　Revised 12/01, 11/04, 3/06, 1/08, 5/09

Developed: 11/01   Revised: 12/03, 1/05, 5/06, 10/07, 9/08, 3/09

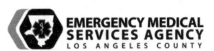

**EMERGENCY MEDICAL
SERVICES AGENCY**
LOS ANGELES COUNTY

CARDIAC EMERGENCY / CARDIOPULMONARY RESUSCITATION
ADULT - 1 RESCUER CPR
Supplemental Information

DEFINITIONS:
- *Recovery position* – Patient is turned onto the side with the arm underneath bent at the elbow and hand near the head. The hand of the upper arm is near the cheek, and the upper leg is bent to stabilize the patient. No single position is perfect for all patients, but the recovery position is preferred to maintain a patent airway and spinal stability, minimize risk of aspiration, and limit pressure on bony prominences and nerves. It also allows for visualization of respirations and skin color, and provides access for needed interventions.

INDICATIONS:
- Patients that are unresponsive, apneic, and pulseless.

CONTRAINDICATIONS:
None when above conditions apply.

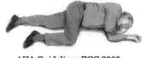

AHA Guidelines ECC 2005

COMPLICATIONS:
- Gastric distention
- Rib fractures
- Sternal fractures
- Separation of ribs from sternum
- Laceration of liver or spleen

- Pneumothorax
- Hemothorax
- Lung and heart contusion
- Fat emboli

NOTES:
- Do not start resuscitation if the patient meets the criteria in Ref. No. 814, 815, and 818.

- The tongue is the most common cause of airway obstruction due to decreased muscle tone.

- The tongue and epiglottis may obstruct the entrance of the trachea due to inspiratory efforts creating negative pressure in the airway.

- Use the jaw thrust maneuver when a head, neck or spine injury is suspected. If the jaw thrust maneuver does not open the airway to allow for adequate ventilation, use the head tilt-chin lift technique.

- Move the patient no more than necessary to maintain an open airway. A second rescuer is needed to maintain in-line axial stabilization if spinal immobilization is required.

- If the patient is in a prone position with suspected trauma, the patient should be turned using log-roll method to avoid flexion or twisting of the neck or back.

- If the patient is breathing adequately with no signs of trauma, place in recovery position as soon as the primary assessment is completed and have suction immediately available. This prevents airway obstruction by the tongue and from mucus or vomitus.

- Remove dentures <u>only</u> if they cannot be kept in place to prevent airway obstruction. Fitted dentures maintain form for a good seal.

- Rescue breathing for an adult is 10-12 breaths/minute. DO NOT hyperventilate patient; this increases intrathoracic pressure, decreases venous return to the heart, and diminishes cardiac output and survival.

- An alternative to checking the carotid pulse is checking the femoral pulse.

- Chest compressions must be performed on a hard surface. If on a soft surface, place a board under the patient or move the patient to the floor.

- Start compressions if unsure if patient has a pulse. Unnecessary CPR is less harmful than if CPR is not performed when indicated.

- The <u>compression rate</u> for CPR is 100/minute (speed of compressions) but delivers fewer than 100/minute due to interruption in providing ventilations. The actual number is determined by the accuracy and consistency of the compression cycle. (Thirty [30] compressions should be delivered within 23 seconds.)
- Five (5) compression cycles of 30:2 should take approximately 2 minutes.

- Continue CPR until AED or additional EMS personnel arrive.

- CPR cycle ends with ventilations and begins with compressions.

- Insert an oropharyngeal or nasopharyngeal airway when using a BVM device for ventilation.

- Priority patients are patients who have abnormal vital signs, signs/symptoms of poor perfusion, or if there is a suspicion that the patient's condition may deteriorate.

- Current law allows for emergency medical personnel to perform a "reasonable search" for organ donor documentation in unresponsive patients who may die prior to arrival at a hospital. HOWEVER, IN NO EVENT SHOULD A SEARCH BE CONDUCTED IF THAT EFFORT WILL DELAY LIFE-SAVING CARE OR TRANSPORT.

POLICIES:
- Reference No. 814 - Determination/Pronouncement of Death in the Field
- Reference No. 815 - Honoring Prehospital Do-Not-Resuscitate (DNR) Orders
- Reference No. 818 - Honoring Advance Health Care Directive (AHCD)
- Reference No. 819 - Organ Donor Identification.
- Reference No. 821 – Physician Orders for Life Sustaining Treatment (POLST)

CARDIAC EMERGENCY / CARDIOPULMONARY RESUSCITATION
ADULT – 1 RESCUER CPR

PERFORMANCE OBJECTIVE

Assess signs of cardiopulmonary arrest in an adult patient and demonstrate competency in performing cardiopulmonary resuscitation and managing a full arrest.

CONDITION

Assess and perform cardiopulmonary resuscitation for an adult patient who appears to be unresponsive. Necessary equipment will be adjacent to the manikin or brought to the field setting.

EQUIPMENT

Adult CPR manikin, bag-valve-mask device, O₂ connecting tubing, oxygen source with flow regulator, AED, oropharyngeal and nasopharyngeal airways appropriate for manikin, silicone spray, water-soluble lubricant, goggles, various masks, gown, gloves, timing device.

PERFORMANCE CRITERIA

- Items designated by a diamond (♦) must be performed successfully to demonstrate skill competency.
- Items identified by double asterisks (**) indicate actions that are required, if indicated.
- Items identified by (§) should be practiced.
- Ventilations and compressions must be performed at the minimum rate required.

PREPARATION	
Skill Component	**Key Concepts**
♦ Take body substance isolation precautions	• Mandatory personal protective equipment – gloves
♦ Assess scene safety/scene size-up ** *Consider spinal immobilization - if indicated*	• If unknown as to possible trauma, treat as trauma (determined by environment and information obtained from bystanders).
♦ Evaluate additional BSI needs	• Situational - goggles, masks, gown
• Approach the patient and introduce yourself to the caregivers	

PROCEDURE	
Skill Component	**Key Concepts**
♦ Establish unresponsiveness, open the airway, and check to see if the patient is breathing • <u>Medical</u> - head-tilt/chin-lift • <u>Trauma</u> – jaw thrust	• Tap or gently shake and shout and look for obvious breathing. • Agonal gasps are not normal breathing. Agonal gasps may be present in the first minutes after sudden cardiac arrest. • DO NOT start CPR in patients who meet the criteria for Reference No. 814, 815, 818. • If determined that resuscitation is not to be initiated, check for organ/tissue donor status as per Reference No. 819 - Organ Donor Identification.
♦ Activate the emergency response system or call for additional EMS personnel - *if indicated* **Request an AED - *if available*	• Call for help prior to starting resuscitation • If second rescuer is present, he/she should contact ALS and get the AED

Skill Component	Key Concepts
◆ Check for carotid pulse - 5-10 seconds: 　• If pulse is present, secure and manage the airway 　• If there is no *definite* pulse, start the CAB sequence: Compressions, Airway, Breathing ** ***Provide rescue breathing (10-12/minute) - if indicated*** ** ***Attach AED - if available/indicated*** ** ***Start compression cycle - if indicated***	• Check carotid pulse on same side as the rescuer. DO NOT reach across neck. • An alternative to checking carotid pulse is checking the femoral pulse. • Start compressions if there is no DEFINITE pulse. Unnecessary CPR is less harmful than if CPR is not performed when indicated. • The viability of organs is directly affected by perfusion and oxygenation. The longer a patient is without CPR, the greater the damage to vital organs. • An AED should be applied if available and indicated. • If the patient is breathing adequately with no signs of trauma, place in recovery position as soon as initial assessment is completed. This prevents airway obstruction by the tongue, mucus or vomitus. • Rescue breathing for an adult is 1 breath every 5-6 seconds (10-12 breaths/minute). DO NOT hyperventilate patient; this increases intrathoracic pressure, decreases venous return to the heart, and diminishes cardiac output and survival.
◆ Place patient on hard surface if no pulse	• Chest compressions must be performed on a hard surface. If on a soft surface, place a board under the patient or move the patient to the floor.
◆ Perform 30 chest compressions - *if indicated*: 　• Lower half of sternum (center of chest between nipples) 　• Heel of one hand on the sternum and other hand on top of the 1st 　• Depth: at least 2 inches 　• Rate: at least 100/min (push hard and fast) ** ***DO NOT compress on or near the xiphoid process.*** ** ***Allow for chest recoil.***	• Compression landmark – 　- Place the heel of 1 hand on the lower half of sternum between the nipples. • Compression method: push hard and fast 　- place the heel of one hand on top of the 1st 　- fingers may be extended or interlaced, but must be kept off chest 　- shoulders directly over hands 　- arms straight and elbows locked - delivers force of compression straight down in order to be more effective 　- allow chest to return to normal position (full recoil) after down stroke to allow blood to flow into the chest and heart (50% of time for down stroke and 50% for chest relaxation) • Compressions need to be hard and fast to be effective. • Compression rate of at least 100/minute (speed of compressions) delivers fewer than 100/minute due to interruption of providing ventilations. The actual number is determined by the accuracy and consistency of the compression cycle (30 compressions should be delivered within 23 seconds).
◆ Deliver 2 rescue breaths – *if indicated* 　• Maintain patent airway during ventilations with a head-tilt chin-lift (medical) or jaw-thrust (trauma) 　• give 2 breaths with BVM device or pocket mask (1 second/breath) 　• insert an oral airway or nasopharyngeal airway - *if indicated* 　• ensure adequate chest rise ***If unable to ventilate, reposition head, attempt ventilation and initiate obstructed airway procedures - if indicated***	• Use *only* enough force to allow for good chest rise. Over-inflation causes gastric distention which will affect tidal volume by elevating the diaphragm. • Using a BVM by a single rescuer is difficult and may not be as effective as a pocket mask due to an inadequate seal and may reduce the number of compressions delivered per minute. • To prevent airway obstruction, remove dentures *only* if they cannot be kept in place. Fitted dentures maintain form for a good seal.
◆ Complete 5 compression cycles of 30:2 　　***[end with ventilations]*** ****Attach AED after 5 cycles of CPR—*if available and indicated***	• Five (5) compression cycles should take approximately 2 minutes.

Skill Component	Key Concepts
	• Continue CPR until AED or additional EMS personnel arrive.
	• CPR cycle ends with ventilations and begins with compressions.
	NOTE: When using the AED, after an initial shock and two minutes of CPR are delivered, there may be a "no shock advised" command. Resume CPR (starting with compressions) and if there are 2 or more rescuers present, a pulse check may be performed during the ventilation phase of the cycles of 30:2
	Pulse check must NOT delay resumption of compressions
♦ Reassess patient every 60 seconds if there is a return of spontaneous circulation (ROSC): • Check for: - unresponsiveness - breathing - pulse ****Obtain baseline vital signs**	• The main considerations post-resuscitation are: - Perform pulse check every 60 seconds - Perform an initial and focused assessment every 5 minutes. • If a pulse is present and the patient is not breathing adequately, start BVM ventilations. • If a pulse is present and the patient is unresponsive and breathing adequately, place in recovery position.

REASSESSMENT
(Ongoing Assessment)

Skill Component	Key Concepts
♦ Perform pulse check every 60 seconds—*if indicated*	
♦ Reassess the patient at least every **5 minutes once the patient has return of spontaneous respirations and circulation (ROSC):** • Primary assessment • Relevant portion of the secondary examination • Vital signs	• This is a priority patient and must be re-evaluated at least every 5 minutes or sooner, if any treatment is initiated, medication administered, or condition changes.
♦ Evaluate response to treatment	♦ The patient must be re-evaluated at least every 5 minutes if any treatment was initiated or medication administered.
♦ Evaluate results of reassessment and compare to baseline condition and vital signs ****Manage patient condition as indicated**	• Evaluating and comparing results assists in recognizing if the patient is improving, responding to treatment or condition is deteriorating.
§ Explain the care being delivered and the transport destination to the patient/caregivers	• Communication is important when dealing with the patient, family or caregiver. This is a very critical and frightening time for all involved and providing information helps in decreasing the stress they are experiencing.

PATIENT REPORT AND DOCUMENTATION

Skill Component	Key Concepts
§ Give patient report to equal or higher level of care personnel	• Report should consist of all pertinent information regarding the assessment finding, treatment rendered and patient's response to care provided.
§ Verbalize/Document: • Arrest witnessed by EMS personnel or citizen • Time last seen alive • CPR initiated by citizen or EMS personnel • Pulses palpated/not palpated with compressions • Response to CPR	• EMS Personnel are defined as EMTs and paramedics. • Law enforcement personnel for documentation purposes are considered citizens when performing CPR. • Time of arrest cannot be determined in an unwitnessed arrest, but information as to when the patient was last seen may be helpful. • When assessing for pulses with CPR, have an additional rescuer check pulse.

• Organ/Tissue Donor - *if able to obtain information*	• If pulses are not felt with compressions this may be due to either inadequate compressions or hypovolemia. • Response to CPR – patient regains pulse and/or respirations or remains pulseless and/or apneic. • Documentation must be on either the Los Angeles County EMS Report or departmental Patient Care Record form. • Documentation element on EMS Report form asks for: Witnessed by: ☐ Citizen ☐ EMS CPR by: ☐ Citizen ☐ EMS.

Developed: 11/01
Revised: 12/03, 1/05, 5/06

CARDIAC EMERGENCY / CARDIOPULMONARY RESUSCITATION
CHILD - 1 RESCUER CPR

PERFORMANCE OBJECTIVES

The examinee will demonstrate proficiency in performing cardiopulmonary resuscitation and/or rescue breathing for a child.

CONDITION

The examinee will be requested to assess and perform cardiopulmonary resuscitation and/or rescue breathing for a child who is found unresponsive. The manikin will be placed on a raised surface or on the floor. Necessary equipment will be adjacent to the manikin.

EQUIPMENT

Child CPR manikin, bag-valve-mask device, O₂ connecting tubing, oxygen source with flow regulator, oropharyngeal and nasopharyngeal airway appropriate for manikin, silicone spray, water-soluble lubricant, towels for positioning, goggles, masks, gown, gloves, timing device.

PERFORMANCE CRITERIA

- 100% accuracy required on all items designated by a diamond (♦) for skills testing and must manage successfully all items indicated by double asterisks (**).
- Documentation, identified by the symbol (§), must be practiced, but is not a required test item.
- Appropriate body substance isolation precautions must be instituted.
- Ventilations and compressions must be at least at the minimum rate required.

PREPARATION	
Skill Component	**Key Concepts**
♦ Take body substance isolation precautions	• Mandatory personal protective equipment – gloves
♦ Assess scene safety/scene size-up ** *Consider spinal immobilization - if indicated*	• If unknown as to possible trauma, treat as trauma (determined by environment and information obtained from bystanders). • Depending on the size of the child and if spinal immobilization is required, an additional rescuer is needed to maintain in-line axial stabilization.
♦ Evaluate additional BSI needs	• Situational - goggles, masks, gown
♦ Approach the child and introduce yourself to the child and caregivers	

PROCEDURE	
Skill Component	**Key Concepts**

♦ Establish unresponsiveness, open the airway, and check to see if the patient is breathing
 	
  • <u>Medical</u> - head-tilt/chin-lift
 	
  • <u>Trauma</u> – jaw thrust
 	
** Activate the emergency response system or call for additional EMS personnel - *if indicated and additional personnel are available*
 	
** Call for an AED - *if available*
	• Tap or gently shake and shout.
	• Use the jaw thrust maneuver when a head, neck or spine injury is suspected
	• If the jaw thrust maneuver does not open the airway to allow for adequate ventilation, use the head tilt-chin lift technique.
	• If the child is breathing adequately and has no signs of trauma, place in recovery position as soon as initial assessment is completed. This prevents airway obstruction by the tongue, mucus or vomit. There is no universal recovery position for children.
	• DO NOT start CPR in patients who meet the criteria for: Reference No. 814, 815, 818.
	• If determined that resuscitation is not to be initiated, check for organ/tissue donor status as per Reference No. 819.
	• The second rescuer should contact ALS and get the AED.
	• A pediatric adapted AED device should be used on all children 1 to 8 years-of age.

Skill Component	Key Concepts

◆ Check for carotid pulse - 5-10 seconds:
 	
  • If pulse is present, secure and manage the airway
  • If there is no *definite* pulse, OR pulse<60 beats/minute with poor perfusion start the CAB sequence: Compressions, Airway, Breathing
 	
** Provide rescue breathing (12 -20/minute) - _if indicated_
 	
** Attach AED–_if available/indicated_
 	
** Start compressions - _if indicated_
	• Check carotid pulse on same side as the rescuer. DO NOT reach across neck.
	• An alternative to checking carotid pulse is checking the brachial/femoral pulse depending on the size of the child.
	• Rescue breathing for a child is 1 breath every 3-5 seconds (12-20 breaths/minute). DO NOT hyperventilate patient; this increases intrathoracic pressure, decreases venous return to the heart, and diminishes cardiac output and survival.
	• Start CPR if the heart rate is less than 60/minute with poor perfusion. Even though the child has a pulse, the slow rate causes the cardiac output to be insufficient for adequate perfusion and cardiac arrest may be imminent.
	• Start compressions if unsure if patient has a pulse. Unnecessary CPR is less harmful than if CPR is not performed when indicated.
	• The viability of organs is directly affected by perfusion and oxygenation. The longer a patient is without CPR, the greater the damage to vital organs.
	• An AED should be applied if available and indicated.

◆ Place patient on a hard surface if no pulse	• Chest compressions must be performed on a hard surface. If on a soft surface, place a board under the patient or move the patient to the floor.

◆ Perform chest compressions - *if indicated*:
 	
  • Lower half of sternum (center of chest between nipples)
  • Use 1 or 2 hands:
    - 1 hand - heel of hand on sternum
    - 2 hands – heel of one hand on sternum with the other hand on top of the 1st hand
  • Depth: At least ⅓ of anterior-posterior depth of chest or APPROXIMATELY 2 inches (5cm)
  • Rate: at least 100/minute (hard and fast)
  • Ratio cycle: 30 compressions to 2 ventilations
	• <u>Compression landmark</u> - center of the chest between the nipples:
	• <u>Compression method</u>: push hard and fast
	
	  Use 1 or 2 hands:
	    - 1 hand - heel of hand on sternum
	    - 2 hands – heel of one hand on the sternum with other hand on top of the 1st hand.
	  - fingers may be extended or interlaced, but must be kept off chest
	  - shoulders directly over hands
	  - arms straight and elbows locked - delivers force of compression straight down in order to be more effective
	  - allow chest to return to normal position after down stroke to allow blood to flow into the chest and heart (50% of time for down stroke and 50% for chest relaxation)
	• DO NOT compress on or near the xiphoid process.
	• Compressions need to be hard and fast to be effective.
	• <u>Compression rate</u> of at least 100/minute (speed of compressions) delivers fewer than 100/minute due to interruption of providing ventilations. The actual number is determined by the accuracy and consistency of the compression cycle (30 compressions should be delivered within 23 seconds).

◆ Deliver 2 rescue breaths – *if indicated*
 	
  • Maintain patent airway during ventilations with a head-tilt chin-lift (medical) or jaw-thrust (trauma)
  • give 2 breaths with BVM device or pocket mask (1 second/breath)
  • insert an oral airway or nasopharyngeal airway - *if indicated*
  • ensure adequate chest rise
 	
** If unable to ventilate, reposition head, attempt ventilation and initiate obstructed airway procedures - if indicated
	• Use shoulder padding to maintain proper airway and spinal alignment.
	• The tongue and epiglottis may obstruct the entrance of the trachea due to inspiratory efforts creating negative pressure in the airway.
	• The child's airway is more compliant and may collapse during respiratory effort. The airway is easily obstructed by mucus, blood, pus, edema, external compression and hyperextension.
	• Move the patient no more than necessary to maintain an airway.
	• To ventilate use *only* enough force to allow for good chest rise. Over-inflation causes gastric distention which will affect tidal volume by elevating the diaphragm.
	• Using a BVM by a single rescuer is difficult and may not be as effective as a pocket mask due to an inadequate seal and may reduce the number of compressions delivered per minute.
	• If the airway is open and it is difficult to compress the bag and air leaks around the seal, an airway obstruction is present.
	• *Most rescuers have a tendency to ventilate too rapidly.*

Skill Component	Key Concepts
♦ Complete 5 compression cycles of 30:2 　　　*[end with ventilations]* **** Attach AED after 5 cycles of CPR – if available and indicated**	• Five (5) compression cycles should take approximately 2 minutes.
♦ Activate the emergency response system or call for additional EMS personnel - *if indicated and not already done* ****Call for an AED - *if available and not already sent for***	• A child, for the use of an AED, is defined as 1-8 years of age. • In an **unwitnessed pediatric** arrest, it is important to provide oxygenation and ventilation. CPR for 5 cycles (2 minutes) should be performed prior to the use of the AED. 　　Child 1 rescuer CPR = 30:2 ratio 　　Child 2 rescuer CPR = 15:2 ratio • For children, use a defibrillator with a child key/switch, pediatric pads, or adult pads with a pediatric dose-attenuator. If an attenuator system is not available, use adult pads and AED.
	• Continue CPR until AED or additional EMS personnel arrive. • CPR cycle ends with ventilations and begins with compressions. **NOTE:** When using the AED, after an initial shock and two minutes of CPR are delivered, there may be a "no shock advised" command. Resume CPR (starting with compressions) and if there are 2 or more rescuers present, a pulse check may be performed during the ventilation phase of the cycles of 30:2 Pulse check must NOT delay resumption of compressions
♦ Reassess patient every 60 seconds if there is a return of spontaneous circulation (ROSC): 　• Check for: 　• Unresponsiveness 　• Breathing 　• Pulse	• The main considerations post-resuscitation are: 　- Perform pulse check every 60 seconds 　- Perform a focused assessment every 5 minutes. • If a pulse is present and the patient is not breathing adequately, start BVM ventilations. • If a pulse is present and the patient is unresponsive and breathing adequately, place in recovery position.

REASSESSMENT
(Ongoing Assessment)

Skill Component	Key Concepts
♦ Perform pulse check every 60 seconds—*if indicated*	
♦ Reassess the patient at least every **5 minutes once the patient has return of spontaneous respirations and circulation (ROSC):** 　• Primary assessment 　• Relevant portion of the secondary examination 　• Vital signs	• This is a priority patient and must be re-evaluated at least every 5 minutes or sooner, if any treatment is initiated, medication administered, or condition changes.
♦ Evaluate response to treatment	♦ The patient must be re-evaluated at least every 5 minutes if any treatment was initiated or medication administered.
♦ Evaluate results of reassessment and compare to baseline condition and vital signs ****Manage patient condition as indicated**	• Evaluating and comparing results assists in recognizing if the patient is improving, responding to treatment or condition is deteriorating.
§ Explain the care being delivered and the transport destination to the patient/caregivers	• Communication is important when dealing with the patient, family or caregiver. This is a very critical and frightening time for all involved and providing information helps in decreasing the stress they are experiencing.

PATIENT REPORT AND DOCUMENTATION	
Skill Component	**Key Concepts**
§ Give patient report to equal or higher level of care personnel	• Report should consist of all pertinent information regarding the assessment finding, treatment rendered and patient's response to care provided.
§ Verbalize/Document: • Arrest witnessed by EMS personnel or citizen • Time last seen alive • CPR initiated by citizen or EMS personnel • Pulses palpated/not palpated with compressions • Response to CPR • Organ/Tissue Donor - *if able to obtain information*	• EMS Personnel are defined as EMTs and paramedics. • Law enforcement personnel for documentation purposes are considered citizens when performing CPR. • Time of arrest cannot be determined in an unwitnessed arrest, but information as to when the patient was last seen may be helpful. • When assessing for pulses with CPR, have an additional rescuer check pulse. • If pulses are not felt with compressions this may be due to either inadequate compressions or hypovolemia. • Response to CPR – patient regains pulse and/or respirations or remains pulseless and/or apneic. • Documentation must be on either the Los Angeles County EMS Report or departmental Patient Care Record form. • Documentation element on EMS Report form asks for: Witnessed by: ☐ Citizen ☐ EMS CPR by: ☐ Citizen ☐ EMS.

Developed: 4/03   Revised: 06/11

CARDIAC EMERGENCY / CARDIOPULMONARY RESUSCITATION
INFANT - 1 RESCUER CPR

DEFINITIONS:

* _Newborn_ - Neonate in the first minutes to hours after birth.

* _Neonate_ - Infant in first month after birth (28 days).

* _Infant_ – Newborn to 1 year (0 - 12 months).

* _Phone fast_ - for breathing difficulties. In infants and children, the most common cause of arrest is an inadequate airway, complete 1 sequence to remove obstruction or provide 5 cycles (30:2) of CPR, before leaving the pediatric patient to call for EMS personnel.

INDICATIONS:

* Infants who are unresponsive, apneic, and pulseless.

CONTRAINDICATIONS:

* None when above conditions apply.

COMPLICATIONS:

* Gastric distention
* Rib fractures
* Sternal fractures
* Separation of ribs from sternum
* Laceration of liver or spleen

* Pneumothorax
* Hemothorax
* Lung and heart contusion
* Fat emboli

NOTES:

* Do not start resuscitation if the patient meets the criteria in Ref. No. 814, 815, 818.

* Start compression cycle if an infant has no pulse or signs of circulation or if a newborn has a pulse < 60 beats/minute. Even though the newborn or infant has a pulse, the low rate and cardiac output is insufficient to provide for adequate perfusion.

* The viability of organs is directly affected by perfusion and oxygenation and the longer a patient is without CPR, the greater the damage to vital organs.

* Use shoulder padding to maintain proper airway and spinal alignment.

* Move the infant no more than necessary to ensure an open airway. A second rescuer is needed to maintain in-line axial stabilization if spinal immobilization is required.

* If the infant is in a prone position with suspected trauma, the patient should be turned using log-roll method to avoid flexion or twisting of the neck or back.

* The recovery position is not recommended for an infant unless the head is adequately supported since the airway may become obstructed. Have suction readily available to prevent airway obstruction by mucus or vomit.

* Other signs of circulation - breathing, coughing or movement in response to rescue breaths. This is checked in conjunction with checking for a pulse.

* An alternative to checking the brachial pulse is checking for a femoral pulse.

* Chest compressions must be performed on a hard surface, if on a soft surface place a board under the infant or move the infant to a table, etc.

* CPR cycle begins with compressions and ends with ventilations.

* Use an oropharyngeal airway when providing positive pressure ventilations.

POLICIES:

* Reference No. 814 - Determination/Pronouncement of Death in the Field
* Reference No. 815 - Honoring Prehospital Do-Not-Resuscitate (DNR) Orders
* Reference No. 818 - Honoring Advanced Health Care Directives
* Reference No. 819 – Organ Donor Identification

Developed: 8/01
Revised: 7/04, 6/06

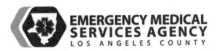

EMS SKILL

CARDIAC EMERGENCY: CARDIOPULMONARY RESUSCITATION INFANT - 1 RESCUER CPR

PERFORMANCE OBJECTIVES
Assess signs of cardiopulmonary arrest in an infant and demonstrate competency in performing cardiopulmonary resuscitation and managing a full arrest.

CONDITION
Assess for signs of cardiopulmonary arrest and perform resuscitative measures as needed for an infant who appears to be unresponsive. Necessary equipment will be adjacent to the manikin or brought to the field setting.

EQUIPMENT
Infant CPR manikin, bag-valve-mask device, O₂ connecting tubing, oxygen source with flow regulator, AED, oropharyngeal airway appropriate for manikin, silicone spray, water-soluble lubricant, 10cc syringe, goggles, masks, gown, gloves, emergency resuscitation tape, timing device.

PERFORMANCE CRITERIA
- Items designated by a diamond (♦) must be performed successfully to demonstrate skill competency.
- Items identified by double asterisks (**) indicate actions that are required if indicated.
- Items identified by (§) should be practiced.
- Ventilations and compressions must be at least at the minimum rate required.

PREPARATION	
Skill Component	**Key Concepts**
♦ Take body substance isolation precautions	• Mandatory personal protective equipment – gloves
♦ Assess scene safety/scene size-up ** *Consider spinal immobilization - if indicated*	• If unknown as to possible trauma, treat as trauma (determined by environment and information obtained from bystanders). • Depending on the size of the child and if spinal immobilization is required, an additional rescuer is needed to maintain in-line axial stabilization.
♦ Evaluate additional BSI needs	• Situational - goggles, masks, gown
♦ Approach the infant and introduce yourself to the caregivers	

PROCEDURE	
Skill Component	**Key Concepts**
♦ Establish unresponsiveness ** *Call for additional resources – if needed* ** *Consider an AED - if available*	• Tap bottom of feet or gently shake and shout. • DO NOT start CPR in infants who meet the criteria for: Reference No. 814, 815, 818, 821. • If determined that resuscitation is not to be initiated, check for organ/tissue donor status as per Reference No. 819. • The second rescuer should contact ALS and get the AED.

♦ Open/Maintain a patent airway:
• <u>Medical</u> - head-tilt/chin-lift
• <u>Trauma</u>
  - jaw-thrust
  - neutral position (tragus of ear level with top of shoulder)
 	
** *Clear/suction airway - if indicated*
 	
** *Consider oropharyngeal airway - if indicated*
	• Use shoulder padding to maintain proper airway and spinal alignment.
	• The tongue is proportionately large in size to the oropharynx and may cause partial or complete airway obstruction in infants.
	• The infant's airway is more compliant and may collapse during respiratory effort. The airway is easily obstructed by mucus, blood, pus, edema, external compression and hyperextension.
	• Infants have limited lung expansion and depend more on diaphragm movement to generate a tidal volume.
	• If suspected trauma, the head and torso should be turned as a unit.
	• A second rescuer is needed to maintain in-line axial stabilization if spinal immobilization is required.

Skill Component	Key Concepts
◆ Assess for adequate breathing 5-10 seconds: • Look • Listen • Feel	• Look at chest for adequate tidal volume and rate. • Check breathing for at least 5 seconds and no more than 10 seconds.

◆ Manage ventilations:
 	
 • If breathing is adequate:
    - medical - place in recovery position
    - trauma - maintain spinal immobilization - *if indicated*
 	
 • If breathing is absent or inadequate:
    - give 2 breaths with BVM device or pocket mask - (1 second/breath)
    - insert an oral airway - *if indicated*
    - ensure visible chest rise
 	
 ** *If unable to ventilate, reposition head, attempt ventilation and initiate obstructed airway procedures - if indicated*
 	
 ** *Provide rescue breathing 1 breath every 3-5 seconds (12 - 20/minute) - if indicated*
	• The recovery position is not recommended for an infant unless the head is adequately supported since the airway may be obstructed. Have suction readily available to prevent airway obstruction by mucus or vomit.
	• Rescue breathing is 1 breath every 3 - 5 seconds (12 – 20/minute).
	• To ventilate, use *only* enough force to produce visible chest rise. Over-inflation causes gastric distention and elevating the diaphragm which will affect tidal volume.
	• If the airway is open and it is difficult to compress the bag and air leaks around the seal, an airway obstruction is present.

◆ Palpate for brachial pulse 5-10 seconds:	• Check for other signs of circulation - breathing, coughing or movement in response to rescue breaths. This is done in conjunction with palpating for a pulse. • Palpate brachial pulse on same side as the rescuer, inside of the upper arm and between the elbow and shoulder. • An alternative to checking the brachial pulse is checking a femoral pulse in neonates and infants or at the base of the umbilical cord in the newborn.

◆ Place patient on hard surface if no pulse
 	
 ** *Start compression cycle - if indicated*
    - no pulse or signs of circulation
    - pulse < 60 beats/minute with poor perfusion
	• Chest compressions must be performed on a hard surface. Can be placed on a table or on rescuer's thigh.
	• Start CPR if the heart rate is less than 60/minute with poor perfusion. Even though the child has a pulse, the slow rate causes the cardiac output to be insufficient for adequate perfusion and cardiac arrest may be imminent.
	• Start compressions if unsure if the infant has a pulse. Unnecessary CPR is less harmful than if CPR is not performed when indicated.
	• The viability of organs is directly affected by perfusion and oxygenation. The longer an infant is without CPR, the greater the damage to vital organs.

◆ Perform chest compressions - *if indicated*:
 	
 • *2 finger technique* – 1 rescuer
    - Location: lower 1/2 of sternum (1 finger width below nipple line)
    - Depth: 1/3 to 1/2 of chest circumference
    - Rate: at least 100/minute
    - Ratio cycle: 30 compressions to 2 ventilation
 	
 • *2 Thumb-encircling technique* – 2 rescuer
    - Location: center of the chest just below nipple line
    - Depth: 1/3 to 1/2 of chest circumference
    - Rate: at least 100/minute
    - Ratio cycle: 15 compressions to 2 ventilation
 	
 ** *DO NOT compress on or near the xiphoid process*
 ** *Allow for chest recoil*
	• Technique for chest compressions when performing CPR :
	    - *2 finger technique* - 2 finger pads of either index & middle finger or middle & ring finger of one hand on lower 1/2 of sternum.
	    - *2 thumb-encircling technique* (2 rescuer CPR) – Use both thumbs side by side
	• Compression method – push hard and fast
	• Compression/ventilation rates for infant:
	    Infant 1 rescuer CPR = 30:2 ratio
	    Infant 2 rescuer CPR = 15:2 ratio
	• Compression rate of 100/minute (speed of compressions) delivers fewer than 100/minute due to interruption of providing ventilations. The actual number is determined by the accuracy and consistency of the compression cycle.
	• Slightly elevate chest so that head and neck remain in neutral position and the neck is not flexed or hyperextended.

Skill Component	Key Concepts
◆ Provide 2 minutes of CPR ** ***Attach AED after 5 cycles of CPR – if available and indicated***	• CPR cycle begins with compressions and ends with ventilations.
◆ Activate the emergency response system or call for additional EMS personnel - *if indicated and not already done* **Call for an AED - *if available and not already sent for***	• A child, for the use of an AED, is defined as an infant -8 years of age. • In a pediatric arrest, it is important to provide oxygenation and ventilation. CPR for 5 cycles (2 minutes) should be performed prior to the use of the AED. • For infants, use a defibrillator with a child key/switch, pediatric pads, or adult pads with a pediatric dose-attenuator. If an attenuator system is not available, use adult pads and AED.
◆ Reassess brachial pulse and other signs of circulation: • If circulation present, but breathing is absent or inadequate - continue with rescue breathing – 1 breath every 3-5 seconds (12-20/minute) • If no circulation present – continue CPR ratio of 30:2 for 1 rescuer OR CPR ratio of 15:2 for 2 rescuers ** ***Start compressions - if heart rate is less than 60/minute with poor perfusion*** ***[begin with compressions]***	• Continue CPR until additional EMS personnel arrive. • Other signs of circulation include normal breathing, coughing, or movement. • CPR cycle begins with compressions and ends with ventilations.
◆ Reassess infant every 60 seconds after return of spontaneous circulation (ROSC): • Check for: - responsiveness - breathing - pulse ** ***Obtain baseline vital signs***	• The main considerations post-resuscitation are: - Perform pulse check every 60 seconds - Perform a focused assessment every 5 minutes. • If a pulse is present and the infant is not breathing adequately, start ventilations.

REASSESSMENT
(Ongoing Assessment)

Skill Component	Key Concepts
◆ Perform pulse check every 60 seconds	
§ Repeat an ongoing assessment at least every **5 minutes**: • Initial assessment • Relevant portion of the focused assessment • Evaluate response to treatment • Compare results to baseline condition and vital signs	• This is a priority patient and must be re-evaluated at least every 5 minutes or sooner if any treatment is initiated; medication administered, or condition changes. • Priority patients are infants who have abnormal vital signs, signs/symptoms of poor perfusion, or if there is a suspicion that the infant's condition may deteriorate.
◆ Evaluate response to treatment:	• Patients must be re-evaluated at least every 5 minutes if any treatment was initiated or medication administered.
◆ Evaluate results of on-going assessment and compare to baseline condition and vital signs **Manage infant's condition as indicated.**	• Evaluating and comparing results assists in recognizing if a patient is improving, responding to treatment or condition is deteriorating.
§ Explain the care being delivered and the transport destination to caregivers	• Communication is important when dealing with the patient, family or caregiver. This is a very critical and frightening time for all involved and providing information helps in decreasing the stress they are experiencing.

Skill Component	Key Concepts
§ Give patient report to equal or higher level of care personnel	• Report should consist of all pertinent information regarding the assessment finding, treatment rendered and patient response to care provided.

§ Verbalize/Document:
 	
• Arrest witnessed by
  - EMS or citizen
  - time last seen to onset of CPR
• Citizen CPR
• Time of onset of Rescuer CPR
• Approximate time patient was without CPR
• Pulses palpated/not palpated with compressions
• Response to CPR
• Organ/Tissue Donor - *if able to obtain information*
	• EMS Personnel are defined as EMTs and paramedics.
	• Law enforcement personnel for documentation purposes are considered citizens when performing CPR.
	• Time of arrest cannot be determined in an unwitnessed arrest, but information as to when the infant was last seen may be helpful.
	• If pulses are not felt with compressions this may be due to either inadequate compressions or hypovolemia.
	• Response to CPR – infant regains pulse and/or respirations or remains pulseless and/or apneic.
	• Documentation must be on either the Los Angeles County EMS Report or departmental Patient Care Record form.

Developed: 8/01   Revised: 12/03, 7/04, 6/06, 12/07, 12/08, 5/09

CIRCULATION EMERGENCY
BLEEDING CONTROL

DEFINITION:

- <u>Dowel</u> - stick, rod, or any object that can be inserted under loop of tourniquet and used to twist tourniquet tight

TYPES OF BLEEDING:

Arterial

- Blood is bright red in color and oxygen rich.
- Arterial bleeding is the most difficult to control due to the pressure that is within the arteries.
- Blood spurts from the wound, but as the blood pressure drops, the spurting becomes less forceful.

Venous

- Blood is dark red in color and oxygen poor.
- Venous bleeding is easier to control than arterial bleeding due to lower venous pressure.
- Blood flows at a steady stream and may be minor or profuse depending on the size of the vessel.

Capillary

- Blood is dark red in color; site of oxygen and carbon dioxide gas exchange.
- Blood oozes from capillaries and usually clots spontaneously.

TOURNIQUET FACTS:

- A tourniquet is used when all other methods have failed. It has the potential to cause damage to nerves, muscle, blood vessels, and soft tissue resulting in loss of the extremity.
- DO NOT apply tourniquet over a joint, but as close to the injury as possible.
- Use a wide bandage and secure tightly to prevent cutting into the skin and underlying tissue.
- Once a tourniquet is applied, it should not be loosened or removed without approval of a physician.
- Apply tourniquet proximal to bleeding site as distal as possible on extremity.

TOURNIQUET APPLICATION:

- Pad skin by wrapping 6-8 layers of a 4" bandage around the extremity twice
- Tie another dressing loosely around extremity
- Insert dowel under last loop of last dressing applied
- Rotate the dowel (to tighten tourniquet) until the bleeding stops
- Secure the dowel in position when the bleeding stops

NOTES:

- Direct pressure may involve just the finger tips or may require hand pressure.
- Elevation of an extremity may be used secondary to and in conjunction with direct pressure.
- Continue to reinforce dressing if bleeding does not stop. DO NOT remove original dressing. Removing the original dressing will increase bleeding if clot formation has begun.
- Pressure points for bleeding control are only found in the extremities. The most commonly used points are the brachial and femoral.
- Motion reduction of bone ends will reduce amount of tissue damage and bleeding associated with a fracture.
- Pneumatic pressure devices include air splints, blood pressure cuff, and the pneumatic antishock garment (PASG). Air splints do not have enough pressure to control an arterial bleed. Blood pressure cuffs often leak air and thus may be ineffective.
- EMTs are able to use the pneumatic antishock garment (PASG) as a pneumatic device on a lower extremity for bleeding control.

Developed 1/02
Revised 9/04

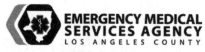

EMERGENCY MEDICAL SERVICES AGENCY
LOS ANGELES COUNTY

EMS SKILL

CIRCULATION EMERGENCY
BLEEDING CONTROL/SHOCK MANAGEMENT

PERFORMANCE OBJECTIVES
Demonstrate proficiency in controlling external venous and/or arterial bleeding.

CONDITION
Assess and control external venous and/or arterial bleeding by appropriate methods. Necessary equipment will be adjacent to the manikin or brought to the field setting.

EQUIPMENT
Manikin or live model, bag-valve-mask device, O_2 connecting tubing, oxygen source with flow regulator, stethoscope, blood pressure cuff, pen light, timing device, 4"x4" dressings, roller gauze, 6" absorbent gauze roll, elastic wraps, constricting band and dowel or commercial tourniquet, tape, clipboard, pen, goggles, masks, gown, gloves.

PERFORMANCE CRITERIA
- Items designated by a diamond (♦) must be performed successfully to demonstrate skill competency.
- Items identified by double asterisks (**) indicate actions that are required if indicated.
- Items identified by (§) should be practiced.

PREPARATION	
Skill Component	**Key Concepts**
♦ Take body substance isolation precautions	• Mandatory personal protective equipment - gloves
♦ Assess scene safety/scene size-up ** ***Consider spinal injury precautions - if indicated***	• If unknown as to possible spinal trauma, treat as spinal trauma (determined by environment and information obtained from bystanders).
♦ Assess type of bleeding: • Arterial • Venous • Capillary	
♦ Evaluate additional BSI needs	• Situational - long sleeves, goggles, masks, gown
♦ Remove enough clothing to expose entire wound	

PROCEDURE	
Skill Component	**Key Concepts**
♦ Manage bleeding by applying direct pressure to wound	• Direct pressure may involve just the finger tips or may require hand pressure. • Tourniquets may be used early on if the EMS provider determines that the arterial or venous bleeding cannot be controlled with other measures.

♦ Manage uncontrollable bleeding by :
 	
 • Apply a tourniquet as distal as possible on the extremity
   - inflated blood pressure cuff
       OR
   - commercial device
       OR
   - constricting band and dowel
	• Pneumatic pressure devices include air splints, blood pressure cuff, and the pneumatic antishock garment (PASG). Air splints do not have enough pressure to control an arterial bleed. Blood pressure cuffs often leak air and thus may be ineffective.
	
	 • Tourniquets may be a commercial product or by using a constricting band that is at least 2 inches wide and a dowel (rod).
	
	 • A tourniquet is used when all other methods have failed or early on when it is determined that other control methods would not control the arterial or venous bleeding.
	   - Caution must be taken to prevent potential damage to nerves, muscle, blood vessels, and soft tissue which may result in loss of the extremity.
	
	 (Continued)

Skill Component	Key Concepts
	- DO NOT apply tourniquet over a joint, but as close to the injury as possible.
	• Use a wide bandage and secure tightly to prevent cutting into the skin and underlying tissue.
	• If blood pressure cuff is used, check pressure frequently and re-inflate to maintain consistent pressure.
	• Once a tourniquet is applied, it should NOT be loosened or removed without approval of a physician.
	• Blood loss reduces perfusion and oxygen to tissues, supplemental oxygen is essential. However, never stop bleeding control in attempt to set up oxygen.
♦ Manage bleeding by using dditional methods *as indicated* by: • Elevate extremity - *if indicated* • Apply additional dressing – *if indicated* • Apply pressure dressing - *if indicated* • Splinting extremity - *if indicated*	• Elevation of an extremity may be used secondary to and in conjunction with direct pressure. • Continue to reinforce dressing if bleeding does not stop. DO NOT remove original dressing. Removing the original dressing will increase bleeding if clot formation has begun. • Motion reduction of bone ends will reduce amount of tissue damage and bleeding associated with a fracture. • Elevation of an extremity may be used secondary to and in conjunction with direct pressure.

SHOCK MANAGEMENT

Skill Component	Key Concepts
♦ Institute shock management measures: • Administer oxygen via mask • Properly position patient • Initiate steps to prevent heat loss • Initiate immediate transportation	

REASSESSMENT
(Ongoing Assessment)

Skill Component	Key Concepts
♦ Reassess the patient at least every **5 minutes or sooner:** • Primary assessment • Relevant portion of the secondary assessment • Vital signs	• This is a priority patient and must be re-evaluated at least every 5 minutes or sooner, if any treatment is initiated, medication administered, or condition changes.
♦ Evaluate response to treatment	
♦ Evaluate results of reassessment and note any changes from patient's condition and vital signs ****Manage patient condition as indicated.**	• Evaluating and comparing results assists in recognizing if the patient is improving, responding to treatment or condition is deteriorating.

MEDICATION ADMINISTRATION
BRONCHODILATOR METERED DOSE INHALER (MDI)

ASSESSMENT: RESPIRATORY DISTRESS:

Onset	Gradual vs. sudden (when it began)
Provokes	Causative event, (allergy, exertion, drugs, etc)
Quality	Effective ventilations, tidal volume, difficulty getting air in or air out
Rate	Fast, slow, normal, respiratory pattern
Recurrence	Initial vs. repeated episodes (time of last episode)
Relief	Constant vs. intermittent (what makes it better or worse)
Severity	Mild, moderate, severe - used to rate initial event or compare to previous episode or ongoing assessment, accessory muscle use, stridor, position, etc.
Time	Duration

Distress level considerations for chief complaint of shortness of breath (SOB)	
Mild	Tachypnea, normal position, answers in full sentences
Moderate	Tachypnea, upright position if possible, answers in partial sentences
Severe	Tachypnea, tripod position, answers in 2-3 words only

INDICATIONS:
- Bronchospasm caused by:
  - asthma
  - COPD
  - bronchitis

CONTRAINDICATIONS:
- Patient does not meet indication or criteria for administration
- Medication not prescribed for patient
- Maximum inhalation dose taken before EMS arrival

ADVERSE EFFECTS:
- *Cardiovascular*   - tachycardia, hypertension
- *Neurological*   - tremors, nervousness, headache, dizziness
- *Respiratory*   - cough, wheezing
- *Gastrointestinal*   - nausea

ADMINISTRATION:
- As prescribed by physician. This information can <u>usually</u> be obtained on the side of the actual box that the medication was in, or on the actual inhaler-cartridge. If neither of these can be obtained, ask the patient or family historian of patient for the accurate-dosage administration.

DEFINITIONS:
- Hypoxemia - decreased oxygen level in arterial blood
- Pursed lips - lips made smaller by puckering. This decreases resistance to air flow by dilating small bronchi.

NOTES:
- EMTs may not a carry bronchodilator inhaler, they may <u>only</u> assist with administration of a patient's prescribed bronchodilator inhaler.
- In life-threatening situations, an ALS Unit <u>must</u> be enroute or BLS should consider transport if ALS arrival is longer than transport time.
- Symptoms of asthma include: shortness of breath, wheezing, coughing (usually dry and irritative), distressed breathing, and difficulty speaking.
- When in a cold environment, warm the canister by rolling it between your hands before use. This results in smaller particles of medication being inhaled and better distribution and absorption by the lungs.
- Patient should not stop inhaling once the dose is delivered, but continue to inhale as long as possible. This effectively mixes the medication with the incoming air and pulls it into the lungs slowly.
- If using a spacer, there may be a whistling sound if the patient inhales too rapidly.
- Avoid spraying into patient's eyes or vision will be temporarily blurred

REFERENCE:
- Reference 802 - Emergency Medical Technician-I Scope of Practice
  Developed: 1/02

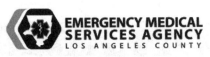

EMS SKILL

MEDICATION ADMINISTRATION
BRONCHODILATOR METERED DOSE INHALER (MDI)

PERFORMANCE OBJECTIVES
The examinee will demonstrate proficiency in recognizing the indications, contraindications, criteria, and assist the patient with the administration of a prescribed bronchodilator inhaler.

CONDITION
The examinee will be requested to establish that a simulated patient who is complaining of difficulty breathing meets the criteria for administration of a bronchodilator inhaler. The examinee will assist the patient with administering the medication with or without using a spacer device. Necessary equipment will be adjacent to the simulated patient.

EQUIPMENT
Simulated patient, oxygen tank with a flow meter, oxygen mask, blood pressure cuff, stethoscope, placebo bronchodilator inhaler cartridge with a plastic mouthpiece, spacer device, timing device, clipboard, pen, goggles, masks, gown, gloves.

PERFORMANCE CRITERIA
- 100% accuracy required on all items designated by a diamond (♦) for skills testing and must manage successfully all items indicated by double asterisks (**).
- Documentation, identified by the symbol (§), must be practiced, but is not a required test item.
- Appropriate body substance isolation precautions must be instituted.

PREPARATION	
Skill Component	**Key Concepts**
♦ Take body substance isolation precautions	• Mandatory personal protective equipment - gloves • Situational - long sleeves, goggles, masks, gown

♦ Complete an initial assessment:
  • General impression
  • Life-threatening condition
  • Assess mental status/stimulus response (AVPU)
  • Assess/Manage airway
  • Assess/Manage breathing
 	
** *Administer 100% oxygen*
	• Any patient complaining of difficulty breathing should be placed on oxygen as soon as possible.
	• If in respiratory distress, patients with a history of COPD should be placed on 15 Liters/minute via mask. DO NOT withhold oxygen from these patients.
	• Use the most effective oxygen delivery system that can be tolerated by the patient.

♦ Verbalize the criteria for assisting patients with medications:
 	
  • Medication prescribed by a physician
  • Medication prescribed for patient
  • Meets indication for administration
  • No contraindications are present for administration
	• EMTs may <u>only</u> assist with administration of a bronchodilator inhaler as per Reference 802 - Emergency Medical Technician-I Scope of Practice.
	• EMTs may NOT carry bronchodilator inhalers, but may assist with the patient's <u>own</u> prescribed medication.
	• In life-threatening situations, an ALS Unit <u>must</u> be enroute or BLS should consider transport if ALS arrival is longer than transport time.

♦ Verbalize the <u>indications</u> for assisting the patient with a bronchodilator inhaler:
 	
  • Symptoms of respiratory distress
    - shortness of breath
    - wheezing
    - coughing
    - difficulty speaking.
	• Symptoms include: shortness of breath, wheezing, coughing (usually dry and irritative), distressed breathing, and difficulty speaking.

♦ Verbalize the <u>contraindications</u> for administration of a bronchodilator inhaler:
 	
  • Patient does not meet indication or criteria for administration
  • Patient has taken maximum prescribed dose before EMS arrival
  • Patient is unable to follow directions or use the inhaler
	• One dose is defined as the number of puffs (sprays) that is prescribed by the physician. This information is obtained from the physician's order which is found on the box or inhaler cartridge.

Skill Component	**Key Concepts**
◆ Check medication for: • Drug name • Integrity of container/medication • Concentration/Dose • Clarity • Expiration date	• <u>Drug name</u> - Trade and generic names include: albuterol, Proventil, Ventolin, Alupent, Metaprel, Brethaire, Brochometer, etc NOT ALL INHALERS are bronchodilators, EMTs are only allowed to assist with bronchodilators. • <u>Integrity of container/medication</u> - Make sure container is NOT broken • <u>Concentration/Dose</u> - dose of a bronchodilator is the number metered sprays administered. (Concentration only refers to liquid form of medications.) • <u>Clarity</u> -if container is transparent, the liquid should be clear • <u>Expiration date</u> - not to be administered after this date
◆ Prepare Medication: • Remove the mouthpiece cover Shake inhaler 5-6 times ** ***Insert cartridge into plastic mouthpiece case - <u>if not done previously</u>*** ** ***Attach spacer - <u>if needed</u>***	• Inhaler cartridge should be already placed in the mouthpiece. Teach student how to connect if first time use for medication. • Always check mouthpiece to make sure there are no foreign objects lodged in mouthpiece that may either be inhaled or plug dispenser. • If the inhaler has not been used for several days "test spray" it into the air before use.
◆ Instruct patient to breath out normally (not forcefully)	

◆ Position the inhaler:
 	
• Hold inhaler 2 finger-widths in front of open mouth
        OR
Place inhaler inside of mouth, past the teeth, above the tongue
        OR
Attach a spacer to the mouth piece and close lips around spacer
	• Ensure that spray opening is pointed toward patient
	
	• The cartridge should be on top and the mouthpiece on the bottom.
	
	• Not everyone is able to use an inhaler effectively. Spacers may be used by patients who are older, have arthritis, or just cannot coordinate inhalation and medication administration activity.

◆ Instruct patient to take a slow, deep breath and take in as much air as possible <u>on command</u>	
◆ Instruct patient to inhale: **Without Spacer** • Inhale for 5-7 seconds and press the inhaler 1 time (1 spray or puff) **With Spacer** • Press inhaler 1 time and have patient breath in and out normally 3-4 breaths ** **May repeat sprays as prescribed - <u>if needed</u>**	• Patient should not stop inhaling once the spray is delivered, but continue to inhale as long as possible (usually 5-7 seconds). • This time frame mixes the medication with the incoming air and pulls it into the lungs slowly. • If using a spacer, there may be a whistling sound if the patient inhales too rapidly. • Avoid spraying into patient's eyes or vision will be temporarily blurred. • Dose of a bronchodilator is the numbered metered sprays that were administered.
◆ Instruct patient to hold breath for as long as comfortable or up to 10 seconds before breathing out slowly through pursed lips	
◆ Remove inhaler and replace oxygen	• Administer supplemental O_2 before and after treatment to decrease hypoxemia.
◆ Reassess respiratory function, breath sounds and patient's response after 3 minutes	• Medication will take effect in within 5 minutes and last 4-6 hours depending on medication administered.
◆ Monitor pulse periodically for irregularity	• Hypoxic patients may experience dysrhythmias.

Skill Component	Key Concepts
§ Repeat an ongoing assessment every **5 minutes**: • Initial assessment • Relevant portion of the focused assessment • Evaluate response to treatment • Compare results to baseline condition and vital signs	• The initial and focused examination is repeated every 15 minutes for stable patients and every 5 minutes for priority patients. • Every patient must be re-evaluated at least every 5 minutes, if any treatment was initiated or medication administered, unless changes in the patient's condition are anticipated sooner. • Priority patients are patients who have abnormal vital signs, signs/symptoms of poor perfusion or if there is a suspicion that the patient's condition may deteriorate.

DOCUMENTATION

Skill Component	Key Concepts

§ Verbalize/Document
• Assessment findings before and after administration
• Drug
  - name
  - dose
  - route
  - site
  - time
  - who administered medication
• Repeat dose - *if indicated*
• Patient's response to medication
• Respiratory status
• Cardiovascular status
• Mental status
• Vital signs
	• Documentation must be on either the Los Angeles County EMS Report or departmental Patient Care Record form.
	• On the Los Angeles County EMS Report, document administration <u>only</u> in the comment section. Mark the box "EMT Medication Assist" and write out all pertinent information.
	• Documenting reassessment information provides a comprehensive picture of patient's response to treatment.
	• Last reassessment information (before patient care is transferred) should be documented in the section of the EMS form that is called "Reassessment after Therapies and/or Condition on Transfer".

Developed: 1/02   Revised: 6/06

MEDICATION ADMINISTRATION
EPINEPHRINE

DEFINITIONS:

- Anaphylaxis - an allergic reaction that may present as a mild allergic reaction to cardiovascular collapse and respiratory arrest.
- Patient assist - assisting patients with medications means that the EMT may:
  - allow the patient to self-administer prescribed medications in the presence of BLS providers
  - assist the patient in taking prescribed medications if the patient has difficulty with self-administration
  - administer the prescribed medication to the patient if the patient is physically incapable of administering the medication

ASSESSMENT: ALLERGIC REACTION / ANAPHYLAXIS / ENVIRONMENTAL EMERGENCY:

- *Onset* - history of allergy
- *Substance* - type of substance
- *Exposure* - ingestion, inhalation, absorption, envenomization
- *Time* - duration
- *Effect* - general vs local c rash, hives, itching, respiratory problems, nausea, vomiting, etc
- *Progression* - initial symptom to current condition
- *Relief* - treatment initiated prior to EMS

ASSESSMENT: RESPIRATORY DISTRESS:

- **O**nset - gradual vs sudden (when it began)
- **P**rovokes - causative event (e.g. allergy, exertion, drugs, etc)
- **Q**uality - effective ventilations, tidal volume, difficulty getting air in or air out
- **R**ate - fast, slow, normal, respiratory pattern
- **R**ecurrence - initial vs repeated episodes, time of last episode
- **R**elief - constant vs intermittent; what makes it better or worse
- **S**everity - mild, moderate, severe - used to rate initial event or compare to previous episode or ongoing assessment, accessory muscle use, stridor, position, etc.
- *Time* - duration

  Distress level considerations for chief complaint of shortness of breath (SOB)
  - *Mild* B tachypnea, normal position, answers in full sentences
  - *Moderate* B tachypnea, upright position if possible, answers in partial sentences
  - *Severe* B tachypnea, tripod position, answers in 2-3 words only

INDICATIONS:

- Severe anaphylaxis with either shock and/or respiratory distress

CONTRAINDICATIONS:

- Patient does not meet indication or criteria for administration

ADVERSE EFFECTS:

- *Cardiovascular* - tachycardia, hypertension, chest pain, ventricular fibrillation
- *Neurological* -seizures, cerebral hemorrhage, headache, tremors, dizziness, anxiety
- *Gastrointestinal* - nausea, vomiting

ADMINISTRATION:

- Adult   - (Epinephrine auto-injector) 0.3mg IM in the upper-outer thigh as a 1 time dose. May NOT repeat.
- Pediatric -(Epinephrine auto-injector junior) 0.15mg IM in the upper-outer thigh as a 1 time dose. May NOT repeat.

NOTES:

- EMTs may not carry epinephrine, they may *only* assist with administration of a patient=s prescribed epinephrine auto-injector.
- In life-threatening situations, an ALS Unit must be enroute or BLS should consider transport if ALS arrival is longer than transport time.
- Anaphylaxis may be caused by insect stings or bites, foods, drugs, other allergens, exercise, or may be spontaneous.
- Signs/symptoms of anaphylaxis: flushed skin, nervousness, syncope, tachycardia, thready or unobtainable pulse, hypotension, convulsions, vomiting, diarrhea, abdominal cramps, urinary incontinence, wheezing, stridor, difficulty breathing, itching, rash, hives, and generalized edema.
- Patients may have been instructed that they can use EpiPen through clothing. This is not recommended for healthcare providers.
- DO NOT inject into buttocks, hands, feet, or intravenously (IV). Injection into the buttocks, hands or feet may result in loss of blood flow to these areas and result in delayed absorption and tissue necrosis. IV injection may cause an acute myocardial infarction or cerebral hemorrhage. Deltoid injection is NOT recommended in Los Angeles County.
- The EpiPen contains 2ml (2mg) of epinephrine. the auto-injector delivers 0.3ml (0.3mg). approximately 1.7ml remains in the pen after activation.

REFERENCE: Reference 802 - Emergency Medical Technician-I Scope of Practice.
Developed 1/02

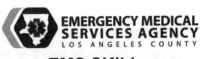

**EMERGENCY MEDICAL
SERVICES AGENCY**
LOS ANGELES COUNTY

MEDICATION ADMINISTRATION
EPINEPHRINE

PERFORMANCE OBJECTIVES
The examinee will demonstrate proficiency in recognizing the indications, contraindications, criteria, and assist the patient with the administration of the prescribed epinephrine using an auto-injector device.

CONDITION
The examinee will be requested to establish that a simulated patient complaining of a severe allergic reaction with respiratory distress meets the criteria for administration of epinephrine and will assist the patient by administering 0.3mg IM using an auto-injector device. Necessary equipment will be adjacent to the simulated patient.

EQUIPMENT
Simulated patient, oxygen tank with a flow meter, oxygen mask, blood pressure cuff, stethoscope, placebo epinephrine in an auto-injector device or auto-injector trainer, biohazard container, alcohol wipes, adhesive bandage, timing device, clipboard, pen, goggles, masks, gown, gloves.

PERFORMANCE CRITERIA
- 100% accuracy required on all items designated by a diamond (♦) for skills testing and must manage successfully all items indicated by double asterisks (**).
- Documentation, identified by the symbol (§), must be practiced, but is not a required test item.
- Appropriate body substance isolation precautions must be instituted.

PREPARATION	
Skill Component	**Key Concepts**
♦ Take body substance isolation precautions	• Mandatory personal protective equipment - gloves • Situational - long sleeves, goggles, masks, gown
♦ Complete an initial assessment: • General impression • Life-threatening condition • Assess mental status/stimulus response (AVPU) • Assess/Manage airway • Assess/Manage breathing ** *Administer 100% oxygen*	• Any patient complaining of difficulty breathing should be placed on oxygen as soon as possible. • If in respiratory distress, patients with a history of COPD should be placed on 15 Liters/minute via mask. DO NOT withhold oxygen from these patients.
♦ Verbalize the criteria for assisting patients with medications: • Medication prescribed by a physician • Medication prescribed for patient • Meets indication for administration • No contraindications present for administration	• EMTs may _only_ assist with administration of epinephrine using an auto-injector device as per Reference 802 - Emergency Medical Technician-I Scope of Practice. • EMTs may NOT carry epinephrine auto-injectors, but may assist with the patient's _own_ prescribed medication. • In life-threatening situations, an ALS Unit <u>must</u> be enroute or BLS should consider transport if ALS arrival is longer than transport time.
♦ Verbalize the <u>indications</u> for assisting the patient with epinephrine auto-injector • Severe anaphylaxis with symptoms of either shock and/or respiratory distress	• Patients may choose to administer their own medication with lesser signs/symptoms. EMTs may assist when there are signs/symptoms of shock and/or respiratory distress. • Symptoms of respiratory distress may include; tightness of throat, wheezing, difficulty speaking, shortness of breath, use of accessory muscles etc. • History of rapid respiratory deterioration is also considered when administering epinephrine.
♦ Verbalize the <u>contraindications</u> for administration of epinephrine: • Patient does not meet indication or criteria for administration	

Skill Component	Key Concepts
◆ Check medication for: • Drug name • Integrity of container/medication • Concentration/Dose • Clarity • Expiration date	• <u>Drug name</u> - Trade and generic names include: adrenalin and EpiPen. EMTs may only use auto-injectors. AnaKits may be used by paramedics since medication requires manual injection of the medication. • <u>Integrity of container/medication</u> - Make sure container is NOT broken • <u>Concentration/Dose</u> - dose of epinephrine is 1 metered dose of 0.3mg for adults and) 0.15mg for pediatric patients per individual injection. (Concentration only refers to liquid form of medications.) • <u>Clarity</u> - if container is transparent, the liquid should be clear • <u>Expiration date</u> - not to be administered after this date
◆ Identify location of injection site: • Remove clothing from thigh area • Locate site - upper-outer thigh	• Patients may have been instructed that they can use EpiPen through clothing. <u>This is not recommended for healthcare providers.</u> • Location of upper-outer thigh is best explained as midway between waist and knee. Deltoid injection is NOT recommended in Los Angeles County. • <u>DO NOT inject into buttocks, hands, feet, or intravenously (IV).</u> Injection into the buttocks, hands or feet may result in loss of blood flow to these areas and result in delayed absorption and tissue necrosis. IV injection may cause an acute myocardial infarction or cerebral hemorrhage.
◆ Cleanse injection site with alcohol wipe	
◆ Remove the safety cap from auto-injector	
◆ Place tip of auto-injector hard against injection site	• Place the auto-injector at a right-angle to the thigh for IM injection. • Pressure on the tip of the injector is required to activate the spring-loaded needle.
◆ Hold the injector in place for 10 seconds until the medication is injected	• It may take up to 10 seconds for the medication to be injected.
◆ Remove the injector and place in biohazard container	• Caution must be taken with auto-injectors, the needle does not retract.
◆ Massage injection site for 10 seconds with alcohol wipe ** *Apply adhesive bandage - if indicated*	• Massage site for 10 seconds, this helps to disperse medication in the muscle.

◆ Evaluate response to epinephrine administration:
 	
• Respiratory status
  - rate
  - tidal volume
  - lung sounds
 	
• Cardiovascular status
  - pulse
  - blood pressure
  - skin vitals
 	
• Mental status
 	
** *Treat for shock - if indicated*
 	
** *Initiate BLS Procedures (CPR, AED) - if indicated*
	• Medication will take effect within 5-10 minutes and last up to 20 minutes.

ONGOING ASSESSMENT	
Skill Component	**Key Concepts**
§ Repeat an ongoing assessment every **5 minutes**: • Initial assessment • Relevant portion of the focused assessment • Evaluate response to treatment • Compare results to baseline condition and vital signs	• The initial and focused examination is repeated every 15 minutes for stable patients and every 5 minutes for priority patients. • Every patient must be re-evaluated at least every 5 minutes, if any treatment was initiated or medication administered, unless changes in the patient's condition are anticipated sooner. • Priority patients are patients who have abnormal vital signs, signs/symptoms of poor perfusion or if there is a suspicion that the patient's condition may deteriorate.

DOCUMENTATION	
Skill Component	**Key Concepts**

§ Verbalize/Document
• Assessment findings before and after administration
• Drug
  - name
  - dose
  - route
  - site
  - time
  - who administered medication
• Patient's response to medication
• Respiratory status
• Cardiovascular status
• Mental status
• Vital signs
	• Documentation must be on either the Los Angeles County EMS Report or departmental Patient Care Record form.
	
	• On the Los Angeles County EMS Report, document administration <u>only</u> in the comment section. Mark the box "EMT Medication Assist" and write out all pertinent information.
	
	• Documenting reassessment information provides a comprehensive picture of patient's response to treatment.
	
	• Last reassessment information (before patient care is transferred) should be documented in the section of the EMS form that is called "Reassessment after Therapies and/or Condition on Transfer".

Developed: 1/02

MEDICATION ADMINISTRATION
NITROGLYCERIN

DEFINITIONS:

- <u>Sublingually</u> - medication administration under the tongue

- <u>Transmucosal</u> - medication route on top of tongue or mucus membrane in the mouth (buccal cavity)

ASSESSMENT: PAIN / DISCOMFORT (non-traumatic)<u>:</u>

- *Onset* - when the pain/discomfort first began (minutes - weeks); what makes it better or worse
- *Provokes* - causative event or what increases pain/discomfort
- *Quality* - type of pain, i.e. sharp, ache, squeezing, burning, etc
- *Region* - area focal vs diffuse pain/discomfort
- *Radiation*, - pain moves to another area away from its origin;
- *Relief* - constant vs intermittent; what makes it better or worse
- *Severity* - mild, moderate, severe or 1-10 scale used to rate initial event or compare to previous episode or ongoing assessment
- *Time* - duration

INDICATIONS:

- Chest pain/discomfort

CONTRAINDICATIONS:

- Patient does not meet indication or criteria for administration
- Patient has taken 3 doses before EMS arrival within the last 5 minutes
- Last dose was < 5 minutes ago
- Systolic blood pressure < 100mm/Hg
- Administration of "erectile-dysfunction" medications such as "Viagra" or "Levitro", do not administer if patient has taken <u>within 24 hours.</u> In addition, do not administer Nitroglycerin if patient has taken the "erectile-dysfunction" drug "Cialis" <u>within 36 hours.</u>

ADVERSE EFFECTS:

- *Cardiovascular* - hypotension, bradycardia, reflex tachycardia, rebound hypertension
- *Neurological* - throbbing headache, dizziness/faintness, confusion, blurred vision
- *Gastrointestinal* - nausea, vomiting, dry mouth
- *General* - flushed skin, sublingual burning

ADMINISTRATION:

- Adult   -1 tablet or 1 spray as a 1 time dose of 0.4mg. May not repeat.

- Pediatric - Not recommended for prehospital care

NOTES:

- EMTs may not carry nitroglycerin, they may <u>*only*</u> assist with administration of a patient=s prescribed nitroglycerin.

- In life-threatening situations, an ALS Unit <u>must</u> be enroute or BLS should consider transport if ALS arrival is longer than transport time.

- Nitroglycerin may cause hypotension due to vasodilation. Always take blood pressure before administration and 5 minutes after administration.

- Instruct patient not to swallow the nitroglycerin tablet, it will change the absorption rate and the amount of drug absorbed. Sublingual absorption is faster than gastrointestinal absorption.

- Instruct patient not to inhale nitroglycerin spray, it will change the absorption rate and the amount of drug absorbed. Sublingual absorption is faster and more accurate than inhaling medication into lungs.

- DO NOT shake nitroglycerin spray container or dose delivered will be altered. One spray delivers 0.4mg of nitroglycerin.

REFERENCE:

- Reference 802 - Emergency Medical Technician-I Scope of Practice.

Developed 1/02

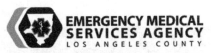

EMERGENCY MEDICAL SERVICES AGENCY
LOS ANGELES COUNTY

EMS SKILL

MEDICATION ADMINISTRATION
NITROGLYCERIN

PERFORMANCE OBJECTIVES
The examinee will demonstrate proficiency in recognizing the indications, contraindications, criteria, and assist the patient with the administration of the prescribed medication nitroglycerin.

CONDITION
The examinee will be requested to establish that a simulated patient complaining of substernal chest discomfort meets the criteria for administration of nitroglycerin and will assist the patient by administering either the nitroglycerin spray or tablet or two different patients may be selected to demonstrate both methods of administration. Necessary equipment will be adjacent to the simulated patient.

EQUIPMENT
Simulated patient, oxygen tank with a flow meter, oxygen mask, blood pressure cuff, stethoscope, placebo nitroglycerin spray and tablets, timing device, clipboard, pen, goggles, masks, gown, gloves.

PERFORMANCE CRITERIA
- 100% accuracy required on all items designated by a diamond (♦) for skills testing and must manage successfully all items indicated by double asterisks (**).
- Documentation, identified by the symbol (§), must be practiced, but is not a required test item.
- Appropriate body substance isolation precautions must be instituted.

PREPARATION	
Skill Component	**Key Concepts**
♦ Take body substance isolation precautions	• Mandatory personal protective equipment - gloves • Situational - long sleeves, goggles, masks, gown
♦ Complete an initial assessment and pertinent vital signs: • General impression • Life-threatening condition • Assess mental status/stimulus response (AVPU) • Assess/Manage airway • Assess/Manage breathing • Blood pressure ** *Administer 100% oxygen* ** *Obtain blood pressure*	• Any patient complaining of difficulty breathing should be placed on oxygen as soon as possible. • If in respiratory distress, patients with a history of COPD should be placed on 15 Liters/minute via mask. DO NOT withhold oxygen from these patients. • Any patient complaining of chest pain should be placed on oxygen as soon as possible. • Nitroglycerin may cause hypotension due to vasodilation. Always take blood pressure before administration and 5 minutes after administration.
♦ Verbalize the criteria for assisting patients with medications: • Medication prescribed by a physician • Medication prescribed for patient • Meets indication for administration • No contraindications are present for administration	• EMTs may _only_ assist with administration of nitroglycerin as per Reference 802 - Emergency Medical Technician-I Scope of Practice. • EMTs may NOT carry nitroglycerin tablets or spray, but may assist with the patient's _own_ prescribed medication. • In life-threatening situations, an ALS Unit <u>must</u> be enroute or BLS should consider transport if ALS arrival is longer than transport time.
♦ Verbalize the <u>indications</u> for assisting the patient with nitroglycerin: • Symptoms of chest pain/discomfort • Systolic blood pressure > 100mm/Hg	• Any degree of chest pain/discomfort should be treated with Nitroglycerin regardless how the patient rates the pain.
♦ Verbalize the <u>contraindications</u> for administration of nitroglycerin: • Patient does not meet indication or criteria for administration • Patient has taken 3 doses before EMS arrival within the last 5 minutes • Last dose was < 5 minutes ago • Systolic blood pressure < 100mm/Hg • Administration of Sildenafil citrate (Viagra®) or similar medication within 24 hours	• If last dose of nitroglycerin exceeds 5 minutes, nitroglycerin may be administered. • If the patient insists on taking nitroglycerin and it meets the <u>contraindications criteria</u>, EMTs should NOT assist in the administration.

PROCEDURE

Skill Component	Key Concepts
◆ Check medication for: • Drug name • Integrity of container/medication • Concentration/Dose • Clarity • Expiration date	• <u>Drug name</u> - Trade names for nitroglycerin may include: Nitrolingual Spray®, Nitrobid®, Nitrostat® • <u>Integrity of container/medication</u> - Make sure container is NOT broken and tablet is whole • <u>Concentration/Dose</u> - dose of nitroglycerin is 0.4mg (grain 1/150) per tablet. (Concentration only refers to liquid form of medications.) • <u>Clarity</u> - not applicable to tablets or unable to see liquid in spray container • <u>Expiration date</u> - not to be administered after this date
◆ Prepare Medication: **Tablet** • Remove tablet from container and check that it is intact **Spray** • Remove top of spray canister	**Tablet** • Make sure that tablet is intact for administration of correct dose. • DO NOT contaminate medication. Pour tablet into lid of container then into the palm for administration. Gloves should be worn when administering nitroglycerin. **Spray** • One spray delivers 0.4mg of nitroglycerin. DO NOT shake container or it will alter the dose. • Ensure that spray opening is pointed toward patient
◆ Remove oxygen mask and instruct patient to open mouth and lift tongue	
◆ Administer medication: **Tablet** • Place tablet under patient's tongue • Instruct patient to allow tablet to dissolve and NOT to swallow **Spray** • Deliver one spray sublingually or transmucosal • Instruct patient NOT to inhale spray	**Tablet** • If patient swallows the tablet it will change the absorption rate and the amount of drug absorbed. Sublingual absorption is faster than gastrointestinal absorption. **Spray** • If patient inhales the spray it will change the absorption rate and the amount of drug absorbed. Sublingual absorption is faster and more accurate than inhaling medication into lungs.
◆ Replace oxygen mask	
◆ Reassess blood pressure and pain response in 5 minutes ** ***Place patient in shock position - if indicated***	• Use the pain scale of mild, moderate, severe or the 1-10 scale. • Nitroglycerin may cause hypotension due to vasodilation. Always take blood pressure before administration and 5 minutes after administration. • EMTs may only administer 1 nitroglycerin dose. Nitroglycerin administration is for <u>EMERGENCY SUPPORTIVE THERAPY ONLY</u> and is not a substitute for immediate medical care. • In life-threatening situations, an ALS Unit <u>must</u> be enroute or BLS should consider transport if ALS arrival is longer than transport time.

ONGOING ASSESSMENT

Skill Component	Key Concepts
§ Repeat an ongoing assessment every **5 minutes**: • Initial assessment • Relevant portion of the focused assessment • Evaluate response to treatment • Compare results to baseline condition and vital signs	• The initial and focused examination is repeated every 15 minutes for stable patients and every 5 minutes for priority patients. • Every patient must be re-evaluated at least every 5 minutes, if any treatment was initiated or medication administered, unless changes in the patient's condition are anticipated sooner. • Priority patients are patients who have abnormal vital signs, signs/ symptoms of poor perfusion or if there is a suspicion that the patient's condition may deteriorate.

Skill Component	Key Concepts

§ Verbalize/Document
 	
• Assessment findings before and after administration
• Blood pressure before administration
• Drug
  - name
  - dose
  - route
  - site
  - time
  - who administered medication
• Patient's response to medication
• Blood pressure 5 minutes after administration
	• Documentation must be on either the Los Angeles County EMS Report or departmental Patient Care Record form.
	
	• On the Los Angeles County EMS Report, document administration only in the comment section. Mark the box "EMT Medication Assist" and write out all pertinent information.
	
	• Last reassessment information (before patient care is transferred) should be documented in the section of the EMS form that is called "Reassessment after Therapies and/or Condition on Transfer".

Developed: 1/02

MEDICATION ADMINISTRATION
ORAL GLUCOSE

INDICATIONS:

- A diabetic or suspected diabetic patient with an altered level of consciousness

CONTRAINDICATIONS

- Patients that are unresponsive.
- Patients that have no gag reflex (Los Angeles County).
- Patients complaining of nausea.

COMPLICATIONS:

- Aspiration
- Nausea and vomiting
- Hyperglycemia

NOTES:

- The DOT considers "unresponsiveness" as a contra-indication for oral glucose administration. The County of Los Angeles considers "diminished gag reflex" as a contra-indication.
- Oxygen should be co-administered with glucose and the patient placed in a left lateral position until full orientation is established.
- Patients receiving oral glucose require ALS or ED follow-up in the County of Los Angeles regardless of full recovery.
- Glucose is absorbed in the gastro-intestinal system. It must be swallowed because it is not absorbed sublingually or buccally.[1]

[1] Prehospital Drug Therapy; Mosby 1994

Developed 7/07

MEDICATION ADMINISTRATION
ADMINISTRATION OF ORAL GLUCOSE

PERFORMANCE OBJECTIVES
The examinee will demonstrate proficiency in administering oral glucose.

CONDITION
The examinee will be requested to properly administer oral glucose on a simulated patient with an altered level of consciousness.

EQUIPMENT
Adult live model, instant glucose paste, dextrose solution, mask, gown, gloves, goggles'

PERFORMANCE CRITERIA
- 100% accuracy required on all items designated by a diamond (♦) for skills testing and must manage successfully all items indicated by double asterisks (**).
- Documentation, identified by the symbol (§), must be practiced, but is not a required test item.
- Appropriate body substance isolation precautions must be instituted.

ADMINISTRATION OF ORAL GLUCOSE PREPARATION	
Skill Component	**Teaching Points**
♦ Take body substance isolation precautions	• Mandatory personal protective equipment - gloves • Situational - long sleeves, goggles, masks, gown
♦ Explain Procedure to patient	• Maintain patient rapport

PROCEDURE	
Skill Component	**Teaching Points**
Dextrose Carbonated Solution:	
♦ Instruct patient to hold bottle and drink entire contents	Patient must be alert enough to self administer liquid.
♦ Reassess and record patient status every five minutes	
♦ Dispose of contaminated equipment using universal precautions	
Glucose Paste:	
♦ Turn patient to left lateral position or tilt backboard to side if spinal immobilization procedures have been implemented and patient has an altered LOC	
♦ Apply approximately 1" of glucose paste between the patient's cheek and gum	Have patient swallow paste if possible.
♦ Reassess and record patient status every five minutes	
♦ Dispose of contaminated equipment using universal precautions	

ONGOING ASSESSMENT	
Skill Component	**Teaching Points**
§ Continue to reassess patient	

Skill Component	Teaching Points
§ Verbalize/Document: • Reason for intervention • Time, dose, and method oral glucose was administered • Other treatment provided	

Developed 7/07

MUSCULOSKELETAL INJURY
BIPOLAR TRACTION DEVICE - HARE SPLINT

INDICATIONS:

- Single long bone fracture of the lower extremity:
  - Isolated, mid-shaft femur fracture

CONTRAINDICATIONS:

- Pelvic fracture
- Hip injury
- Knee injury
- Lower third (near the ankle) of a lower extremity injury
- Ankle and foot fractures
- Distal end of femur fracture
- Partial amputation or avulsion of the lower extremity
- More than one fracture of the same extremity

COMPLICATIONS:

- Neurovascular compromise if traction splint is applied incorrectly.
- Injury to genitals if groin strap is not positioned correctly.

SPLINTING PRINCIPLES:

- <u>**Priorities in managing a patient with an extremity fractures:**</u>
  - 1st - life-threatening conditions
  - 2nd - limb-threatening conditions
  - 3rd - all other conditions

- <u>**General management for suspected fractures:**</u>
  - Stop bleeding and treat for shock
  - Support area of injury
  - Immobilize joints above and below injury site

- <u>**General splinting principles:**</u>
  - Pad rigid splints to adjust for anatomic shapes and patient comfort
  - Remove jewelry to prevent neurovascular compromise with increased swelling
  - Evaluate extremity before and after immobilization for neurovascular function

SPLINTING ERRORS:

- Splinting before life-threatening injuries are addressed. *(Treat life-threatening injuries first, then splint.)*

- Delaying transport for critical patients in order to splint extremity.

- Improper splinting extremity:
  - Splints applied too tight will compromise circulation and can cause nerve and muscle damage.
  - Splints applied too loosely may result in further soft-tissue damage or convert a closed fracture into an open fracture.

- Applying an incorrect splint device - not appropriate to the severity of the patient=s condition and method of transport.

- Not realigning long bones when an extremity is pulseless and cyanotic.

- Attempting to realign joints. *(May increase damage to soft tissue, nerves, and muscles.)*

NOTES:

- Traction splints may be used on open or closed femur fractures, especially when there is neurovascular compromise, uncontrollable bleeding and severe pain due to muscle spasm.

- Femur fractures result from major force and in children is commonly the result of child abuse.

- Purpose of traction splint is to prevent overriding of the bone ends, decrease pain, relax muscle spasm, reduces blood loss.

- There can be a significant blood loss with a femur fracture, 500-1000 or even more if it is an open fracture.

- The Hare splint is a bipolar device because it uses two (2) pole-like sides to initiate countertraction against the ischial tuberosity. It elevates and stabilizes the extremity when the patient is moved.

NOTES (Continued):

• DO NOT secure straps before traction has been established. This may interfere with pulling traction along the entire length of the lower extremity and can cause angulation and excessive tightening of the strap resulting in compromised circulation.

• Adequate traction is applied when the injured lower extremity is the same length as the other lower extremity or the patient feels relief.

• Never apply a Pneumatic Anti-shock Garment (PASG) over a rigid splint. The metal shaft of the splint produces a void between the PASG and the extremity allowing for continued internal or external bleeding. This may also press the splint into the extremity causing tissue damage, circulatory compromise, or puncture the PASG resulting in sudden dangerous deflation.

• Never release the mechanical traction unless manual traction is re-established. The release of traction may cause additional injury to the lower extremity.

Developed 11/01

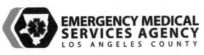

EMERGENCY MEDICAL SERVICES AGENCY
LOS ANGELES COUNTY

EMS SKILL

MUSCULOSKELETAL INJURY
BIPOLAR TRACTION DEVICE - HARE SPLINT

PERFORMANCE OBJECTIVES
Demonstrate competency in applying a bipolar traction device - Hare splint.

CONDITION
Apply a traction splint on a patient who has sustained an isolated lower extremity fracture. There are no contraindications for application of a traction splint. Necessary equipment will be adjacent to the patient or brought to the field setting.

EQUIPMENT
Adult CPR/trauma manikin or live model, assistant, Hare splint, long spine board, all necessary straps, sterile dressings, 1" tape, goggles, masks, gown, gloves.

PERFORMANCE CRITERIA
* Items designated by a diamond (♦) must be performed successfully to demonstrate skill competency.
* Items identified by double asterisks (**) indicate actions that are required if indicated.
* Items identified by (§) are not skill component items, but should be practiced.

PREPARATION	
Skill Component	**Key Concepts**
♦ Establish body substance isolation precautions	• Mandatory personal protective equipment - gloves
♦ Assess scene safety	
♦ Evaluate additional BSI needs	• Situational - long sleeves, goggles, masks, gown
♦ Determine if patient sustained possible spinal injury ** ***Institute spinal immobilization - if indicated***	• If unknown of possible spinal injury, institute spinal immobilization (determined by environment and information obtained from bystanders).
♦ Direct assistant to stabilize lower extremity	• To apply the Hare splint requires 2 rescuers; Rescuer #1 to apply splint and Rescuer #2 to stabilize the extremity, apply and maintain manual traction.
♦ Expose the injured extremity: • Cut clothes away - *if indicated* • Remove shoes and socks • Remove extremity and toe jewelry	• Femur fractures result from major force and in children is commonly the result of child abuse. • The lower extremity is generally shortened, externally rotated with midthigh swelling due to hemorrhage. • Shoes must be removed to assess for pulse and sensation and prevent interference with the stability of the ankle harness. • Jewelry must be removed prior to swelling of the foot and therefore not compromise circulation. • Fractures of the tibia/fibula generally do not require traction splints since the calf muscles are not strong enough to override the bone fragments.
♦ Assess extremity distal to injury for: • Circulation • Motor movement/function • Sensation	• <u>Pulse</u> - palpate either the popliteal or pedal pulse and mark location of the pulse with an "X". • <u>Circulation</u> - check for color, temperature, capillary refill. • <u>Motor movement</u> - have patient move toes. • <u>Sensation</u> - determine numbness or tingling and sensitivity to touch of the lower extremity including toes.

Skill Component	Key Concepts
◆ Cover wound with sterile dressing and secure in place - *if indicated*	• Blood loss from femoral fractures may exceed 500-1000 ml. This may be doubled if the fracture is an open fracture.
◆ Determine if traction splint should be applied ** ***Consider rapid transport - if patient is critical***	• If the patient is critical, splinting should be limited to securing the fractured limb to a long spine board and rapid transport. • Splinting minimizes pain, reduces hemorrhage, risk of a closed fracture converted to an open fracture, blood vessel and nerve damage, and fat emboli.

PROCEDURE

Skill Component	Key Concepts
◆ Apply the ankle harness above the ankle and adjust harness to ensure a snug fit	• Depending on patient's condition, traction may need to be applied first before splint is ready. It takes several minutes for spasm and pain to ease after traction is applied. Therefore, traction is recommended as soon as possible. • It is easier, faster and more stable to apply the harness before applying traction. This prevents the conflict of working around hands that are holding traction. • The bottom edge of the side flaps of the harness should be about 1" above the lateral protrusions of the ankle. • Make sure that side flaps do not cross over the top of the foot, but at the ankle so that traction will be pulled against the ankle and not the top of the foot.
◆ Direct assistant to initiate and maintain manual traction: • Hold the harness (ring strap) in one hand • Place other hand under the extremity and above the harness • Slowly pull the extremity until pain is reduced and/or circulation improves	• The amount of traction applied should be enough to reduce pain and/or improve circulation if compromised. • Manual traction must be maintained until the splint has been applied. • The assistant should position self without interfering with sliding the splint in place. • The assistant should keep arms straight and lean backward using the weight of the upper torso maintaining consistent traction. • The fracture site must be supported consistently throughout procedure. • DO NOT put fingers in D-rings. Fingers may get stuck as extremity is moved.
◆ Unlock collet sleeves	
◆ Measure splint for length: • Place against lateral aspect of the uninjured extremity • Extend splint approximately 8"-12" beyond the heel	• The uninjured extremity is used for splint measurement. Using the injured extremity would give an <u>inaccurate</u> splint measurement due to being shortened and externally rotated. • It is better to go with an increased splint length then having it too short. If splint is too short, appropriate traction cannot be applied.
◆ Relock collet sleeves	• It is important that the splint does not shorten when traction is applied. This may lead to increased bleeding and cause muscle, nerve and vascular damage.
◆ Fold down heel stand and lock in place	
◆ Place splint next to the injured lower extremity and prepare support straps: • 1st above fracture site • 2nd above knee • 3rd below knee • 4th above ankle	• Straps may be placed over the fracture site, but not over the knee.

Skill Component	Key Concepts
♦ Support the fracture site under thigh with one hand	
♦ Direct assistant to lift the extremity while maintaining manual traction • Slowly elevate the foot 10"-12" off the ground for stable alignment. ** *Ensure that the fracture site is supported*	• The foot should be elevated approximately 10"-12" off the ground for stable alignment. • Both rescuers must lift the extremity at the same time. If the extremity is not kept in alignment, the movement will increase pain and possibly additional injury.
♦ Slide the splint under the affected extremity until it seats against the ischial tuberosity	• Make sure that the half ring is seated well against the ischial tuberosity.
♦ Direct assistant to lower the extremity onto the splint while maintaining manual traction ** *Ensure that the fracture site is supported*	• Both rescuers must lower the extremity at the same time. If the extremity is not kept in alignment, the movement will increase pain and possibly additional injury.
♦ Pad the groin area as needed	• Use trauma dressing or equivalent for padding. • Make sure pressure is NOT directly applied to the external genitalia or bony areas.
♦ Secure the groin strap high around the upper thigh of the injured extremity	
♦ Hook the D-ring(s) into the "S" hook	
♦ Adjust the traction by turning the winch until manual traction has been equaled	• Adequate traction is achieved when patient feels some relief.
♦ Direct assistant to slowly release manual traction	
♦ Secure the 4 support straps: • 1st above fracture site • 2nd above knee • 3rd below knee • 4th above ankle	• DO NOT secure straps before traction has been established: - may interfere with pulling traction along the entire length of the extremity - may cause angulation and excessive tightening of the strap resulting in compromised circulation
♦ Re-assess extremity distal to injury for: • Circulation • Motor movement/function • Sensation	
♦ Secure patient and splint to backboard	• Securing the patient and splint to the backboard will stabilize the hip joint and prevent movement of the splint during transport. • The kick stand must be secured to prevent collapse and additional pain and injury to the patient. • Move the patient on the backboard toward the top of the gurney if there is a concern that the door will not shut. • Apply an ice pack for pain relief and to minimize additional swelling.

Skill Component	Key Concepts
◆ Reassess the patient at least every **5 minutes or sooner:** • Primary assessment • Relevant portion of the secondary assessment • Vital signs	• This is a priority patient and must be re-evaluated at least every 5 minutes or sooner, if any treatment is initiated, medication administered, or condition changes.
◆ Evaluate response to treatment	
◆ Evaluate results of reassessment and note any changes from patient's condition and vital signs ****Manage patient condition as indicated.**	• Evaluating and comparing results assists in recognizing if the patient is improving, responding to treatment or condition is deteriorating.

PATIENT REPORT AND DOCUMENTATION

Skill Component	Key Concepts
§ Verbalize/Document: • Mechanism of injury • Description of injury • Treatment provided • Patient response to treatment • Circulation before and after splinting • Motor movement before and after splinting • Sensation before and after splinting	• Documentation must be on either the Los Angeles County EMS Report or departmental Patient Care Record form.

Developed 11/01,   Revised 12/09

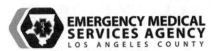

Supplemental Information
MUSCULOSKELETAL INJURY / SPLINTS
RIGID & CONFORMING SPLINTS

INDICATIONS:

- Protect and maintain the position of an injured extremity:
    - fracture
    - sprain/strain
    - dislocation

COMPLICATIONS:

- Neurovascular compromise if splint is applied incorrectly.

SPLINTING PRINCIPLES:

- **Priorities in managing a patient with extremity fractures:**
    - 1st - life-threatening conditions
    - 2nd - limb-threatening conditions
    - 3rd - all other conditions

- **General management for suspected fractures:**
    - Stop bleeding and treat for shock
    - Support area of injury
    - Immobilize joints above and below injury site

- **General splinting principles:**
    - Pad rigid splints to adjust for anatomic shapes and patient comfort
    - Remove jewelry to prevent neurovascular compromise with increased swelling
    - Evaluate extremity before and after immobilization for nerve and vascular function

SPLINTING ERRORS:

- Splinting before life-threatening injuries are addressed. *(Treat life-threatening injuries first, then splint.)*

- Delaying transport of critical patients in order to splint an extremity.

- Improper splinting technique:
    - Splints applied too tight will compromise circulation and can cause nerve and muscle damage.
    - Splints applied too loosely may result in further soft-tissue damage or convert a closed fracture into an open fracture.

- Applying an incorrect splinting device that is inappropriate for the severity of the patient's condition and method of transport.

- Not realigning long bones when an extremity is pulseless and cyanotic.

- Attempting to realign joints. *(May increase damage to soft tissue, nerves, and muscles.)*

NOTES:

- Rigid splints include: board splints (wood, plastic or metal), air splints, traction splints, pre-formed specific area splints, and spine board (long board).

- Conforming splints include: cardboard splints, ladder splints, SAM splints, vacuum splints, malleable metal finger splints, blanket rolls, and pillows.

- There are two situations when an extremity must be splinted in the position found:
    - dislocations
    - when resistance or extreme pain is encountered during the attempt to realign a long bone fracture

- Splinting minimizes pain, reduces hemorrhage and the risk of converting a closed fracture into an open fracture, prevents blood vessel and nerve damage, and fat emboli.

- Immobilizing the joint above and below the fracture site ensures stabilization of the fracture.

- Shimming involves padding the extremity in the splint to decrease any movement of the extremity. Make sure there is even pressure and contact. Pad all bony prominences.

- For lower extremity fractures, patient should be supine and the extremity elevated about 6" to minimize swelling.

- Always apply a layer of protection between an ice pack and the skin to reduce the possibility of frostbite or further injury to underlying tissue.

- Always splint the hand in the position of function. DO NOT tape fingers flat or cause angulation of the wrist.

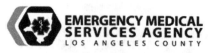

MUSCULOSKELETAL INJURY / SPLINTS
RIGID & CONFORMING SPLINT

PERFORMANCE OBJECTIVES
Demonstrate proficiency in applying either a rigid or conforming splint.

CONDITION
Apply either a rigid or a conforming splint on a patient who has sustained an isolated extremity fracture. Necessary equipment will be adjacent to the manikin or brought to the field setting.

EQUIPMENT
Adult CPR/trauma manikin or live model, various rigid and conforming splints, long spine board, all necessary straps, sterile dressings, 2"-3"roller gauze, 1" tape, goggles, masks, gown, gloves.

PERFORMANCE CRITERIA
- Items designated by a diamond (♦) must be performed successfully to demonstrate skill competency.
- Items identified by double asterisks (**) indicate actions that are required if indicated.
- Items identified by (§) are not skill component items, but should be practiced.

PREPARATION	
Skill Component	**Key Concepts**
♦ Take body substance isolation precautions	• Mandatory personal protective equipment - gloves
♦ Assess scene safety	
♦ Evaluate additional BSI needs	• Situational - long sleeves, goggles, masks, gown
♦ Determine if patient sustained possible spinal injury ** ***Institute spinal immobilization - if indicated***	• If unknown as to possible spinal injury, institute spinal immobilization (determined by environment and information obtained from bystanders).
♦ Stabilize and expose the injured extremity: • Cut clothes away - *if indicated* • Remove shoes and socks - *if indicated* • Remove extremity and toe/finger jewelry	• Shoes must be removed to assess for pulse and sensation. • Some extremities may be readily exposed and do not require that clothes are cut. • Jewelry must be removed prior to swelling of extremity or digits and therefore not compromise circulation.
♦ Assess extremity distal to injury for: • Circulation • Sensation • Motor movement ** ***Consider realignment of extremity - if distal part of extremity is pulseless and cyanotic***	• <u>Pulse</u> - palpate pulses distal to injury and mark with an "X". • <u>Circulation</u> - check for pulse characteristics, color, temperature, capillary refill. • <u>Motor movement</u> - have patient wiggle fingers or toes. • <u>Sensation</u> - determine numbness or tingling and sensitivity to touch. • <u>If fracture of long bone with severe deformity</u> - realign extremity using constant, gentle manual traction to realign extremity. • <u>If extremity resistant to realignment</u> - splint in position found.
♦ Cover wound with sterile dressing and secure in place - *if indicated*	
♦ Determine if splint should be applied ** ***Consider rapid transport - if patient is critical***	• If the patient is critical, splinting should be limited to securing the fractured limb to a long spine board and rapid transport. • Splinting minimizes pain, reduces hemorrhage and the risk of a closed fracture converted to an open fracture, blood vessel and nerve damage, and fat emboli.
♦ Select the proper splint for stabilization and immobilization	• The splint selected should achieve the goal of stabilization and immobilization of the joint above and below the fracture site.

Skill Component	Key Concepts
◆ Prepare and pad the splint - *as needed*	• The splint should be measured, cut or bent prior to being placed on the patient to avoid jostling the injured extremity. • When immobilizing the lower leg, cut or mold a cardboard or ladder splint 10"-12" longer than the desired length to allow for forming the splint at a perpendicular angle to support the foot.

PROCEDURE

Skill Component	Key Concepts	
◆ Support the fracture site and maintain manual immobilization: ** *Insert a 2"-3" wide roller bandage into patient's cupped palm - if indicated*	◆ Select the proper splint for stabilization and immobilization	• The imm(
◆ Lift the extremity	• Lift the limb only far enough to slide the splint under the injured extremity.	
◆ Slide the splint under the extremity		
◆ Lower the extremity into the splint		
◆ Secure the splint: • Bone - immobilize the joint above and below the fracture site • Joint - immobilize the bones above and below the injured joint • Make sure extremity is properly shimmed ** *Elevate extremity slightly above the level of the heart* ** *Consider application of ice packs - if swelling is present*	• Immobilizing the joint or bone above and below the site ensures stabilization of the fracture or injury. • Shimming involves padding the extremity in the splint to decrease any movement of the extremity. Make sure there is even pressure and contact. Pad all bony prominences. • For lower extremity fractures, patient should be supine and the extremity elevated about 6" to minimize swelling. • Always apply a layer of protection between an ice pack and the skin to reduce the possibility of frostbite or further injury to underlying tissue.	
◆ Re-assess extremity distal to injury for: • Pulse/Circulation • Motor movement • Sensation		

REASSESSMENT
(Ongoing Assessment)

Skill Component	Key Concepts
§ Repeat an ongoing assessment every **5-15 minutes**: • Initial assessment • Relevant portion of the focused assessment • Evaluate response to treatment • Compare results to baseline condition and vital signs	• The initial and focused examination is repeated every 15 minutes for stable patients and every 5 minutes for priority patients. • Every patient must be re-evaluated at least every 5 minutes, if any treatment was initiated or medication administered, unless changes in the patient's condition are anticipated sooner. • Priority patients are patients who have abnormal vital signs, signs/symptoms of poor perfusion or if there is a suspicion that the patient's condition may deteriorate.

PATIENT REPORT AND DOCUMENTATION

Skill Component	Key Concepts
§ Verbalize/Document • Mechanism of injury • Description of injury • Treatment provided • Type of splint • Pulse/Circulation before and after splinting • Motor movement before and after splinting • Sensation before and after splinting	• Documentation must be on either the Los Angeles County EMS Report or departmental Patient Care Record form.

MUSCULOSKELETAL INJURY / SPLINTS
Sling and Swathe

INDICATIONS:

• Suspected fracture of the clavicle or humorous

CONTRAINDICATIONS

• None

COMPLICATIONS:

• If swathe is applied to tight it may impair breathing

NOTES:

• Keep the knot from the sling from pressing on the patient's neck
• Swathe should not restrict the patient's uninjured arm

Developed 7/07

MUSCULOSKELETAL INJURY / SPLINTS
SLING AND SWATHE

PERFORMANCE OBJECTIVES
The examinee will demonstrate proficiency in applying a sling and swathe

CONDITION
The examinee will be requested to apply a sling and swathe to a patient with a suspected clavicle injury

EQUIPMENT
Adult CPR/trauma manikin or live model, all necessary bandages including cravats, gloves,

PERFORMANCE CRITERIA
- 100% accuracy required on all items designated by a diamond (♦) for skills testing and must manage successfully all items indicated by double asterisks (**).
- Documentation, identified by the symbol (§), must be practiced, but is not a required test item.
- Appropriate body substance isolation precautions must be instituted.

SLING AND SWATHE PREPARATION	
Skill Component	**Teaching Points**
♦ Take body substance isolation precautions	• Mandatory personal protective equipment - gloves • Situational - long sleeves, goggles, masks, gown
♦ Explain Procedure to patient	• Maintain patient rapport
♦ Check bilateral, distal circulation, sensory and motor function	
♦ Instruct patient to support arm of injured extremity if not done already	

PROCEDURE	
Skill Component	**Teaching Points**
♦ Place the base of sling (triangle) under the wrist of injured extremity with upper and over the opposite shoulder (apex toward the elbow of the injured extremity)	
♦ Lift lower end of sling over the forearm and shoulder of the injured extremity	
♦ Tie ends together to the side of the neck padding if possible	• Make sure that knot does not press against the back of the patients neck
♦ Fold apex of sling around elbow and secure	
♦ Tie ends together to the side of the neck padding if possible	
♦ Place swathe under uninjured extremity and over the injured extremity and rap around body. Secure	• Swathe should not restrict the patient's uninjured arm
♦ Arm must be immobilized against the chest wall utilizing swathe with minimum width of 1 inch and not compromising the patient's ability to breathe	
♦ Recheck distal circulation, sensory and motor function of injured arm	

Skill Component	Teaching Points
§ Recheck distal circulation, sensory and motor function of injured arm every fifteen minutes	• Student need only to state

DOCUMENTATION

Skill Component	Teaching Points
§ Verbalize/Document: • Reason for intervention • Distal vascular and neurological functions • Treatment provided	

Developed 7/07

MUSCULOSKELETAL INJURY
UNIPOLAR TRACTION DEVICE - SAGER SPLINT

INDICATIONS:
- Long bone fracture of the lower extremity:
  - Isolated, mid-shaft femur fracture

CONTRAINDICATIONS:
- Pelvic fracture
- Hip injury
- Knee injury
- Lower third (near the ankle) of a lower leg injury
- Ankle and foot fractures
- Distal end of femur fracture
- Partial amputation or avulsion of the leg
- More than one fracture of the same extremity

COMPLICATIONS:
- Neurovascular compromise if traction splint is applied incorrectly.
- Injury to genitals if "T-bar" and groin strap are not positioned correctly.

SPLINTING PRINCIPLES:

- **Priorities in managing a patient with an extremity fractures:**
  - 1st - life-threatening conditions
  - 2nd - limb-threatening conditions
  - 3rd - all other conditions

- **General management for suspected fractures:**
  - Stop bleeding and treat for shock
  - Support area of injury
  - Immobilize joints above and below injury site

- **General splinting principles:**
  - Pad rigid splints to adjust for anatomic shapes and patient comfort
  - Remove jewelry to prevent neurovascular compromise with increased swelling
  - Evaluate extremity before and after immobilization for neurovascular function

SPLINTING ERRORS:
- Splinting before life-threatening injuries are addressed. *(Treat life-threatening injuries first, then splint.)*
- Delaying transport of critical patients in order to splint an extremity.
- Improper splinting technique:
  - Splints applied too tight will compromise circulation and can cause nerve and muscle damage.
  - Splints applied too loosely may result in further soft-tissue damage or convert a closed fracture into an open fracture.
- Applying an incorrect splinting device that is inappropriate for the severity of the patient's condition and method of transport.
- Not realigning long bones when an extremity is pulseless and cyanotic.
- Attempting to realign joints. *(May increase damage to soft tissue, nerves, and muscles.)*

NOTES:
- Traction splints may be used on open femur or closed fractures, especially if there is neurovascular compromise, uncontrollable bleeding and severe pain due to muscle spasm.
- Femur fractures result from major force and in children is commonly the result of child abuse.
- Purpose of traction splint is to prevent overriding of the bone ends, decrease pain, relax muscle spasm, and reduce blood loss.
- There can be a significant blood loss with a femur fracture, 500-1000 or even more if it is an open fracture.
- The Sager splint is a unipolar device because it uses a single pole to initiate countertraction against the ischial tuberosity. It does not elevate or stabilize the lower extremity when the patient is moved. Additional support and splinting is required which is accomplished by securing both legs together.
- The Sager allows splinting of both legs with one splint if needed. Attach groin strap and ankle harness to the most serious fracture if only one ankle harness is available.

MUSCULOSKELETAL INJURY
UNIPOLAR TRACTION DEVICE - SAGER SPLINT

NOTES (Continued):

- The Sager splint may be applied by a single rescuer, the 2nd rescuer generally stabilizes the lower extremity to prevent movement. It does not require manual traction and elevation of the leg.

- DO NOT secure cravats (elastic straps) before traction has been established. This may interfere with pulling traction along the entire length of the leg and can cause angulation and excessive tightening of the strap resulting in compromised circulation.

- Never apply a Pneumatic Anti-shock Garment (PASG) over a rigid splint. The metal pole of the Sager splint produces a void between the PASG and the lower extremity allowing for continued internal or external bleeding. This may also press the splint into the extremity causing tissue damage, circulatory compromise, or puncture the PASG resulting in sudden dangerous deflation.

- The spring within the pole of the Sager splint allows for some automatic self-adjustment to maintain the proper level of traction once the splint has been applied when changes in muscle spasms occur.

- Never release the mechanical traction unless manual traction is re-established. The release of traction may cause additional injury to the leg.

- An "Infant" traction splint is used for neonates and children up to 6-years-of-age.

Developed 10/01

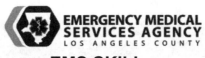

EMERGENCY MEDICAL SERVICES AGENCY
LOS ANGELES COUNTY

EMS SKILL

MUSCULOSKELETAL INJURY
UNIPOLAR TRACTION DEVICE - SAGER SPLINT

PERFORMANCE OBJECTIVES
Demonstrate competency in applying a unipolar traction device - Sager splint.

CONDITION
Apply a traction splint on a patient who has sustained an isolated mid-shaft femur fracture. There are no contraindications for application of a traction splint. Necessary equipment will be adjacent to the patient or brought to the field setting.

EQUIPMENT
Adult CPR/trauma manikin or live model, Sager splint, long spine board, all necessary straps/cravats, sterile dressings, 1" tape, goggles, masks, gown, gloves.

PERFORMANCE CRITERIA
- Items designated by a diamond (♦) must be performed successfully to demonstrate skill competency.
- Items identified by double asterisks (**) indicate actions that are required if indicated.
- Items identified by (§) are not skill component items, but should be practiced.

PREPARATION	
Skill Component	**Key Concepts**
♦ Establish body substance isolation precautions	• Mandatory (minimal) personal protective equipment – gloves
♦ Assess scene safety/scene size-up ** ***Consider spinal immobilization - if indicated***	• Spinal immobilization should be initiated when spinal trauma is suspected by taking bystander information and mechanism of injury into consideration.
♦ Evaluate need for additional BSI precautions	• Situational - goggles, mask, gown
♦ Stabilize and expose the injured lower extremity: • Cut clothes away - *if indicated* • Remove shoes and socks • Remove extremity and toe jewelry	• Femur fractures usually result from significant force; therefore, there is an increased risk for additional injuries. • Femur fracture most commonly present with mid-thigh swelling and generally the lower extremity is shortened and externally rotated. • Shoes must be removed to assess for pulse and sensation and prevent interference with the stability of the ankle harness. • Jewelry must be removed prior to swelling of the foot which may compromise circulation.
♦ Assess the lower extremity distal to injury for: • Circulation • Motor movement/function • Sensation *PMS*	• <u>Pulse</u> - palpate either popliteal or pedal pulses and mark location of pulse with an "X" <u>Circulation</u> - check for color, temperature, capillary refill. • <u>Motor movement</u> - have patient wiggle toes. • <u>Sensation</u> - determine numbness or tingling and sensitivity to touch of the lower extremity and toes.
♦ Cover wound with dry sterile dressing and secures in place - *if indicated*	• Blood loss from femoral fractures may exceed 1000 ml or more. This may be doubled if the fracture is an open fracture.
♦ Determine if traction splint should be applied ** ***Consider rapid transport - if patient is critical***	• If the patient is critical, splinting should be limited to securing the fractured limb to a long spine board and rapid transport. • Splinting minimizes pain, reduces hemorrhage and reduces the risk of a closed fracture being converted to an open fracture, blood vessel and nerve damage, and fat emboli.

Skill Component	Key Concepts
◆ Place splint on ground with the top of the padded "T-bar" in-line with the patient's groin	• The Sager Splint may be applied by a single rescuer; the 2nd rescuer generally stabilizes the lower extremity to prevent movement. • The Sager provides countertraction against the pubic bone and the ischial tuberosity (sitting bone) of the pelvis. *A common application mistake that is made is that the bar is placed too high into the groin area and not seated against the pubic bone and the ischial tuberosity.* • The "T-bar" fits like a bicycle seat. • The Sager allows splinting of both lower extremities with one splint if needed. However, there must be provision for 2 ankle harnesses. The groin strap will allow for traction of both lower extremities.

◆ Measure splint for length:
  • Place against medial aspect of the injured or uninjured lower extremity
  • Extend pole to the level of the heel
	• The splint may have either a pulley wheel, a perpendicular "L", or a cross bar for bilateral splinting.
	
	• The spring, within the shaft of the distal section, allows for some automatic self-adjustment to maintain proper traction when muscles spasm.

◆ Seat the padded "T-bar" firmly against:
  • Medial side of the thigh of the injured lower extremity and genitalia at the ischial tuberosity and the pubic bone
 OR
  • Outside of the injured lower extremity
	• Remove bulky clothing and pad area if necessary.
	
	• Ensure that genitals are not compressed.
	
	• Use groin strap to maintain traction against the pubis when placing the splint on the outside of the injured lower extremity.
	
	• The "outside" method does not pull traction as well as the "inside" method. However, it is more comfortable. The "T-bar" is extremely uncomfortable after a brief period of time for both male and female patients.

◆ Pad the groin area and between the lower extremity and pole of the splint - *if indicated*	• Pad the groin area and make sure no pressure is directly on external genitalia or bony areas.
◆ Secure groin (ischial) strap high around the upper thigh of the injured lower extremity	• The groin strap should be angled up toward patient's hip to prevent strap from slipping down when traction is applied. • The groin strap must be placed next to the side of the injured lower extremity.
◆ Size ankle harness just above the ankle for a secure fit: • Fold the extra ankle pads out - *if not needed*	• To maintain foot in proper alignment: - place the fixed padded part of the ankle harness under the posterior aspect of the ankle - ensure that the harness strap pulls from the underside of the foot

◆ Tighten the ankle harness above the ankle:
  • Bring end of harness up
  • Cross velcro closures one end over the other
  • Pull strap down to the sole of the foot
	• The ankle harness can be temporarily disconnected from the splint for easier application of the harness around the lower extremity.

◆ Attach the ankle harness to the splint and tighten - *if not already attached*	• Reduce slack in the traction strap. Failure to reduce the slack may result in inadequate traction and separation of the metal pole when traction is applied. • DO NOT attempt to apply an ankle harness to the second lower extremity if traction has already been applied.

◆ Extend the splint's inner pole to apply traction about 10% of body weight to maximum of 15 lbs:
  • Hold the upper portion of the metal pole while pulling traction
  • Apply countertraction to the groin
  • Align red arrow with the proximal weight marker
  • Stabilize upper part of splint to prevent movement of the injured lower extremity
	• Manual traction must be applied if the lower extremity is raised. The ankle harness may be used to assist in elevating the lower extremity.
	
	• Recommended traction applied is <u>10% of body weight per femur fracture</u> with maximum of 15 lbs. per lower extremity. If both femurs require traction, apply maximum of 30 lbs.
	
	<div align="center">(Continued)</div>

Skill Component	Key Concepts
	• Maximum traction for <u>lower extremity fractures</u> is 10 lbs. However, traction is generally not indicated for lower extremity fractures unless the limb has neurovascular compromise. • DO NOT over stretch the limb, this may cause further injury. • Adequate traction is applied when the injured lower extremity is the same length as the other lower extremity or until the patient feels relief. • Most patients will not get pain relief until the splint has been applied for several minutes and the muscle spasm subsides.
♦ Release pull on the distal section and ensure ratchet is locked	
♦ Check groin strap and tighten as needed for snug fit	• If the strap slips and traction is released this will result in increased damage to tissue, nerves and blood vessels.

♦ Secure the splint to lower extremity(s) with the cravats (elastic straps) at the level of the:
 	
• Thigh(s)
• knee(s)
• Lower extremity(s) - above the ankle harness
• Both extremities together - *if extra long (figure 8) strap is available*
	• May secure one lower extremity or both extremities at the same time.
	
	• Avoid excessive pressure on knees if possible when securing the cravats.
	
	• DO NOT secure cravats before traction has been established:
	  - may interfere with pulling traction along the entire length of the lower extremity
	  - may cause angulation and excessive tightening of the strap resulting in compromised circulation
	
	• Use the hollow of the knee to initially place the cravats and then move into proper position to minimize lower and midlimb movement. Stack cravats on top of the other in order of use.
	
	• Slide cravats into position starting with the one closest to the ground.
	
	• The Sager does not elevate or stabilize the lower extremity when the patient is moved and additional support and splinting is required. This is accomplished by securing both extremities and feet together.
	
	• Secure both feet together with figure 8 strap - *if not already secured*:
	  • Place strap under ankles
	  • Cross straps and bring between both feet
	  • Bring crossed straps under soles of feet
	  • Bring straps over top of feet
	  • Secure straps

♦ Secure patients to long spine board	• All traction splints must be used with a long spine board to prevent lateral and posterior movement of the lower torso and distal lower extremity by securing the pelvis and distal end of the traction device.
♦ Re-assess both extremities distal to injury for: • Circulation • Motor movement/function *PMS* • Sensation	• Since the uninjured lower extremity is also secured, it is important to make sure that nerves and circulation are not compromised in either lower extremity.
§ Make an effort to explain the care being delivered and the transport destination to the patient/caregivers	• Communication is extremely important when dealing with the patient, family or caregiver. This is a very critical and frightening time for all involved and providing information helps in decreasing the stress they are experiencing.

REASSESSMENT
(Ongoing Assessment

Skill Component	Key Concepts
♦ Reassess the patient at least every **5 minutes or sooner:** • Primary assessment • Relevant portion of the secondary assessment • Vital signs	• This is a priority patient and must be re-evaluated at least every 5 minutes or sooner, if any treatment is initiated, medication administered, or condition changes.
♦ Evaluate response to treatment	
♦ Evaluate results of reassessment and note any changes from patient's condition and vital signs ***Manage patient condition as indicated.**	• Evaluating and comparing results assists in recognizing if the patient is improving, responding to treatment or condition is deteriorating.

PATIENT REPORT AND DOCUMENTATION

Skill Component	Key Concepts
§ Verbalize/Document: • Mechanism of injury • Description of injury • Treatment provided • Patient responds to treatment • Pounds of traction applied • Pulse/Circulation before and after splinting • Motor movement before and after splinting • Sensation before and after splinting	• Documentation must be on either the Los Angeles County EMS Report or departmental Patient Care Record form.

Developed 10/01   Revised 10/09

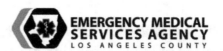

NEUROLOGICAL EMERGENCY / SPINAL IMMOBILIZATION
VEST–TYPE EXTRICATION DEVICE FOR THE SEATED PATIENT
Supplemental Information

INDICATIONS:
- Suspected spinal injury or when patient is found in a confined space, in a sitting position, and needs to be extricated.
  Immobilization Algorithm:
  - Mechanism of injury - if high suspicion of spinal injury with negative findings
  - <u>Unresponsive</u> or <u>history</u> of loss of consciousness
  - Not alert/disoriented with GCS <15
  - Communication barrier
  - Recent history of loss of consciousness
  - Suspected ETOH/Drug intoxication
  - Spinal pain/tenderness with or without motion
  - Spinal deformity
  - Neurological deficit
  - Painful or distracting injury

CONTRAINDICATIONS FOR ATTEMPTING NEUTRAL IN-LINE POSITION OF THE HEAD:
- If head is grossly misaligned (no longer extends from midline)
- If moving the head into a neutral in-line position results in:
  - compromising airway or ventilation
  - initiating or increasing muscle spasms of the neck
  - increasing neck pain
  - initiating or increasing neurological deficits
  - encountering resistance when attempting to move the head of an unconscious patient

COMPLICATIONS:
- Hypoventilation
- Aspiration
- Positional asphyxia

COMMON MISTAKES:
- Inadequate immobilization – leads to movement within the device if the device is not adequately secured.
- Lack of appropriate padding under occiput for adults and older children – results the head to be hyperextended.
- Lack of appropriate padding under shoulders and torso in toddlers and infants – results the head to be hyperflexed.
- Failure to immobilize penetrating trauma of the head, neck or torso – may result in neuro deficits due to injury of the spinal cord.
- Failure to reassess patients for circulation, sensation, motor movement, airway compromise and inadequate chest expansion – may result in increased neuro deficits or death.
- Taping or placing straps across the chin – may cause aspiration resulting in airway obstruction.
- Improper materials used for head immobilization such as IV bags and sandbags – may cause further injury if the patient's position is shifted or is moved.
- Sizing cervical collars in place – may jostle the patient's head and neck resulting in additional discomfort or spinal compromise.

TIGHTENING THE STRAPS:
- Remove excess slack from the strap after removing from storage position and before placing device on the patient.
- To secure a fractured pelvis use the lower portion of the extrication device.
- When groin injuries are suspected, use the same side configuration or DO NOT use leg straps
- Use caution in placing leg straps if patient has a possible hip or femur fracture – lower legs cannot be secured.
- Use the feed-and-pull technique to snug or tighten straps so that the patient's torso is not jostled during the immobilization process.
  <u>Feed-and-pull technique:</u>
  - Grasp the portion of the strap and create a little slack in the strap.
  - Feed the slack into the buckle with the other hand.
  - Repeat until the strap is snug or tight.

ORDER FOR SECURING AND TIGHTENING THE STRAPS (some devices have color coded straps)
- <u>Torso</u> – middle strap
- <u>Torso</u> – bottom strap
- <u>Leg</u> straps
- <u>Head</u> – upper strap
- <u>Neck</u> – bottom head strap – **must be removed prior to securing patient's head to the back board.**
- <u>Torso</u> – top strap – **may initially be buckled, but do not tighten until patient is ready to be transferred to a long spine board.**

VEST–TYPE EXTRICATION DEVICE FOR THE SEATED PATIENT
Supplemental Information (Continued)

TRANSFERRING PATIENT TO THE LONG SPINE BOARD
- Pivot, tilt and lift patient until his/her back is toward the outside of the vehicle. Both rescuers must be on the same side of the vehicle.
- Slide the spine board between the patient and the seat
- Lift vest and patient out of vehicle and onto long spine board
- Loosen the top torso strap. Loosening the top torso strap allows the patient more chest expansion. Decreased chest expansion results in positional asphyxia.
- Remove bottom neck strap.
- Keep remaining straps tightened to provide stability during the starts, stops and cornering of the ambulance ride.
- Patient must be well padded if leg straps are removed or have loosened – leg straps will loosen if applied correctly once patient is placed on the backboard.

ADAPTING EXTRICATION DEVICE FOR A PREGNANT PATIENT
- Fold 2 slats inward of each torso flap inward to leave abdomen free.
- Straps can be positioned to lie beneath the breasts but above the abdomen.
  - Two strap method – fasten bottom strap in the middle buckle and middle strap in bottom buckle.
  - Three strap method – fasten middle strap in its own buckle, bottom strap in top buckle, and top strap in bottom buckle.

ADAPTING EXTRICATION DEVICE FOR PEDIATRIC PATIENTS
- Child's size and condition determines how the extrication device can be adapted.
- If legs are longer than the extrication device, the child is placed in the device and then onto a long spine board.
- If extra padding is needed due to a small size, a folded blanket can be placed on the child so the torso flaps can be wrapped and fastened normally.
- Keep children in the car seat if they are stable; car seats provide an excellent immobilization device if no damage to it has been sustained.

ADAPTING EXTRICATION DEVICE FOR AN ANGULATED NECK
- Fold the head flaps inward, position a rolled towels as needed.
- Place head strap across forehead and secure strap to the fastening strips.

ADAPTING EXTRICATION DEVICE WHEN USING AN AED OR MANUAL DEFIBRILLATOR AND PLACING ECG LEADS
- Fold 2 slats of each torso flap inward to provide more chest exposure. Loosening 2 of the 3 torso straps allows defibrillation without losing immobility.

ADAPTING THE EXTRICATION DEVICE FOR HIP AND FEMUR STABLIZATION
- Place the extrication device on a long spine board with the head portion of the device toward the foot end.
- Center the torso portion of the device slightly above the waist.
- Secure the torso flaps around the patient.
- Wrap the head flaps around the injured leg and secure with the head straps.

ADAPTING THE EXTRICATION DEVICE FOR PELVIC STABILIZATION
- Place the extrication device on a long spine board with the head portion of the device toward the foot end.
- Center the torso portion of the device slightly above the waist.
- Secure the torso flaps around the patient's pelvic area.
- Wrap the head flaps around both legs and secure with the head straps.

NOTES:
- Cervical collars DO NOT completely immobilize; they allow for 25-30% of flexion and extension and up to 50% for other types of motion.
- When securing a patient in the sitting position, the torso is immobilized first, the legs second and the head last.
- Restriction of chest movement and increasing intra-abdominal pressure may result in positional asphyxia. Pediatric patients are especially susceptible to this.
- Immobilize the head and neck in or near the position found if a contraindication for instituting neutral in-line position of the head is present.
- Pain management may improve a patient's tolerance for spinal immobilization.

Developed: 2/05,   Revised: 9/09

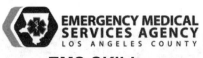

EMERGENCY MEDICAL SERVICES AGENCY
LOS ANGELES COUNTY

EMS SKILL

NEUROLOGICAL EMERGENCY / SPINAL IMMOBILIZATION
VEST–TYPE EXTRICATION DEVICE FOR THE SEATED PATIENT

PERFORMANCE OBJECTIVES
Demonstrate competency in performing and directing team members in spinal immobilization using an extrication device for the seated patient.

CONDITION
Perform and direct team members to secure a simulated patient using an extrication device used for the seated patient. There is no need for rapid extrication. Necessary equipment will be adjacent to the patient or brought to the field setting.

EQUIPMENT
Live model or manikin, chair or car, various sizes of rigid cervical collars, extrication device for the seated patient, long spine board, straps or binders, head-neck immobilizer, padding material, 2-3" cloth tape, 2-3 assistants, goggles, masks, gown, gloves.

PERFORMANCE CRITERIA
- Items designated by a diamond (♦) must be performed successfully to demonstrate skill competency.
- Items identified by double asterisks (**) indicate actions that are required if indicated.
- Items identified by (§) are not skill component items, but should be practiced.

PREPARATION	
Skill Component	**Key Concepts**
♦ Take body substance isolation precautions	• Mandatory (minimal) personal protective equipment – gloves
♦ Assess environment for safety	• Check if airbags have been deployed. If not, use caution during assessment and extrication. Request additional help to inactivate air bag system. • Make sure electrical vehicles are turned off. Unable to hear if idling since they are silent.. • Ensure that area is safe from falling debris in confined space.
♦ Evaluate additional BSI needs	• Situational - goggles, mask, gown
♦ Approach the patient from the front side	• Approaching the patient from the front side, minimizes the potential that the patient will turn his/her head to look at the EMS provider.
♦ Direct patient not to move or turn head: • Explain importance of remaining still • Explain immobilization procedure	• Keeping the head still and not moving will prevent any further injuries. • Spinal immobilization is restrictive and uncomfortable. Explaining the procedure will decrease anxiety and elicit a greater degree of cooperation.
♦ Place patient's head in neutral in-line position to initiate axial stabilization – *unless contraindicated* *NOTE: Spinal immobilization procedure is also called the spinal motion restriction (SMR) system*	• Depending on the situation, the rescuer who initiates and/or maintains axial stabilization may be positioned behind the patient r at the side of the patient. • The team leader is responsible for patient assessment and for directing patient care and should NOT be the rescuer to <u>physically maintain</u> spinal immobilization. • The sole focus of the rescuer immobilizing the head and neck should be to maintain axial stabilization throughout the procedure. • Spinal immobilization begins with manual control of the head and neck. The C-collar is applied <u>after</u> the primary assessment is completed. • NEVER apply traction when stabilizing the neck. • DO NOT attempt to move the head into an in-line position if the head is grossly misaligned (no longer extends from midline). Moving the head may result in: - compromising the airway or ventilation - initiating or increasing muscle spasms of the neck - increasing neck pain - initiating or increasing neurological deficits - encountering resistance when attempting to move the head of an unconscious patient

Skill Component	Key Concepts
◆ Prepare the extrication device	• Remove the leg straps at this point since they are usually secured behind the head of the device. If they are not freed at this time, further manipulation of the patient's spine will occur. *If the leg straps are not to be used, leave them attached in the storage configuration so they will not interfere with the extrication device.* • Leg straps are placed after the torso has been secured.
◆ Direct assistant to maintain manual immobilization of head and neck ** **Team leader should relinquish manual spinal immobilization to another EMS provider as soon as possible** ** **Ensure that manual stabilization is maintained at all times**	• Axial stabilization of the neck results in manual stabilization of the head and neck. • Maintain manual stabilization of the patient's head and neck until the patient's head is immobilized by a cervical collar and the extrication device.
◆ Assess all extremities for: • Circulation • Motor movement/function • Sensation	• Condition of the extremities must be assessed prior to moving the patient and when immobilization procedure has been completed.
◆ Assess neck/cervical spine • Assess for DCAP/BTLS: - Deformity (visible and palpated) - Contusions - Abrasions - Penetrations / Punctures - Burns/bruises - Tenderness - Lacerations - Swelling / Scars • Palpate for: - Tenderness - Instability - Crepitus • Additional Assessment Elements - Track marks and tattoos - Medical alert tags - Jugular vein distention (JVD) - Tracheal deviation - Accessory muscle use - Carotid pulses - Subcutaneous emphysema (crepitus) - Stoma • Medical Devices: - Tracheostomy - Central venous catheters ** **Apply occlusive dressing - if puncture wound to neck**	• DCAP/BTLS is a mnemonic used for rapid trauma assessment. The assessment elements given in the skills component incorporate the elements of the mnemonic and additional assessment information specific to each body part. • Most cervical collars have an opening at the anterior neck, which allows for only limited examination. Therefore, the neck must be thoroughly assessed before application of the cervical collar.
◆ Size and apply cervical (extrication) collar ** **Ensure that the cervical collar does not obstruct the airway and hinder mouth opening, ventilation or circulation**	• DO NOT attempt to apply a cervical collar if the head is not in an in-line position. Cervical collars do not accommodate an angulated or rotated head. • DO NOT apply a cervical collar if a stoma is present, but immobilize head and neck with a head immobilizer. *Placing a cervical collar on a patient who has a stoma will compromise the airway.* • Cervical collars DO NOT immobilize. They allow for 25-30% of motion by flexion and extension and up to 50% for other types of motion. (Continued)

Skill Component	Key Concepts
	A unique function of the cervical collar is to rigidly maintain a minimum distance between the head and neck to eliminate intermittent compression of the cervical spine.
	Cervical collars help to prevent significant movement of the head toward the neck during transport when the ambulance accelerates or decelerates or bounces due to pavement irregularities.
	• An incorrectly sized cervical collar may cause hyperflexion, hyperextension, or compression of the trachea/carotid arteries/large veins of the neck, and increased patient discomfort.
	• A cervical collar that hinders mouth opening may result in aspiration if the patient vomits.
	• A cervical collar sized improperly may result in unnecessary complications if:
	- **too loose** it is ineffective and can cover the anterior chin, mouth, and nose resulting in airway obstruction
	- **too tight** it can compress the carotid arteries and neck veins
	- **too short** it will not protect the cervical spine from compression and allows for significant flexion
	- **too tall** it will cause hyperextension of the head and neck
◆ Sit the patient forward as a unit and remove any articles and debris behind the patient ** ***Ensure spinal alignment is not compromised***	• Articles and debris can interfere with sliding the extrication device between the patient and the seat or cause additional trauma to patient's torso. • Moving the patient slightly forward (i.e. a hand's thickness) will assist in placing the extrication device appropriately and reducing friction. • To avoid jostling the patient's head, coordinate moving the patient slightly forward while maintaining axial stabilization.

◆ Tilt the extrication device at a 45° angle and slide the device behind the patient until aligned with patient's spine	• Place the velcro and buckle side against the seat and away from the patient.
	
	• Tilt the extrication device at about a 45-degree angle and use the lift handles to slide it behind the patient. Tilting the device:
	  - prevents the extrication device from rolling up
	  - allows the extrication device to clear a roofline

◆ Pull the extrication device up vertically until the torso flaps are positioned securely in both axillas ** ***Ensure that the patient's head is not jostled during this maneuver*** ** ***Ensure that the device is centered alongside the patients spine***	• The rescuer stabilizing the head lifts his/her elbow slightly to provide clearance for the extrication device and taking care not to move the head. • Use the lift handles to center the extrication device behind the patient.
◆ Adjust the patient's position and lean patient back against the device	• To check and adjust patient's position, the rescuer behind the patient continues to stabilize the head and neck and the rescuer on the side of the patient gently presses the patient's chest just below the cervical collar to ensure contact with the device. *Some patients may not be able to sit fully back into the device.* • Positioning the patient as close as possible against the device <u>minimizes</u> the amount of padding needed between the head, neck and shoulders, and the extrication device.
◆ Wrap both torso flaps around the patient just below axillas ** ***Ensure that the extrication device is in contact with the patients back as much as possible.*** ** ***Ensure that the top edges of the torso flaps press firmly into both axillas*** ** ***Fold 2 slats of each torso flap inward for pregnant patients***	• Use the lift handles to raise and adjust the extrication device torso flaps under both axillas to keep the device in place until the straps can be buckled. • It is important that the extrication device is snug under both axillas to make sure the patient's weight is suspended and prevent the patient slipping down when lifted.

Skill Component	Key Concepts

◆ Fasten the torso straps using the feed-and-pull tightening technique
 	
• <u>First</u> fasten and snug the <u>middle</u> strap
 	
• <u>Second</u> fasten and snug the <u>bottom</u> strap
 	
** *Ensure that the top strap is not fastened at this time, but is clear and __not__ under the middle or bottom strap*
 	
** *Criss-cross middle and bottom straps to keep abdominal area free for pregnant patient*
 	
Note: *The top strap is <u>secured</u> and the rest of the torso straps are <u>tightened</u> just before the patient is transferred to a long spine board.*
	• <u>Feed-and-pull tightening technique</u>
	  - Grasp the portion of the strap and create a little slack in the strap.
	  - Feed the slack into the buckle with the other hand.
	  - Repeat until the strap is snug or tight.
	
	• The <u>middle strap</u> secures the greatest possible area of the extrication device.
	
	• Snug the middle and bottom straps leaving a space between the strap and patient's chest by placing 2-3 fingers flat between the strap and the patient's chest.
	
	• Straps must never be twisted; this may compromise the patient's stability in the devise or cause additional discomfort and skin breakdown.

◆ Apply leg straps
 	
<u>Criss-cross configuration</u>
• Cross straps at the groin and buckle the straps opposite their sides of origin
 	
    OR
 	
<u>Same-side configuration</u>
• Do not cross straps at the groin, but buckle them on their sides of origin
 	
** *Ensure that straps lie flat from their anchor point and are as close as possible to the body's midline*
	• For suspected groin injury, the EMS provider should determine if the use of leg straps will cause further injury.
	
	• <u>Applying leg straps:</u>
	  - pass one leg strap between the leg and car seat "see-saw" strap into position under the patient's leg and buttock
	
	• Straps in either the criss-cross configuration or same-side configuration must be positioned as close as possible to the body's midline (straight down) from their anchoring points on the back before passing beneath the buttocks.
	
	• To prevent pressure on the groin when using the same-side configuration, extra care must be taken to correctly position the leg straps close to the body midline. *This requires a more focused effort because the tendency is to place the straps away from the midline.*

◆ Fasten and snug the leg straps	• Snug both straps leaving a space between the leg and strap by placing 2-3 fingers flat between the strap and the patient's leg.
◆ Place padding behind patient's head and neck - *if* <u>*indicated*</u> ** **Place padding without hyperextending or flexing the neck**	• The amount of padding depends on the patient's medical condition, body structure, and head shape. *Some patents may not need padding when they are placed in the extrication device correctly* • Placing padding behind the head and neck ensures neutral alignment of the spine. Can use the Adjusta-Pad or other suitable padding.
◆ Wrap the head flaps around the patient's head	

◆ Secure patient's head:
 	
<u>Upper strap (head)</u>
• Center the rubber padded strap or tape over the patient's forehead (tape must adhere to skin)
 	
• Position strap ends or tape at a downward angle and secure them to the fastening straps on the head flaps
 	
<u>Bottom strap (neck)</u>
• Place strap or tape against a rigid area beneath the "chin" of the cervical collar and above the neck opening
 	
• Position the strap ends or tape horizontally and secure them to the head flaps
 	
** *Ensure tape adheres to the skin.*
	• <u>If the upper strap contains a rubber pad:</u>
	  - grasp the strap with both hands
	  - turn the pad fully inside-out exposing the rubber pad
	  - center the pad at the patient's forehead with the rubber against the skin
	
	• Placing the head strap or tape at a downward angle minimizes the chance that the strap will slip upward on the forehead. The rubber or tape keeps the strap from sliding.
	
	• A patient should not be able to move his/her head if properly restrained. Therefore, DO NOT use gauze or folded tape over the forehead.
	
	• If there is a gap between the extrication device and the patient's head, cervical collar or shoulders, padding needs to be placed without hyperextending or flexing the neck.
	
	• The Adjusta-Pad can be folded or other padding materials used if additional thickness is needed.

Skill Component	Key Concepts
◆ Fasten and snug the <u>top</u> torso strap using the feed-and-pull tightening technique	• Snug both straps leaving a space between the chest and strap by placing 2-3 fingers flat between the strap and the patient's chest.
◆ Evaluate device application and readjust as needed	• Check that the flaps are securely in both axillas, head is in the in-line position, and straps and pads are secure.

◆ Tighten all straps to transfer patient to the long spine board.
 	
** **Reassess airway and chest expansion**
	• Straps should be tighten in the following order:
	  - middle torso strap
	  - bottom torso strap
	  - leg straps
	  - top torso strap
	• Ask patient to inhale and exhale to adjust torso straps. Assess chest expansion to prevent chest constriction and hypoventilation.
	• Head straps are already secured and do not need to be tightened and further.

◆ Reassesses airway and chest expansion	
◆ Reassess all extremities for: • Circulation • Motor movement/function • Sensation	
◆ Remove the patient from the vehicle using appropriate extrication technique	• Remove patient by using the side lifting handles and supporting the legs which minimizes the need to use the extremities or clothing to move the patient.
◆ Place the patient on a long spine board	
◆ Loosen the top torso strap without unfastening the buckle	• Decreased chest expansion results in positional asphyxia. Loosening the top torso strap allows the patient more chest expansion.
◆ Keep remaining straps tightened ** ***Ensure patient is well padded if leg straps were not applied, removed or have loosened and not retightened***	• Keeping the remaining straps tightened provides stability during transport. • Patient must be well padded if leg straps were not applied, removed, or have loosened and not retightened. *Leg straps will loosen if applied correctly and need to be tightened when patient is on long spine board.*
◆ Secure patient's torso and legs to spine board	• Securing the patient to the spine board prevents further injury if patient needs to be tilted or rolled to the side.
◆ Remove bottom head strap (neck)	• DO NOT use a chin strap to immobilize the head. The patient may aspirate if he/she cannot open his/her mouth in case of vomiting. Also, compression of the trachea and carotid arteries may occur.
◆ Secure patient's head and neck with a head immobilizing device using appropriate technique ** ***Ensure that device does* not *compromise patient's airway, carotid arteries or neck veins*** ** ***Reduce or remove occipital and neck padding - if indicated.***	• Always secure head last to spine board since the body weighs more and may pull the spine out of alignment if the body is not secured first. • Re-evaluate padding to ensure axial stabilization is maintained and it does not compromise the airway. • Reducing or removing the occipital and neck padding prevents hyperflexion of neck if padding is not needed.
◆ Secure spine board to gurney	
◆ Remove shoes and socks	• When shoes and socks are left on the patient, assessing feet for circulation, motor movement/function and sensation, cannot be properly assessed.
◆ Reassess all extremities for: • Circulation • Motor movement/function • Sensation ** ***Correct area of circulatory compromise – if needed***	• Condition of the extremities must be reassessed prior to moving the patient and when immobilization procedure has been completed. • Once a patient has been placed in spinal immobilization, only a physician should determine if the patient can be removed from the immobilization device.
◆ Secure the arms	• Secure arms with backboard straps or tape to prevent injury when transporting patient.

Skill Component	Key Concepts
♦ Evaluate device application and readjust as needed	
§ Explain the care being delivered and transport destination to the patient/caregiver	• Communication is important when dealing with the patient, family or caregiver. This is a very critical and frightening time for all involved and providing information helps in decreasing the stress they are experiencing.

REASSESSMENT
(Ongoing Assessment)

Skill Component	Key Concepts
♦ Repeat assessment at least every **5 minutes for priority** patients and every **15 minutes for stable** patients. • Primary assessment • Relevant portion of the secondary assessment • Vital signs	• Priority patients are patients who have abnormal vital signs, S/S of poor perfusion, if there is a suspicion that the patient's condition may deteriorate, or when the patient's condition changes.
♦ Evaluate device application and readjust as needed	• Patients must be re-evaluated at least every 5 minutes if any treatment was initiated, medication administered or unless a change in the patient's condition is anticipated.
♦ Evaluate results of reassessment and note any changes from patient's previous condition and vital signs ****Manage patient condition as indicated.**	• Evaluating and comparing results assists in recognizing if the patient is improving, responding to treatment or condition is deteriorating.

PATIENT REPORT AND DOCUMENTATION

Skill Component	Key Concepts
§ Report and document: • Mechanism of injury • Neuro and circulatory findings of all 4 extremities before and after spinal immobilization • Injuries sustained • Treatment rendered and response	• Documentation must be on either the Los Angeles County EMS Report or departmental Patient Care Record form. • Documenting reassessment information provides a comprehensive picture of patient's response to treatment. • Last reassessment information (before patient care is transferred) should be documented in the section of the EMS form that is called "Reassessment after Therapies and/or Condition on Transfer".

Developed: 2/05,   Revised: 9/09

NEUROLOGICAL EMERGENCY / SPINAL IMMOBILIZATION
HELMET REMOVAL

INDICATIONS:

• Inability to assess and/or reassess airway and breathing.
• Helmet prevents effective management of the airway or breathing.
• Excessive patient head movement within helmet.
• Proper spinal immobilization is impaired due to helmet.
• Cardiac or respiratory arrest.

CONTRAINDICATIONS

• No immediate or impending airway or breathing problems.
• Helmet does not interfere with ongoing assessment of airway and breathing.
• Helmet provides snug fit with little movement of head.
• Removal of helmet with result in further injury.

COMPLICATIONS:

• Improper technique may lead to exacerbation of pre-existing cervical spine injury

Developed 7/07

NEUROLOGICAL EMERGENCY / SPINAL IMMOBILIZATION
HELMET REMOVAL

PERFORMANCE OBJECTIVES
The examinee will demonstrate proficiency in removing a helmet from a patient

CONDITION
The examinee will be requested to properly remove a helmet from patient with possible airway complications.

EQUIPMENT
Adult CPR/trauma manikin or live model, motorcycle or football helmet, gloves.

PERFORMANCE CRITERIA
- 100% accuracy required on all items designated by a diamond (♦) for skills testing and must manage successfully all items indicated by double asterisks (**).
- Documentation, identified by the symbol (§), must be practiced, but is not a required test item.
- Appropriate body substance isolation precautions must be instituted.

SPECIFIC SKILL PREPARATION	
Skill Component	**Teaching Points**
♦ Take body substance isolation precautions	• Mandatory personal protective equipment - gloves • Situational - long sleeves, goggles, masks, gown
♦ Explain Procedure to patient	• Maintain patient rapport
♦ Take position above the patient and place hands on each side of the helmet to initiate stabilization	• Ensure that assistant is in proper position
♦ Instruct assistant to provide spinal stabilization by placing hands at side of the neck at the angle of jaw or placing one hand on the lower jaw and the other hand behind the head at the occipital area	• When removing a football helmet it is important to know that the shoulder pads will cause the head to hyperextend. It is helpful to remove the shoulder pads to maintain proper cervical alignment .
♦ Release or cut the chinstraps	
♦ Instruct assistant to maintain in-line spinal stabilization to prevent head movement to assure head is not dropped when helmet is removed	

PROCEDURE	
Skill Component	**Teaching Points**
♦ Remove helmet slowly by pulling out on the sides until the ears are cleared and pulling straight back (full face helmets may be tilted back to clear the nose)	
♦ Place hands on each side of the patient's head with the fingers at the angles of the jaw and the palms over the ears	

ONGOING ASSESSMENT	
Skill Component	**Teaching Points**
§ Continue spinal immobilization procedure	• Manual spinal stabilization should not be released until the patient's head has been properly secured to a long board.

DOCUMENTATION	
Skill Component	**Teaching Points**
§ Verbalize/Document: • Mechanism of injury • Description of injury • Treatment provided	

Developed 7/07

NEUROLOGICAL EMERGENCY / SPINAL IMMOBILIZATION
LONG SPINE BOARD

INDICATIONS:
- Suspected spinal injury when:
  - <u>Unresponsive</u> or <u>history</u> of loss of consciousness
  - Not alert / disoriented with GCS <15
  - Suspected ETOH/Drug use
  - Spinal pain with or without motion
  - Spinal deformity
  - Neurological deficit
  - Painful or distracting injury
  - Mechanism of injury - if high suspicion of spinal injury with negative findings or communication barrier

CONTRAINDICATIONS FOR ATTEMPTING NEUTRAL IN-LINE POSITION OF THE HEAD:
- Head is grossly misaligned (no longer extends from midline)
- Moving the head into a neutral in-line position results in:
  - Compromising airway or ventilation
  - Initiating or increasing muscle spasms of the neck
  - Increasing neck pain
  - Initiating or increasing neurological deficits
  - Encountering resistance when attempting to move the head of an unconscious patient

COMPLICATIONS:
- Aspiration
- Positional asphyxia

COMMON MISTAKES:
- Inadequate immobilization - torso or head not sufficiently secured.
- Immobilization with the head hyperextended in adults and older children - caused by lack of appropriate padding under occiput.
- Immobilization with the head hyperflexed in toddlers and infants - caused by lack of appropriate padding under shoulders and torso.
- Readjusting the torso straps after the head has been secured - results in movement of the head and neck.
- Failure to immobilize penetrating trauma of the head, neck or torso - may result in neuro deficits due to injury to the spinal cord.
- Failure to reassess patients for circulation, sensation, motor movement, airway compromise and inadequate chest expansion - may result in increased neuro deficits or death.
- Taping or placing straps across chin - may cause airway obstruction.

NOTES:
- Cervical collars DO NOT immobilize, they allow for 25-30% of motion by flexion and extension and up to 50% for other type of motion.
- Occipital padding is required for adults and older children. Shoulder or torso padding is required for young children, toddlers and infants.
- When log rolling, the patient's arms should be kept at the side to help splint the body. Placing the patient=s arm above the head interferes with head and neck alignment.

- To prevent aspiration and airway compromise, tape should <u>never</u> be directly applied to chin or collar and then secured to the board without a head-neck immobilizer device in place.

- Securing the torso before securing the head prevents angulating the cervical spine.
- Shim patients well to prevent lateral movement in situations when the patient must be turned on their side:
  - Vomiting
  - 3rd trimester pregnancy the board must be propped 45° toward the left side to prevent compression of the vena cava and thereby prevent compromised venous return to the heart.

- Only approved immobilization devices such as commercial immobilizers, towels, blanket rolls, etc. should be used. Sand bags, IV bags and other heavy objects should not be used as head immobilizing devices which may shift and result in further spinal injury.

- Prolonged backboard immobilization is frequently associated with headache, back pain, mandibular pain and pressure sores. Symptoms develop at point of contact between a bony prominence and the board or cervical collar.

- Helmets should be removed in the field if they are loose, unstable, and if they compromise the ability to control the airway. Sports helmets should not be removed unless necessary and then the patient must be padded appropriately if shoulder pads are in place.

- Patients > 64 years of age have a higher incident of spinal injury, therefore, mechanism of injury should be taken into consideration when deciding if spinal immobilization should be instituted.

- Too much padding under the head or shoulders will result in neck extension and too little padding results in neck flexion.
- Restriction of chest movement and increasing intra-abdominal pressure may result in positional asphyxia. Pediatric patients are especially susceptible to this.

- Immobilize the head and neck in or near the position it was initially found if contraindications for instituting neutral in-line position of the head are present.

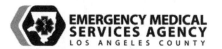

**EMERGENCY MEDICAL
SERVICES AGENCY**
LOS ANGELES COUNTY

EMS SKILL

NEUROLOGICAL EMERGENCY / SPINAL IMMOBILIZATION
LONG SPINE BOARD

PERFORMANCE OBJECTIVES
Demonstrate proficiency in performing and directing team members in spinal immobilization using a long spine board.

CONDITION
Perform and direct team members to apply a cervical collar, log roll and secure a patient onto a long spine board. Necessary equipment will be adjacent to the manikin or brought to the field setting.

EQUIPMENT
Live model or manikin, various sizes of rigid collars, long spine board, straps or binders, head-neck immobilizer, padding material, 2-3" cloth tape, 2-3 assistants, goggles, various masks, gown, gloves.

PERFORMANCE CRITERIA
- Items designated by a diamond (♦) must be performed successfully to demonstrate skill proficiency.
- Items identified by double asterisks (**) indicate actions that are required, if indicated.
- Items identified by (§) should be practiced.

PREPARATION	
Skill Component	**Key Concepts**
♦ Take body substance isolation precautions	• Mandatory personal protective equipment - gloves
♦ Assess environment for safety	
♦ Evaluate additional BSI needs	• Situational - goggles, masks, gown

PROCEDURE	
Skill Component	**Key Concepts**

♦ Place patient's head in neutral in-line position and maintain axial stabilization throughout procedure - *unless contraindicated*
 	
- If team leader initiates C-spine immobilization first - *relinquish position to an assistant as soon as possible*
- If an assistant is immediately available - *direct assistant to initiate C-spine immobilization*
	• The team leader should not remain at head of patient for C-spine immobilization since he/she is in charge of assessment and directs patient care.
	
	• To prevent extension, flexion, and lateral bending or rotation of the head, place thumbs facing anteriorly just below the zygomatic arches and spread fingertips along the sides of the face with the little fingers touching the base of the occiput. DO NOT apply traction.
	
	• Move head into an in-line position. Immobilize the head and neck in or near the position it was initially found if any of the following conditions are present:
	- head is grossly misaligned (no longer extends from midline)
	- moving the head into a neutral in-line position results in:
	  ~ compromising airway or ventilation
	  ~ initiating or increasing muscle spasms of the neck
	  ~ increasing neck pain
	  ~ initiating or increasing neurological deficits
	  ~ encountering resistance when attempting to move the head of an unconscious patient
	
	• Initially the head of an adult may need to be held off the ground to achieve a neutral position and prevent hyperextension.
	(Continued)

Skill Component	Key Concepts
Continued from page 1	• If patient requires bag-valve-mask ventilation, the rescuer places the patient's head between the rescuers thighs with his knees at the level of the patient's shoulders to maintain in-line stabilization.
◆ Assess all extremities for: • Circulation • Sensation • Motor function *PMS*	• Condition of the extremities must be assessed prior to moving the patient and when immobilization procedure has been completed.
◆ Assess neck for: • Accessory muscle use • Neck vein distention • Tracheal deviation • Medical alert tags • Penetrations/lacerations • Contusions/bruises/abrasions • Deformities (visible and palpated) • Tenderness • Crepitus • Quality of carotid pulse	• Many cervical collars have an opening at the anterior neck, which allows for only limited examination. Therefore, the neck must be thoroughly assessed before application of the collar. • Check for a tracheostomy stoma. If stoma is present, immobilize head and neck with <u>approved</u> head immobilizer device and DO NOT apply cervical collar. *Placing a cervical collar on patients who have a stoma is extremely dangerous due to the possibility of the collar shifting and occluding the airway.*

◆ Apply appropriately sized extrication collar
 	
** ***Ensure that collar does not obstruct the airway, or hinder mouth opening, ventilation or circulation***
	• DO NOT attempt to apply a collar if the head is not in an in-line position. Cervical collars do not accommodate an angulated or rotated head.
	
	• Cervical collars DO NOT immobilize, they allow for 25-30% of motion by flexion and extension and up to 50% for other type of motion.
	
	A unique function of the cervical collar is to rigidly maintain a minimum distance between the head and neck to eliminate intermittent compression of the cervical spine.
	Rigid collars help to prevent significant movement of the head toward the neck during transport when the ambulance accelerates or decelerates or bounces due to pavement irregularities.
	
	• An incorrectly sized collar may cause hyperflexion/extension, or compression of the trachea, carotid arteries and large veins of the neck, and increased patient discomfort.
	
	• A collar sized improperly may result in unnecessary complications if:
	  - <u>too loose</u> it is ineffective and can cover the anterior chin, mouth, and nose resulting in airway obstruction
	  - <u>too tight</u> it can compress the carotid arteries and neck veins
	  - <u>too short</u> it will not protect the cervical spine from compression and allows for significant flexion
	  - <u>too tall</u> it will cause hyperextension of the head and neck
	
	• A collar that hinders mouth opening may cause aspiration if the patient vomits.

◆ Direct one assistant to position long board parallel to the patient (opposite side of rescuers)	

◆ Position team members appropriately to turn patient:
 	
➤ ***4 team members***
  - 1st assistant - remains at head
  - Team leader - near midchest with one hand on patient's shoulder and the other on patient's hip and securing near arm with knees
  - 2nd assistant - by hips with one hand above patient's waist and the other below patient's knee and securing far arm to lateral upper thigh
  - 3rd assistant - by knees with one hand on patient's mid-thigh and the other below patient's calf
	• Four team members are preferable in maintaining proper spinal alignment during a log roll, but three team members may be used if necessary.
	
	• Team leader should not remain at head of patient for C-spine immobilization since he/she is in charge of assessment and total patient care.
	
	• The near and far arm must be controlled during the log-roll. The arms are extended at the sides with palms inward. The patient is rolled onto one arm which provides proper spacing and acts as a splint for the body (turn patient only onto an uninjured arm).
	
	• DO NOT raise the arm above the head or place the arms anteriorly. This interferes with head and neck alignment and results in movement of the spine.

Skill Component	Key Concepts
➢ **_3 team members_** - 1st assistant - remains at head - Team leader - near midchest with one hand on shoulder and other hand on upper thigh and securing near arm with knees - 2nd assistant - near upper legs with one hand on hip and other hand below knee and securing far arm to lateral upper thigh	
◆ Give the signal and roll patient towards team members while maintaining body alignment	• The team leader should give the command to turn the patient. However, if this role is relinquished, the team leader must make it clear as to who gives the command to turn the patient. • Patient must be turned as a unit only far enough to inspect the back and roll patient onto the backboard. (Bring the board to the patient.) • Grasping clothing to turn the patient may result in compromising spinal immobilization during log roll if clothing gives way or tears.
◆ Assess back: • Slide hand holding shoulder to center of back to stabilize patient • Use other hand to palpate for injuries, tenderness and deformity	
◆ Direct assistant near patient's hips to slide board into position next to patient	• Either the team leader at the mid-chest area or assistant at the hip-thigh area may pull board over. However, it is more difficult for the person at the chest area to reach over patient without compromising his position.
◆ Give signal to roll patient onto board maintaining body alignment	• The team leader should give the command to turn the patient. However, if this role is relinquished, the team leader must make it clear as to who gives the command to turn the patient.
◆ Center patient vertically on board angling the patient towards center by sliding patient towards foot of board then towards the head of board	• Sliding the patient in this manner prevents jerking movement and maintains alignment of head, shoulders, hips and legs as patient is centered onto the board.

◆ Fill in spaces between the body and the board or straps with padding - if indicated
 	
• Occipital padding for an adult or older child
 	
• Shoulder padding for a young child, toddler or infant
 	
• Shimming padding for spaces between torso, hips, and legs and the edge of the board or straps
	• Shim patients well to prevent lateral movement in situations when the patient must be turned on the side:
	  - vomiting
	  - 3rd trimester pregnancy - The board must be propped 45° on left side to prevent compression of the vena cava and thereby prevent compromised venous return to the heart.
	• Too much padding under the head or shoulders will result in neck extension and too little padding results in neck flexion in peds patients.
	• A young child is defined as having the body size of less than an average 8-year-old.
	• Geriatric patients often require additional padding due to arthritic changes resulting in abnormal curvature of the spine.

◆ Secure chest, hips and legs to board with straps or binder ** **_Ensure chest expansion is not compromised and intra-abdominal pressure is not increased_**	• Securing the torso before securing the head prevents angulating the cervical spine. • Straps should be placed across chest in manner that does not compromise chest expansion and increase intra-abdominal pressure. The straps should be placed over the shoulder girdle and pelvis and allow insertion of a finger between the chest and straps during full inspiration. • Restriction of chest movement and increasing intra-abdominal pressure may result in positional asphyxia. Pediatric patients are especially susceptible to this. • Straps secured too tightly across the soft abdomen may result in organ damage and internal bleeding.

Skill Component	Key Concepts
♦ Immobilize head and neck with an approved immobilizing device and securing technique ** ***Ensure that device does not compromise patient's airway, carotid arteries or neck veins*** *Cheeseblocks*	• The head cannot be immobilized adequately by using only a strap or tape over the forehead. The sides of the head and neck must be stabilized with an <u>approved</u> head immobilizer, pads, rolled towels or blanket. DO NOT use sandbags or IV bags. • If a stoma is present, immobilize head and neck with an <u>approved</u> head immobilizer device. DO NOT apply a cervical collar. • Straps or 2-3" tape may be used to secure the head immobilizer device. Place strap or tape across the supraorbital ridge. *If tape is used, ensure that person removing the supraorbital tape understands that the tape should be cut between the eyebrows and pulled in the direction that the eyebrows grow (anterior to lateral ridge of orbit) to prevent denuding the hairs.* ☠ **DO NOT use chin cups or straps encircling the chin or tape the chin support of the collar. This will prevent airway obstruction and allows the patient to open the mouth if they need to vomit.** • Tape is used <u>only</u> across the cervical collar and immobilizing device to secure the immobilizing device. It is <u>never</u> applied across the collar alone to secure the neck to the board. (The immobilization device disburses the pressure of the tape.) ***Direct pressure on the anterior neck may result in compression of the trachea/carotid arteries or large veins of the neck.***
♦ Check: • Airway • Chest expansion	• Have patient inhale to check for adequate chest expansion.
♦ Ensure arms are secured prior to transport	• Arms should be secured next to the patient's side or across the torso prior to moving the patient. • The arms should not be included in either the hips or groin loops (if used). If these straps are tight enough to immobilize, they will compromise circulation.
♦ Reassess all extremities for: • Circulation • Sensation • Motor function *PMS*	• Condition of the extremities must be assessed prior to moving the patient and when immobilization procedure has been completed. • Log rolling and securing the patient to the backboard may increase or result in injury to the spine. Also, straps may be too tight and compromise neuro and circulatory functions. *If problem noted, reassess patient and correct area of compromise. If no problem identified, transport patient immediately - DO NOT remove from spinal immobilization.*

ONGOING ASSESSMENT

Skill Component	Key Concepts
§ Repeat an ongoing assessment every **5-15 minutes**: • Initial assessment • Relevant portion of the focused assessment • Evaluate response to treatment • Compare results to baseline condition and vital signs	• The initial and focused examination is repeated every 15 minutes for stable patients and every 5 minutes for priority patients. • Every patient must be re-evaluated at least every 5 minutes, if any treatment was initiated or medication administered, unless changes in the patient's condition are anticipated sooner. • Priority patients are patients who have abnormal vital signs, signs/ symptoms of poor perfusion or if there is a suspicion that the patient's condition may deteriorate.

DOCUMENTATION

Skill Component	Key Concepts
§ Report and document neuro and circulatory findings of all 4 extremities before and after spinal immobilization	• Documentation must be on either the Los Angeles County EMS Report or departmental Patient Care Record form.

Developed 3/01   Revised 8/01, 12/07

OBSTETRICAL EMERGENCY / EMERGENCY CHILDBIRTH
DELIVERY

DEFINITIONS:

- _Baby_ - name used to indicate newborn

- _Newborn_ - neonate in the first minutes to hours after birth

- _Neonate_ - infants in first month after birth (28 days)

- _Infant_ - includes the neonate period to 1 year (12 months)

- Bloody show - watery bloody discharge is normal through out the three stages of labor. During the 1st stage of labor it is the displacement of the mucus plug as the cervix dilates

- _Crowning_ - bulging of the vaginal opening or when the presenting part of the baby is visible. This is the most reliable sign of imminent delivery

- _Duration of the contraction_ - from the beginning of the contraction to its completion

- _Frequency of contractions_ - from the beginning of one contraction until the onset of the next contraction

- Labor pains - pain in addition to the discomfort of the contractions, usually felt in the lower abdomen and back

- _Meconium_ - fetal feces that is normally passed as the baby's first bowel movement. However, during fetal or maternal stress defecation may occur before birth

- _Nuchal cord_ - umbilical cord wrapped around baby's neck

- _Uterine inversion_ - uterus is inverted or turned inside-out. Caused by extensive pressure on the uterus or from pulling on the umbilical cord before the placenta is delivered

COMPLICATIONS AND INTERVENTIONS:

- **Meconium-stained amniotic fluid**

  Problem - will cause pneumonia or other problems
  Intervention - suction mouth and nose aggressively before delivery of the rest of the body

- **Nuchal cord**

  Problem - will choke the baby and the cord may tear during the deliver causing sever hemorrhage in baby and mother
  Intervention - slip the cord around neck or double clamp and cut cord if unable to slip it

STAGES OF LABOR:

- **The three stages of labor are:**
  1st stage (dilation stage) - Starts with regular contractions and thinning and gradual dilation of the cervix
  Ends with complete dilation of the cervix

  2nd stage (expulsion stage) - Starts with baby entering the birth canal
  Ends with the deliver of the baby

  3rd stage (placental stage - Starts with the delivery of the baby
  Ends with the delivery of the placenta

- **Contractions follow the following pattern:**

  Latent (early) phase of 1st stage of labor
  + frequency – every 15-30 minutes
  + duration – 30-40 seconds
  + intensity – mild

  Active phase of 1st stage of labor
  + frequency – every 2-3 minutes
  + duration – average 60 seconds
  + intensity – moderate to strong

ABNORMAL DELIVERIES:

- **Prolapsed cord**
  Problem - cord presents through the birth canal before delivery of the head. This is a serious emergency which endangers the life of the unborn fetus.

  Intervention:
  - Administer high flow oxygen to the mother to increase oxygen delivery to fetus
  - Elevate mother's pelvis on a pillow or inverted bed pan to reduce pressure on cord
  - Elevate presenting part of the baby off the cord to prevent compression of the cord and maintain fetal circulation
  - Cover cord with sterile moist dressings to minimize temperature change and reduce umbilical artery spasm

ABNORMAL DELIVERIES (Continued):

- **Limb presentation**

  Problem - either an arm or leg appears first instead of the head.

  Intervention:
  - Administer oxygen to the mother to increase oxygen delivery to the fetus
  - Elevate mother's pelvis on a pillow or inverted bed pan to reduce pressure on the baby
  - Transport immediately - delivery is impossible

- **Breech presentation**

  Problem - baby's feet or buttocks appear first instead of the head. Every attempt should be made to transport to the hospital. *(It is not uncommon to have meconium in amniotic fluid with breech presentation.)*

  Intervention:
  - Administer oxygen to the mother to increase oxygen delivery to the fetus
  - Let delivery proceed
  - If the head does not deliver within 3 minutes
    - form an airway for the baby by placing the middle and index fingers along the infant's face
    - hold the vaginal wall away from the baby's nose and mouth
    - hold baby's mouth open slightly with finger so that baby can breathe
    - transport rapidly

- **Multiple births**

  Problem - generally both babies are delivered normally, however about 1/3 of the second babies are breech

  Intervention:
  - When the 1st baby is born, clamp the cord to prevent hemorrhage to the 2nd baby
  - If the 2nd baby has not delivered within 10 minutes of the 1st, transport immediately
  - Expect hemorrhage after the 2nd baby has delivered
  - Deliver the placenta or placentas or transport if not delivered when mother and babies are stabilized and ready for transport
  - Keep the babies warm, they are usually small and readily become hypothermic

- **Premature birth**

  Problem - baby is more susceptible to respiratory problems, infections and hypothermia

  Intervention:
  - Keep baby warm with extra insulation
  - Administer supplemental oxygen by blow by
  - Avoid contamination from birth process and DO NOT breath into baby's face

NOTES:
- When the amniotic fluid is stained greenish or brownish-yellow, it indicates that either maternal of fetal distress during labor. This is caused by the release of fetal feces released into the amniotic fluid.
- Aspiration of meconium stained amniotic fluid may cause pneumonia or other breathing problems.
- The mother and newborn should be transported to the same facility.
- BLS units shall call for an ALS unit or transport to the most appropriate hospital as per Reference 511 and 808
- APGAR score is not required in Los Angeles County and is not in the EMT-B DOT Curriculum, but is found in all ECB literature.
- APGAR score is assessed at 1 minute and 5 minutes and if the score is less than 7, it is repeated every 5 minutes for 20 minutes.

Evaluation Factor	Findings	Score
Appearance (color)	- cyanotic or pale - blue hands and feed with pink body - extremities and trunk pink	0 points 1 point 2points
Pulse	- no pulse - < 100/ minute - > 100/minute	0 points 1 point 2 points
Grimace (reflex irritability)	- no reflex to stimulation - slight reflex to stimulation - grimace, cough, sneeze, or cry in response to stimulation	0 points 1 point 2 points
Activity (extremity movement, degree of flexion and resistance to straightening them)	- limp, no extremity movement - some flexion with no movement - actively moving	0 points 1 point 2 points
Respirations	- no respiratory effort - slow, irregular effort with weak cry - good effort with strong cry	0 points 1 point 2 points
7-10 points = normal - provide routine care 4-6 points = moderately depress - provide stimulation and oxygen 0-3 points = severely depressed - provide CPR and BVM ventilations		

REFERENCES: Ref No. 511 - Perinatal Patient Destination   Ref No. 808 - Base Hospital Contact and Transport Criteria.

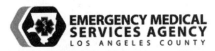

OBSTETRICAL EMERGENCY / EMERGENCY CHILDBIRTH
DELIVERY

PERFORMANCE OBJECTIVES
The examinee will demonstrate proficiency in assisting with a an imminent delivery and perform initial interventions as necessary.

CONDITION
The examinee will be requested to assess and assist in the delivery of a newborn and initiate appropriate interventions as needed using a simulated patient. The pregnancy is full term, the patient is having frequent contractions and the baby's head is crowning. Required equipment will be next to the patient or brought to the scene by the examinee.

EQUIPMENT
Obstetrical manikin with baby, placenta and umbilical cord, 1 assistant, obstetrical kit with cleansing towelettes and germicidal wipes, 4x4s, drapes, sheet, 8 towels, 2 cord clamps, 2 plastic ties, umbilical cord scissors, bulb syringe, obstetrical pad, plastic bag, sterile gloves, baby blanket, oxygen tank with flow meter, oxygen tubing, adult and neonatal oxygen mask, adult and neonatal bag-valve-mask device, nasal cannula, stethoscope, goggles, masks, gown, gloves.

PERFORMANCE CRITERIA
- 100% accuracy required on all items designated by a diamond (♦) for skills testing and must manage successfully all items indicated by double asterisks (**).
- Documentation, identified by the symbol (§), must be practiced, but is not a required test item.
- Appropriate body substance isolation precautions must be instituted.

PREPARATION	
Skill Component	**Key Concepts**
♦ Take body substance isolation precautions	• Mandatory personal protective equipment - gloves • Situational - goggles, masks, gown

♦ Assess mother's history:
 • Last menstrual period (LMP) and/or expected due date (EDD)
 	
 • Prenatal care
 	
 • Diabetes
 	
 • Drug use (street or prescribed)
 	
 • Problems with this pregnancy
 	
 • Vaginal discharge
  - bleeding
  - bloody discharge
  - rupture of amniotic membranes (color and odor)
 	
 • Number of pregnancies and births
 	
 • Type of previous deliveries - *if indicated*
  - vaginal
  - cesarean
	• The LMP (last menstrual period) or EDD (expected due date) is important to determine if baby is premature, term, post term. Determines special needs and problems that may be encountered.
	
	• Vaginal discharge:
	  - frank bleeding may indicate placenta previa.
	  - bloody discharge of mucus is normal in all 3 stages of labor.
	  - amniotic fluid that is greenish or brownish-yellow indicates maternal or fetal distress. Cloudy or foul smelling fluid indicates an infection.
	
	• Diabetes information is important to prepare for a large baby and excessive amniotic fluid (polyhydramnios).
	
	• Drug use information is important to prepare for a possible depressed baby.
	
	• Previous cesarean section may lead to possible uterine rupture during labor.

♦ Assess contractions: • Frequency • Duration • Intensity	• Frequency of contractions is from the onset of one contraction until the onset of the next contraction. • Duration of the contraction is from the onset of one contraction to its completion.
♦ Determine if delivery is imminent: • Crowning present • Contractions 2-3 minutes apart • Mother has urge to push	• Crowning is the most reliable sign of imminent delivery. • May or may not have the urge to push. The urge to push is due to the baby moving into the birth canal and pressing the vaginal wall against the rectum and stimulating the sacral nerves. This may be interpreted as having to have a bowel movement.

Skill Component	Key Concepts
◆ Determine: 　• Additional resources 　• Specialized equipment ** *Consider equipment needed for administration of oxygen to the mother and/or baby*	• Maintaining privacy for the mother is essential. Makeshift protective screens can be improvised with tarps, blankets, sheets, furniture, etc. • Have oxygen with appropriate size masks or cannulas available for mother and baby if needed. • Have emesis basin ready in case mother becomes nauseated and may possibly vomit.
◆ Put on protective equipment: 　• Gown with long sleeves 　• Face mask 　• Goggles 　• Gloves (non-sterile if not already applied)	• Sterile gloves, gown, face mask, goggles should be put on to protect the healthcare providers from splashing blood and bodily fluids during delivery. This protective equipment also protects the mother and baby from contamination.
◆ Position mother: 　• Place in a semi-Fowler's position 　• Elevate buttocks with pillow or blanket 2"- 4" 　• Remove clothing that obstructs perineum 　• Pull up knees and spread apart	• DO NOT touch vaginal area except when actually assisting with the delivery. Always have a team or family member in attendance when touching a woman's perineal area. • If delivering in a car, position mother on the seat with one foot resting on the seat and the other foot resting on the floor. • Mother should be several feet in from the edge to provide support for a slippery infant.
◆ Open Obstetrical kit	• Place on table or chair so that all items are in easy reach.
◆ Cleanse perineum with cleansing towelette and germicidal wipes	• Clean by wiping from the anterior to the posterior area to prevent contaminating the vaginal opening. *(One wipe per towelette.)*
◆ Put on sterile gloves	
◆ Drape mother and establish a sterile field around vaginal opening	• Draping: 　- 1 sheet under the mother's buttocks 　- 1 sheet over abdomen and upper legs 　- 1 towel over each thigh 　- 1 towel under buttocks which can be removed in case of fecal contamination (have additional towels readily available).

PROCEDURE

Skill Component	Key Concepts
◆ Support the baby's head and apply gentle pressure to perineum to prevent explosive delivery: 　• Keep one hand on baby's head 　• Apply pressure to perineum with sterile towel	• Spread fingers evenly around baby's head to prevent concentrated pressure on fontanelles. Be careful not to poke fingers into baby's eyes or fontanelles. • An explosive delivery will cause perineal tears and result in harm to the baby due to the sudden change in pressure to the baby's head.
◆ Rupture the amniotic membranes and pull membranes from baby's mouth and nose - *if not ruptured previously* ** *Note color and odor of amniotic fluid - if membranes were not ruptured previously*	• To rupture membranes, pinch membranes between fingers and twist until membranes tear. DO NOT use an instrument to rupture membranes since this may cause injury to baby's presenting part. • Amniotic fluid that is greenish or brownish-yellow indicates maternal or fetal distress. Cloudy or foul smelling fluid indicates an infection. • The baby is said to have been born with a veil or caul if membranes did not rupture spontaneously prior to this stage.
◆ Check for umbilical cord around neck as soon as head is delivered: ** *If no nuchal cord - continue with delivery* ** *If nuchal cord - loosen cord with 2 fingers and slip over baby's head and if necessary - clamp in 2 places 2"- 3" apart and cut the cord*	• Ask mother NOT to push at this point to prevent tightening of the cord around the baby's neck. • Place 2 fingers under the cord at the back of the baby's neck and gently bring forward over the head. • When the cord cannot be loosened, clamp the cord in 2 places about 2" apart and carefully cut between the clamps. Unwrap the cord from the neck and continue with the delivery.

Skill Component	Key Concepts
◆ Clear the baby's airway: • Suction mouth 2-3 times • Suction each nostril 1-2 times	• Make sure that the bulb syringe is compressed first before inserting in the mouth and nose. • Insert the syringe approximately 1-1½" into the mouth and not more than ½" into the nostrils. Slowly release the bulb to allow fluids to be drawn into the syringe and discharge the contents onto a towel. • Suction the mouth first to prevent the baby from aspirating any accumulated fluid from the mouth and pharynx. Aspiration of fluid, may cause pneumonia or other respiratory complications.
◆ Assist in releasing the shoulders: • Upper shoulder - guide head downward - *if indicated* • Lower shoulder - guide head upward - *if indicated*	• Support the head between both hands and make sure the baby is supported throughout the procedure.
◆ Assist in delivering the rest of the baby	• As the feet are delivered, grasp them to assure a good hold on the baby.

◆ Hold baby securely:
 	
• Place in Trendelenburg position
• Support the head at the level of the mother's perineum
	• This position allows for fluids and mucus to drain from the mouth and nose.
	
	• Keep the baby at the level of the perineum until the cord is cut to prevent critical exchange of blood flow:
	  - <u>above perineum</u> -- siphons the blood from the baby back into the placenta resulting in the baby becoming hypovolemic.
	  - <u>below the perineum</u> – provides too much blood to the baby and results in the baby becoming fluid overloaded.

◆ Wipe and suction the baby's mouth and nose again	• Suctioning should stimulate baby to breathe if no spontaneous respirations.
◆ Stimulate the baby to breathe - *if indicated* • Vigorously rub the back with a towel • Flick the soles of the feet ** ***Ventilate baby with bag-valve-mask - if no response after 5-10 seconds of stimulation***	• In a normal birth, the baby must be breathing on its own before clamps are applied and the cord is cut. Oxygen is still provided through the placenta until the baby takes its first breath.
◆ Double clamp umbilical cord - *if not clamped previously*; • 1st clamp - 6"- 8" from baby • 2nd clamp - 2"- 3" from the 1st clamp toward the mother (10"-12" from the baby)	• The cord need not finish pulsating before it is clamped and cut. Wrapping the infant before clamping and cutting the cord could result in prematurely dislodging the placenta or tearing the cord. • The baby may be placed on sterile surface near the level of the perineum, while clamping and cutting the cord. • Make sure clamps are secure and will not slip or the baby and/or mother may hemorrhage. • Use ties in case of an enlarged umbilical cord.
◆ Cut the umbilical cord between the clamps - *if not cut previously*;	• Use sterile umbilical cord scissors • Periodically check the ends of the cord for bleeding. Control bleeding by placing another clamp or tie proximal to the initial clamp.
◆ Dry and wrap the baby in a blanket or towel	• Newborns become hypothermic very rapidly. This can precipitate hypoglycemia, respiratory problems, increased oxygen demand and bradycardia. • Wrap the baby so only that the face is exposed. They lose most of their heat from the head area.
◆ Direct assistant to monitor and complete initial care of the baby	• If lone rescuer, place baby on its side with head slightly lower than the trunk or give the baby to the mother to hold, if she is able. • If the mother chooses to breast feed, DO NOT put baby to breast until placenta has been delivered. Suckling causes the uterus to contract which may hinder the delivery of the placenta.

Skill Component	Key Concepts
♦ Assess mother's vital signs and check for vaginal bleeding	
♦ Observe for signs of placental separation: • Lengthening of the umbilical cord • Contraction of the uterus (uterus raises into a globular shape) • Gush of blood from the vagina	
♦ Prepare for delivery of the placenta: • Have mother bear down • Have basin ready to receive placenta • Expect a gush of blood after placenta is delivered	• DO NOT pull on umbilical cord. This may result in hemorrhage, an inverted uterus, or retained membranes. • DO NOT delay transport if the placenta has not delivered (may take over 30 minutes). *Transport as soon as the mother and baby are stabilized.* • Up to 500cc of blood may be normally expelled (1-2 cups).
♦ Deliver the placenta: • Grasp the placenta when it appears at the vaginal opening • Rotate the placenta - DO NOT pull on cord • Guide the placenta and membranes from the vaginal opening into basin or towel ** ***Check for integrity of the placenta and cord***	• Retained pieces of the placenta or membranes will cause persistent bleeding and may require surgical intervention.
♦ Place the placenta into plastic bag and transport with the mother	• The placenta is about 7" in diameter and 1" thick. It has a smooth side and a rough side that is divided into lobes. EMTs should wrap the placenta in a towel and then place it in a plastic bag and transport to the hospital where it will be inspected to make sure that it is intact. Paramedics should inspect the placenta prior to being placed in plastic bag and inform hospital personnel if the placenta and cord do not appear to be intact.
♦ Check for perineal lacerations and apply pressure to control bleeding - *if indicted*	• If there is a perineal tear, inform mother that this is normal and will be taken care of by physician in the hospital
♦ Remove the soiled sheets and place in plastic bag	
♦ Place 2 obstetrical pads over the vaginal and perineal area: • Touch only the outer surface of the pads • Place pads from vagina down towards anus • Assist mother in putting thighs together to hold pads in place	• Placing the obstetrical pads from the vagina down toward the anus prevents contamination of perineal lacerations or the vaginal area.
♦ Assess the fundus every 5 minutes and massage - *if indicated* • Place one hand above pubic bone • Place other hand above contracted uterus • Massage (knead) over area using a circular motion until the uterus is firm	• Fundal massage is indicated if there is postpartum hemorrhage or the uterus has not contracted after the placenta has delivered. • Fundal massage: - place the medial aspect of the little finger and palm of the hand above the public bone and inferior part of the uterus - cup the other hand above the superior aspect of the uterus - use the flat of the 4 fingers of the cupped hand and massage the uterus in a circular motion until it the uterus is firm
♦ Provide comfort and support to the mother and transport	• The mother will chill easily after giving birth due to decreasing blood volume. Cover her with a blanket to keep her warm. • The mother and newborn should be transported to the same facility. • BLS units shall call for an ALS unit or transport to the most appropriate hospital as per Reference: - 511 - Perinatal Patient Destination - 808 - Base Hospital Contact and Transport Criteria.
♦ Dispose of contaminated equipment using approved technique	

Skill Component	Key Concepts
§ Repeat an ongoing assessment every **5 minutes**: • Initial assessment • Relevant portion of the focused assessment • Evaluate response to treatment • Compare results to baseline condition and vital signs	• Every patient must be re-evaluated at least every 5 minutes, if any treatment was initiated or medication administered or changes in the patient's condition are anticipated sooner. • Priority patients are patients who have abnormal vital signs, signs/ symptoms of poor perfusion or if there is a suspicion that the patient's condition may deteriorate. • The initial and focused examination is repeated every 15 minutes for stable patients and every 5 minutes for priority patients. This is considered a priority patient.

DOCUMENTATION

Skill Component	Key Concepts
§ Verbalize/Document: • Time of delivery of baby and placenta • LMP and/or EDD • Problems with this pregnancy • Vaginal discharge • Number of pregnancies and births • Type of previous deliveries - *if indicated* • Estimated blood loss • Integrity of the placenta and cord • Condition of the baby • Fundal massage - *if provided*	• Documentation must be on either the Los Angeles County EMS Report or departmental Patient Care Record form. • Two EMS forms are necessary, one for the mother and one for the baby (2 patients). • Time of delivery for the baby is the time when the baby's body is delivered. • Time of delivery for the placenta is when it passes out of the vagina **** The birth certificate should be signed by the "person who attended" the birth. Often the ER physician will sign the birth certificate, however, prehospital personnel may be asked to sign instead or in conjunction with the physician. This may be days or even weeks later and thus accurate information must be documented.

Developed: 12/01   Revised: 9/04

OBSTETRICAL EMERGENCY / EMERGENCY CHILDBIRTH
NEWBORN ASSESSMENT & MANAGEMENT

DEFINITIONS:
- _Baby_ - name used to indicate newborn
- _Newborn_ - neonate in the first minutes to hours after birth
- _Neonate_ - infants in first month after birth (28 days)
- _Infant_ - includes the neonate period to 1 year (12 months)
- _Central cyanosis_ - bluish color on trunk and face
- _Peripheral cyanosis_ - bluish color limited to hands and feet
- _Meconium_ - fetal feces that is normally passed as the baby's first bowel movement. However, during fetal or maternal stress, defecation may occur before birth
- _Oxygen administration_ - administration of free-flow oxygen directly to baby's face by either mask or blow-by method:
  - mask - at least 5 Liters/minute, held loosely over baby's face
  - blow-by with oxygen tubing - at least 5 Liters/minute, held near the nostrils

INDICATIONS FOR BAG-VALVE-MASK VENTILATIONS:
- Apnea, gasping, or inadequate respirations
- Heart rate less than 100 beats/minute
- Persistent central cyanosis unresponsive to administration of oxygen

INDICATIONS FOR CARDIOPULMONARY RESUSCITATION:
- Pulseless
- Heart rate less than 60 beats/minute

NOTES:
- Newborns must make three rapid transitions to the out side world from their protected environment in utero:
  - Changing their circulatory pattern
  - Emptying fluid from their lungs and beginning ventilation
  - Maintaining body temperature
- Four main objectives in caring for the newborn:
  - Provide and maintain warmth. Important to dry and wrap baby with only face exposed, they lose most of their heat from the head area.
  - Continually assess respirations, heart rate and color.
  - Maintain adequate respirations by positioning, suctioning, administration of oxygen, and ventilate with a BVM if indicated
  - Provide cardiac compressions for heart rate < 60
- The mother and newborn should be transported to the same facility.
- BLS units shall call for an ALS unit or transport to the most appropriate hospital as per Reference No. 511 and 808
- Signs of poor perfusion are: weak cry, bradycardia (heart rate < 100 beats/minute), inadequate respirations (< 40 breaths/minute), and cyanosis.
- Hyperextension or flexion of neck may cause an airway obstruction. To maintain in position, place a folded blanket or towel under the neck and shoulders.
- If copious secretions are present, position the baby on the side and slightly extend the neck. This allows the secretions to collect in the mouth and not in the posterior pharynx.
- When ventilating with a BVM, use _only_ enough force to allow for good chest rise. Over-inflation causes gastric distention which will affect tidal volume by elevating the diaphragm
- If ventilating with a bag-valve-mask device, heart rate must be re-assessed every 30 seconds.
- Check pulse by one of the following:
  - auscultate apical pulse
  - palpate pulse at base of umbilical cord
  - palpate brachial or femoral pulse
- Normal newborn heart rate is 120-160 beats/minute.
- Compression to ventilation ratio is 3 compressions to 1 ventilation.
- APGAR score is not required in Los Angeles County and is not in the EMT-I DOT Curriculum, but is found in all ECB literature.
- APGAR score is assessed at 1 minute and 5 minutes and if the score is less than 7, it is repeated every 5 minutes for 20 minutes.

OBSTETRICAL EMERGENCY / EMERGENCY CHILDBIRTH
NEWBORN ASSESSMENT & MANAGEMENT

APGAR SCORE

Evaluation Factor	Findings	Score
Appearance (color)	- cyanotic or pale - blue hands and feed with pink body - extremities and trunk pink	0 points 1 point 2points
Pulse	- no pulse - < 100/ minute - > 100/minute	0 points 1 point 2 points
Grimace (reflex irritability)	- no reflex to stimulation - slight reflex to stimulation - grimace, cough, sneeze, or cry in response to stimulation	0 points 1 point 2 points
Activity (extremity movement, degree of flexion and resistance to straightening them)	- limp, no extremity movement - some flexion with no movement - actively moving	0 points 1 point 2 points
Respirations	- no respiratory effort - slow, irregular effort with weak cry - good effort with strong cry	0 points 1 point 2 points

7-10 points = normal - provide routine care   4-6 points = moderately depress - provide stimulation and oxygen   0-3 points = severely depressed - provide CPR and BVM ventilations

- The <u>inverted pyramid</u> - reflects the frequencies for neonatal resuscitation without meconium stained amniotic fluid

INVERTED PYRAMID STEPS

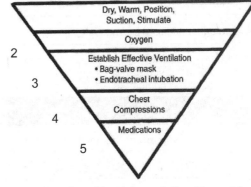

American Heart Association Pyramid

Step 1 - always needed

Step 2 - frequently needed

Step 3 - infrequently needed

Step 4 - infrequently needed

Step 5 - rarely needed

- **Always assess and manage:**
  ~ Temperature (warm & dry)
  ~ Airway (position & suction) ~ Breathing (stimulate to cry)
  ~ Circulation (heart rate & color)

Developed 12/01
Revised 7/04, 5/06

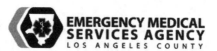

OBSTETRICAL EMERGENCY / EMERGENCY CHILDBIRTH
NEWBORN ASSESSMENT & MANAGEMENT

PERFORMANCE OBJECTIVES
The examinee will demonstrate proficiency in assessing the newborn and performing initial care and interventions as necessary.

CONDITION
The examinee will be requested to assess and perform the initial care of the newborn and intervene as necessary using a simulated patient. The newborn is full term with no major complications during pregnancy. The newborn was suctioned during the birth process, the cord clamped and cut and the baby is wrapped in a blanket. Required equipment will be in the room readily accessible.

EQUIPMENT
Baby manikin with umbilical cord clamped, bulb syringe, baby blankets, oxygen tank with flow meter, oxygen tubing, neonatal oxygen mask, neonatal bag-valve-mask device, stethoscope, goggles, masks, gown, gloves.

PERFORMANCE CRITERIA
- 100% accuracy required on all items designated by a diamond (♦) for skills testing and must manage successfully all items indicated by double asterisks (**).
- Documentation, identified by the symbol (§), must be practiced, but is not a required test item.
- Appropriate body substance isolation precautions must be instituted.
- Ventilations and compressions must be at least at the minimum rate required.

PREPARATION	
Skill Component	**Key Concepts**
♦ Take body substance isolation precautions	• Mandatory personal protective equipment – gloves
♦ Evaluate additional BSI needs	• Situational - goggles, masks, gown
♦ Determine: • Additional resources • Specialized equipment	

PROCEDURE	
Assessment of the newborn is performed after the baby is dried, wrapped, airway cleared, and stimulated	
Skill Component	**Key Concepts**
♦ Assess and support body temperature: • Dry newborn completely - *if not done previously* • Keep wrapped with head covered	• Newborns become hypothermic very easy which can precipitate hypoglycemia, respiratory problems, increased oxygen demand and bradycardia. • Wrap the baby so only the face is exposed, they lose most of their heat from the head area.
♦ Assess and support the airway: • Position on back or side with neck in a neutral position • Suction with bulb syringe - *if needed*	• Hyperextension or flexion of neck may cause an airway obstruction. To maintain in position, place a rolled blanket or towel under the neck and shoulders. • If copious secretions, place baby on the side with the neck slightly extended. This allows the secretions to collect in the mouth and not in the posterior pharynx. • When suctioning with a bulb syringe: - make sure that the bulb syringe is compressed first before placing in the mouth and nose - place the syringe approx. 1"-1 1/2" into the mouth and no more than 1/2" into nostrils, slowly release the bulb drawing fluid into the syringe and discharge contents onto a towel. • Prolonged or deep suctioning of the newborn's oropharynx may cause bradycardia and/or apnea. Never suction longer than 3-5 seconds per attempt.

Skill Component	Key Concepts

◆ Assess breathing:
 	
  • <u>If adequate</u> - continue with assessment
 	
  • <u>If respirations shallow or slow</u> - administer oxygen and stimulate by:
    - vigorously rubbing back with a towel slapping or flicking the soles of the feet
 	
  • <u>If gasping or respirations are inadequate</u> - ventilate with bag-valve-mask at 40-60 breaths per minute
	• Ventilate baby with bag-valve-mask if no response to administration of 100% oxygen and stimulation of 5-10 seconds.
	
	• Oxygen should be administered by:
	  - using a face mask with at least 5 Liters/minute, held loosely over the baby's face
	  - blow-by with oxygen tubing at least 5 Liters/minute, held near the baby's nostrils
	
	• For effective bag-valve-mask ventilations, the mask must be the appropriate size and have a tight seal.
	
	• Use <u>only</u> enough force to allow for good chest rise. Over-inflation causes gastric distention, which will affect tidal volume by elevating the diaphragm.

◆ Assess circulation:
 	
  • **Heart rate**
    If > than 120 beats/minute - continue assessment
    If 100-120 beats/minute -administer oxygen
    If < than 100 beats/minute - ventilate with bag-valve-mask device attached to 100% oxygen
    If < 60 beats/minute - start CPR @ rate of 120 compressions/minute
 	
  • **Color**
    If pink or peripheral cyanosis of hands and feet - no treatment indicated
    If central cyanosis and good respirations and heart rate > 100 beats/minute - administer oxygen
    If generalized pallor or cyanosis and no response to oxygen administration - ventilate with bag-valve-mask device attached to 100% oxygen
	• The heart rate is a reliable indicator of the newborn's distress level.
	
	• Check pulse by one of the following:
	  - palpate pulse at base of umbilical cord
	  - palpate brachial or femoral pulse
	  - auscultate apical pulse
	
	• Normal newborn heart rate is 120-160 beats/minute.
	
	• If ventilating with a bag-valve-mask device, or performing chest compressions the heart rate must be re-assessed every 30 seconds.
	
	• Compression to ventilation ratio is 3 compressions to 1 ventilation.
	
	• Color is the least important indicator of adequate circulation. The newborn must also be assessed for activity, grimace cry, heart rate and respirations.
	
	• DO NOT attempt to obtain an APGAR score if the newborn requires resuscitation measures.
	
	• APGAR score is determined at 1 minute and 5 minutes after birth. If the score is less than 7, it is repeated every 5 minutes for 20 minutes.
	
	• Los Angeles County does not required an APGAR score, nor is the APGAR score part of the National DOT Curriculum. However, EMT and Paramedic textbooks provide this information and many EMS systems use this score as part of the newborn assessment.

◆ Assess umbilical cord for:
 	
  • Bleeding - *apply sterile dressing and direct pressure if indicated*
 	
  • Security of clamps or ties - *use additional clamps or ties as indicated*
	• Make sure clamps are secure and will not slip or the baby may hemorrhage.
	
	• Use ties in case of an enlarged umbilical cord.
	
	• The mother and newborn should be transported to the same facility.
	
	• BLS units shall call for an ALS unit or transport to the most appropriate hospital as per Reference:
	  - 511 - Perinatal Patient Destination
	  - 808 - Base Hospital Contact and Transport Criteria.

ONGOING ASSESSMENT

Skill Component	Key Concepts

§ Repeat an ongoing assessment every **5 minutes**:
 	
  • Initial assessment
  • Relevant portion of the focused assessment
  • Evaluate response to treatment
  • Compare results to baseline condition and vital signs
	• The initial and focused examination is repeated every 15 minutes for stable patients and every 5 minutes for priority patients.
	
	• Every patient must be re-evaluated at least every 5 minutes, if any treatment was initiated or medication administered, unless changes in the patient's condition are anticipated sooner.
	
	• Priority patients are patients who have abnormal vital signs, signs/symptoms of poor perfusion or if there is a suspicion that the patient's condition may deteriorate.

DOCUMENTATION	
Skill Component	**Key Concepts**

§ Verbalize/Document:
  • Time of delivery of baby
  • Problems with this pregnancy
  • Presence of meconium
  • Integrity of the cord
  • Condition of the baby
	• Documentation must be on either the Los Angeles County EMS Report or departmental Patient Care Record form.
	• Time of delivery for the baby is the time when the baby's body is delivered.

Developed 12/01   Revised 7/04

Patient Lifting and Moving
Emergency, Urgent and Non-Urgent Moves

INDICATIONS:

- Emergency Move – immediate danger to the patient or to the rescuer
- Urgent Move – immediate threat to life and the patient must be moved quickly and transported for care.
- Non-Urgent Move – no immediate threat to life exists and the patient can be moved in a normal manner when ready for transport

COMPLICATIONS:

- Caution should be used to protect the rescuers from back injury. Proper use of body mechanics is essential.
- Consider need for neck and back immobilization when performing a patient lift or move.

PATIENT CARRYING DEVICES:

- Basket (Stokes) stretcher
- Flexible stretcher
- Long spine board (backboard)
- Portable (cot/flat) stretcher
- Scoop (orthopedic) stretcher
- Short spine board
- Stair Chair
- Vest-type extrication device (KED)
- Wheeled ambulance stretcher (gurney)

Developed 7/07

Patient Lifting and Moving
Emergency Moves

PERFORMANCE OBJECTIVES

The examinee will demonstrate proficiency in moving a patient that is in immediate danger due to the environment or there is an inability to provide life-saving care due to the patient's position.

CONDITION

The examinee will be requested to demonstrate an emergency move on an adult patient.

EQUIPMENT

Simulated adult patient, blanket, gloves.

PERFORMANCE CRITERIA

- 100% accuracy required on all items designated by a diamond (♦) for skills testing and must manage successfully all items indicated by double asterisks (**).
- Documentation, identified by the symbol (§), must be practiced, but is not a required test item.
- Appropriate body substance isolation precautions must be instituted.

EMERGENCY MOVES PREPARATION	
Skill Component	**Teaching Points**
♦ Take body substance isolation precautions	• Mandatory personal protective equipment - gloves • Situational - long sleeves, goggles, masks, gown
♦ Explain Procedure to patient	• Maintain patient rapport

PROCEDURE	
Skill Component	**Teaching Points**
♦ Armpit – Forearm Drag • Grasp the patient's left forearm with your right hand, the right forearm with your left hand, and drag	• Good move for patients on the ground or floor • Pull the patient in the direction of the long axis of the body
♦ Shirt Drag • Fasten the patient's hands or writs loosely together • Grasp the neck and shoulders of the shirt so that the patient's head rests on your fists • Using the shirt as a handle, pull the patient towards you	• Regular T-Shirt will not work for this move • If possible, link the patient's hands to belt or pants with a small velcro strap or bandage • Be careful not to strangle the patient, the pulling should engage the armpits, not the neck. Reposition your hands if you notice excessive pressure or strain from the shirt on the patient's neck
♦ Blanket Drag • Spread a blanket alongside the patient, gathering about half into lengthwise pleats • Roll the patient away from you onto their side, tucking the pleated part as far beneath the patient as possible • Roll the patient back onto the center of the blanket on onto his back • Wrap the blanket securely around the patient • Grab the part of the blanket that is beneath the patient's head and drag the patient toward you.	• Effective way for a single rescuer to move a patient to safety. • If not blanket is available, use a coat or sheet.

	gluteal muscles.
arms and grasps the patient's wrists being held by the second rescuer. • The second rescuer slips his hands under the patient's knees. • Both rescuers move up to a crouching position • On signal from the first rescuer, both rescuers stand up simultaneously and move with the patient to a stretcher or other patient-carrying device.	

◆ Direct Carry Method
  • Position the gurney perpendicular to the bed, with the head of the device at the foot of the bed
  • Prepare the gurney by unbuckling straps and removing other items.
  • Both rescuers should stand between the bed and gurney, facing the patient.
  • The first rescuer then slides an arm under the patient's neck and cups the patient's shoulder.
  • After the second rescuer slides a hand under the patient's hip and lifts slightly, the first rescuer slides an arm under the patient's back.
  • The second rescuer places his arms under the patient's hips and calves.
  • Slide the patient to the edge of the bed, lift and curl the patient to their chests, and then rotate and place the patient gently onto the gurney.
	• A technique to transfer a supine patient from a bed to a gurney or from any patient carrying device to another.

◆ Draw Sheet Method
  • Loosen the bottom sheet of the bed
  • Position the gurney next to the bed.
  • Prepare the gurney by adjusting the height, lowering rails and unbuckling straps.
  • Reach across the stretcher and grasp the sheet firmly at the patient's head, chest, hips and knees.
  • Slide the patient gently onto the gurney.
	• A technique to transfer a supine patient from a bed to a gurney or from any patient carrying device to another.
	• Use your hip to support yourself against the stretcher, keeping your back straight.
	• Contract your abdominal and gluteal muscles to splint your lower back as you slide the patient to the gurney.

DOCUMENTATION	
Skill Component	**Teaching Points**

§ Verbalize/Document:
  • Type of move utilized to transfer patient
  • Patient's position / location prior to moving	

Developed 7/07

Patient Lifting and Moving
Non-Urgent Moves

PERFORMANCE OBJECTIVES
The examinee will demonstrate proficiency in moving a patient when there is no immediate threat to life.

CONDITION
The examinee will be requested to demonstrate a non-urgent move on an adult patient.
EQUIPMENT
Simulated adult patient, second rescuer, blanket, gurney, gloves.

PERFORMANCE CRITERIA
- 100% accuracy required on all items designated by a diamond (♦) for skills testing and must manage successfully all items indicated by double asterisks (**).
- Documentation, identified by the symbol (§), must be practiced, but is not a required test item.
- Appropriate body substance isolation precautions must be instituted.

EMERGENCY MOVES PREPARATION	
Skill Component	**Teaching Points**
♦ Take body substance isolation precautions	• Mandatory personal protective equipment - gloves • Situational - long sleeves, goggles, masks, gown
♦ Explain Procedure to patient	• Maintain patient rapport

PROCEDURE	
Skill Component	**Teaching Points**
♦ Direct Ground Lift • Two or three rescuers should line up on the same side of the patient. • Each rescuer should kneel on one knee, preferably the same knee for all rescuers. • The second rescuer should place the patient's arms on the patient's chest. • The first rescuer cradles the patient's head by placing one arm under the patient's neck and shoulder. The other arm should be placed under the patient's lower back. • The second rescuer should place one arm under the patient's knees and one arm above the buttocks. • On signal from the first rescuer, the patients should be lifted and placed on the rescuers knees, rolling the patient toward the rescuer's chest. • On signal from the first rescuer, stand and move the patient to the stretcher or other patient-carrying device. • To lower patient, roll the patient away from the rescuer's chest and onto the patient-carrying device.	• Not recommended for extremely heavy patients. • When lifting a patient from the ground, it is usually safer and mechanically more efficient to use a long backboard or a scoop stretcher. • If a third rescuer is available, he should place both arms under the waist. The other two rescuers then should slide their arms either up to the midback or down to the buttocks as appropriate. • Bend at the hips and not the waist, keeping your back straight and lifting with your legs and buttocks.
♦ Extremity Lift • The first rescuer should kneel at the patient's head; the second should kneel at the patient's knees. • The first rescuer should place one hand under each of the patient's shoulders, while the second rescuer grasps the patient's wrists. • The first rescuer slips his hands under the patient's	• Use this lift to move a patient from the ground or a chair to a patient-carrying device. • While lifting the patient, each rescuer must maintain a straight back and contract the abdominal muscles. • The rescuer's head must remain in line with the back. • When lifting the patient, the rescuer should drive upward with leg and

arms and grasps the patient's wrists being held by the second rescuer.	gluteal muscles.
• The second rescuer slips his hands under the patient's knees.	
• Both rescuers move up to a crouching position	
• On signal from the first rescuer, both rescuers stand up simultaneously and move with the patient to a stretcher or other patient-carrying device.	
◆ Direct Carry Method	• A technique to transfer a supine patient from a bed to a gurney or from any patient carrying device to another.
• Position the gurney perpendicular to the bed, with the head of the device at the foot of the bed	
• Prepare the gurney by unbuckling straps and removing other items.	
• Both rescuers should stand between the bed and gurney, facing the patient.	
• The first rescuer then slides an arm under the patient's neck and cups the patient's shoulder.	
• After the second rescuer slides a hand under the patient's hip and lifts slightly, the first rescuer slides an arm under the patient's back.	
• The second rescuer places his arms under the patient's hips and calves.	
• Slide the patient to the edge of the bed, lift and curl the patient to their chests, and then rotate and place the patient gently onto the gurney.	
◆ Draw Sheet Method	• A technique to transfer a supine patient from a bed to a gurney or from any patient carrying device to another.
• Loosen the bottom sheet of the bed	• Use your hip to support yourself against the stretcher, keeping your back straight.
• Position the gurney next to the bed.	
• Prepare the gurney by adjusting the height, lowering rails and unbuckling straps.	• Contract your abdominal and gluteal muscles to splint your lower back as you slide the patient to the gurney.
• Reach across the stretcher and grasp the sheet firmly at the patient's head, chest, hips and knees.	
• Slide the patient gently onto the gurney.	

DOCUMENTATION	
Skill Component	**Teaching Points**
§ Verbalize/Document: • Type of move utilized to transfer patient • Patient's position / location prior to moving	

Developed 7/07

Patient Lifting and Moving
Urgent Moves – Rapid Extrication

PERFORMANCE OBJECTIVES

The examinee will demonstrate proficiency in moving a patient that has been in an automobile collision and must be moved quickly. The patient's condition is such that utilizing the short board or KED would take too much time.

CONDITION

The examinee will be requested to perform and direct team members during a rapid extrication on an adult patient involved in an automobile accident. The patient will have a cervical collar applied, will be rapidly extricated and secured to a long spine board. The patient was found sitting in the front driver's seat of an automobile. The patient has an altered mental status and has critical injuries. Necessary equipment will be adjacent to the manikin.

EQUIPMENT

Live model or manikin, various sizes of rigid collars, long spine board, straps or binders, head-neck immobilizer, padding material, 2-3" cloth tape, 2-3 assistants, goggles, masks, gown, gloves.

PERFORMANCE CRITERIA

- 100% accuracy required on all items designated by a diamond (♦) for skills testing and must manage successfully all items indicated by double asterisks (**).
- Documentation, identified by the symbol (§), must be practiced, but is not a required test item.
- Appropriate body substance isolation precautions must be instituted.

URGENT MOVES – RAPID EXTRICATION PREPARATION	
Skill Component	**Teaching Points**
♦ Take body substance isolation precautions	• Mandatory personal protective equipment - gloves • Situational - long sleeves, goggles, masks, gown
♦ Explain Procedure to patient	• Maintain patient rapport
PROCEDURE	
Skill Component	**Teaching Points**
♦ Bring the patient's head into neutral in-line position	• Best achieved from behind or to the side of the patient
♦ Perform an initial assessment and rapid trauma assessment	
♦ Apply the appropriate size cervical collar	

♦ Bring the patient out of the vehicle with maintaining in-line stabilization
  • Support the patient's thorax
  • Rotate the patient until their back is facing the open car door
  • Bring the patient's legs and feet up onto the car seat
  • Bring the board in line with the patient and under the buttocks.
  • Stabilize the gurney under the board.
  • Lower the patient onto the board
	• Alternative methods should be considered and may need to be utilized when bringing the patient out of the vehicle and attempting to maintain in-line stabilization.
	
	• A pre rolled blanket may be utilized to assist rescuers in extricating the patient from the vehicle.

♦ Continue full body immobilization and rapid transportation	

DOCUMENTATION	
Skill Component	**Teaching Points**
§ Verbalize/Document: • Reason for utilizing urgent move • Patient's position / location prior to moving	

Developed 7/07

PATIENT ASSESSMENT
PEDIATRIC EMERGENCY TAPE - BROSELOW

PURPOSE:

- To estimate weight, drug dosages and correct size of equipment for pediatric patients up to 36kg (79lbs).

INDICATION:

- <u>All</u> infants and children smaller or equal to length of tape.

NOTES:

- The starting or ending point of the foot is the heel and not the extended foot or toes.

- If the child is longer than the tape, stop and estimate weight by using other techniques, i.e.
  Child's weight = 2kg x age in years + 10kg

- Only pediatric resuscitation drugs for shock, hypoglycemia or cardiac arrest are listed on the tape. Other emergency pediatric drugs are not listed. Use the "Los Angeles County Kids" color code chart for all emergency drug dosages.

- Color code for the "newborn and small infant" is grey. Newer tapes have now colored this section, older tapes may have left this section blank. This strip is to be coded as the color *GREY* on the EMS form.
  If this section is not marked Grey - WRITE "GREY" IN THE APPROPRIATE SECTION ON THE TAPE.

PREHOSPITAL DRUGS ON TAPE	PREHOSPITAL DRUGS <u>NOT</u> ON TAPE
Atropine Calcium Chloride $D_{25}W$ Diazepam Dopamine Infusion Epinephrine Lidocaine Naloxone Sodium Bicarbonate	Albuterol Adenosine Dextrose (Oral) Diphenhydramine Epinephrine for Anaphylaxis and Asthma Glucagon Morphine

Upright   Supine

Los Angeles Color Code for Kids

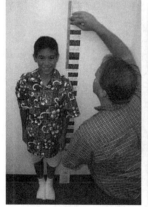

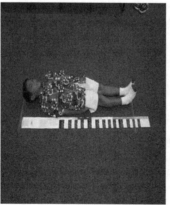

Developed 11/99
Revised1/03, 5/06

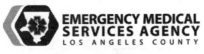

EMERGENCY MEDICAL SERVICES AGENCY
LOS ANGELES COUNTY

EMS SKILL

PATIENT ASSESSMENT
PEDIATRIC EMERGENCY TAPE - BROSELOW

PERFORMANCE OBJECTIVES
The examinee will demonstrate proficiency in the use of a Pediatric Emergency Tape (within their scope of practice) to determine color code, weight, drug dosages, and size of equipment for a simulated pediatric patient.

CONDITION
The examinee will be asked to determine the weight, drug dosage, and/or correct size of equipment for a pediatric patient who is either in an upright or supine position using the Pediatric Emergency Tape. Necessary equipment will be adjacent to the patient.

EQUIPMENT
Simulated pediatric patient or infant/child manikin, Pediatric Emergency Tape, goggles, masks, gown, gloves.

PERFORMANCE CRITERIA
- Items designated by a diamond (♦) must be performed successfully to demonstrate skill competency.
- Items identified by double asterisks (**) indicate actions that are required if indicated.
- Items identified by (§) are not skill component items, but should be practiced.

PREPARATION	
Skill Component	**Key Concepts**
♦ Take body substance isolation precautions	• Mandatory (minimal) personal protective equipment – gloves
♦ Place patient in position for optimal evaluation of body length or height: • Supine • Upright	• Optimal position depends on the infant/child's condition and temperament. • Some children become extremely agitated if placed on their back, but are cooperative if allowed to stand.
♦ Remove tape from package	
♦ Locate red end of tape labeled "Measure From This End"	

PROCEDURE	
Skill Component	**Key Concepts**
♦ Partially unfold tape with the multi-colored strips and kg markings visible	• Tape should be facing up and forward (Kg side up)
♦ Place red end of tape even with the most stable end of patient's body: • Supine - at top of head • Upright - at the heel of the foot	
♦ Hold red end of tape even with the starting point, unfurl tape and stop at the: • Heel - if supine • Head - if Upright	• Extend the tape the full length of the child and ensure that there are no bends or wrinkles in the tape. • Ensure that the child's legs are fully extended. • If the child is longer than the tape, stop and use appropriate technique for obtaining weight and size of equipment. • Place infant supine and extend a leg to measure from the top of the head to the bottom of the heel.

Skill Component	Key Concepts
◆ Note the colored strip and the colored zone that is even with the top of the head or at the bottom of the heel.	• Multi-colored strips identify equipment size and the color code required for documentation.

◆ Read:
  • Color zone on the side of the tape
  • Kg weight
	• Color code for the "newborn or small infant" is grey. Newer tapes have now colored this section, older tapes may have left this section blank. This strip is to be coded as the color _GREY_ on the EMS form.

◆ Use weight range to calculate correct drug dosages - _if applicable and within scope of practice._	• Not all drugs or dosages used in prehospital care are noted on the tape. • NEVER use the color chart independent of the emergency tape. Must actually measure the infant or child to obtain the correct color zone and weight from the emergency tape. • The "Los Angeles Kids Color Chart" should be used for all drug dosages. This is the Los Angeles County prehospital standard.
◆ Use the colored zone to identify the correct size of equipment - _if applicable._	• Colored zones identify airway, vascular access, and B/P cuff sizes applicable to prehospital care.

REASSESSMENT
(Ongoing Assessment)

Skill Component	Key Concepts
§ Keep tape available for equipment or drug information - _if indicated_	• Broselow provides information such as the size of possible airway adjuncts needed.

PATIENT REPORT AND DOCUMENTATION

Skill Component	Key Concepts

§ Verbalize/Document:
  • Color zone
  • Kg in color zone
  • Weight given by caregiver
	• Weight documented on EMS report form must come from the tape.
	• Weight given by caregiver should be documented in the comment section. The two weights obtained may differ since the tape weight is based on lean body weight.
	• Documentation must be on either the Los Angeles County EMS Report form or departmental Patient Care Record form.

Developed 11/99   Revised 7/01, 9/02, 1/03, 2010

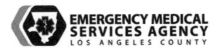

PATIENT ASSESSMENT & MANAGEMENT
Supplemental Information

NOTES:

- The preliminary chief complaint is the reason for summoning EMS to the scene.

- The field impression is determined by EMS personnel utilizing information gathered early in the assessment.

- The final step in securing a patient on a long backboard is to pad (shim) all the areas that are hollow after the straps have been secured to maintain a neutral position and restrict movement on a long spine board:

- Repeat the primary and secondary examination at least <u>every 5 minutes</u> for priority patients and <u>every 15 minutes</u> for stable patients.

- Priority patients are patients who have abnormal vital signs, S/S of poor perfusion, there is a suspicion that the patient's condition may deteriorate, treatment was rendered or when the patient's condition changes.

- Trauma patients with chest injuries and having difficulty breathing or signs of shock should be assessed for bilateral breath sounds during the primary assessment to determine possible tension pneumothorax.

- A patient with a respiratory rate is outside of the normal range and has inadequate tidal volume accompanied by altered level of consciousness and abnormal skin signs needs positive pressure ventilation.

- Capillary refill can be taken at any skin area such as: fingernail bed, palm of the hand, chest, forehead, etc. If using the ball of the foot in pediatric patients, the child must be in a supine position. The most accurate site is a central site, such as the chest wall rather than a peripheral site.

- A patient deemed competent is a person who is alert, oriented, has the ability to understand the circumstances surround their illness or impairment, and the possible risks associated with refusing treatment and/or transport.

- Mental illness, drugs, alcohol intoxication, or physical/mental impairment may affect a patient's competency. A patient, who has attempted or verbalized suicide or is suspected of suicidal intent, should be regarded as being incompetent to make decisions for refusal of treatment and transport.

- Medical and trauma conditions can be evaluated by using the mnemonic OPQRST:
  Onset – activity at time the problem/pain started and did emotional or environmental factors contribute to problem
  Provokes – what makes it worse, **P**alliative – what makes it better, **P**osition – what position is patient found
  Quality – type of discomfort (burning stabbing crushing) and constant or intermittent
  Region – area involved, **R**adiation – does the pain/discomfort spread from origin, **R**ecurrence – has this occurred before
  Severity – pain scale
  Time – when did the problem/pain begin and what is the duration of time

- GCS Eye Opening (awake or unresponsive), verbal response, motor response (Normal 4-5-6)

Los Angeles County Eye Opening (awake or unresponsive), motor response, verbal response (Normal 4-6-5)

Eye Opening	Verbal Response	Motor Response
Stimuli needed for patient to open eyes	Best communication when questioned	Best response to command or stimulus
4 = spontaneous 3 = responds to voice 2 = responds only to painful stimuli 1 = no response	5 = oriented , converses normally 4 = confused, disoriented 3 = inappropriate words or phrases 2 = incomprehensible sounds 1 = makes no sound	6 = obeys commands 5 = localizes stimulus (purposeful) 4 = flexion, withdraws from stimulus 3 = abnormal flexion (spastic) (*decorticate posturing*) 2 = extension (rigid) (*decerebrate posturing*) 1 = makes no movement

PERTINENT CHIEF COMPLAINT QUESTIONS

ABDOMINAL DISCOMFORT / NAUSEA / VOMITING / DIARRHEA

- Causative event and if acute or chronic
- Time of onset
- Duration of event
- Type of expelled GI contents (coffee ground emesis, hemoptysis, bile, melena [black tarry] or hematochezia [bright red bloody] stool, etc.)
- Amount and frequency of expelled GI contents
- Skin temperature/fever
- Pain/discomfort
- Skin color
- Signs of dehydration (skin turgor/tenting, absence of tearing, decreased urinary output, and quality of pulse)

PATIENT ASSESSMENT & MANAGEMENT

Supplemental Information (Continued)

ALLERGIC REACTION / ANAPHYLAXIS / ENVIRONMENTAL EMERGENCY
- Causative event (allergy, heat, cold, water or altitude)
- Type of substance
- Exposure (ingestion, inhalation, absorption, envenomization, injection)
- Duration of exposure
- General vs. local effect (rash, hives, itching, respiratory problems, nausea, vomiting, etc)
- Progression of symptoms
- Treatment initiated prior to EMS
- Response to treatment prior to EMS

ALTERED LEVEL OF CONSCIOUSNESS / SEIZURE / WEAKNESS / DIZZINESS / SYNCOPE
- Causative event and if acute or chronic
- Time of onset
- Duration of event
- Orientation level (name, place, and time)
- Associated symptoms (neuro deficits, pupil response)
- Position found in
- Length of time unconscious
- Incontinence
- Dysrhythmia
- Possible causes: (not all inclusive)
    - **A** alcohol, anoxia, allergic reaction, arrhythmia (dysrhythmia)
    - **E** epilepsy, electrolyte imbalance
    - **I** insulin (hyper-hypo glycemia)
    - **O** overdose
    - **U** uremia, under-dose
    - **T** trauma
    - **I** infection
    - **P** psychiatric, post-ictal, poisoning (ingestion, inhalation), palpitation (dysrhythmias)
    - **S** stroke

BEHAVIORAL EMERGENCY
- Causative event (medical, psychiatric, traumatic event)
- Compliance with medications
- Type of behavior (danger to self or others)

FEVER
- History of fever (highest temperature and latest reading)
- Associated signs/symptoms (nausea, vomiting, diarrhea, pain, cough, urinary symptoms, stiff neck)
- Measures taken to reduce fever
- Last dose of antipyretic (fever reduction) medications (ibuprofen, acetaminophen, aspirin)

OBSTETRICAL / GYNECOLOGICAL EMERGENCY
- Last menstrual period or due date
- Type of birth control used
- Bleeding / discharge / amniotic fluid (rupture of membranes [ROM]) - color, odor, amount (number of saturated pads)
- Pregnant - how far along, number of pregnancies and births
- Prenatal care and anticipated complications
- Multiple births (twins, etc.) expected
- Pain/discomfort - duration, (constant vs. intermittent)
- Labor - time and length of contractions, crowning, urge to push
- Use of legal or illegal substances

PAIN / DISCOMFORT
- When did the pain/discomfort first began (minutes - weeks) and if acute or chronic
- Causative event and what makes it better or worse
- Type of pain, i.e. sharp, ache, squeezing, burning, etc
- Area effected and if focal or diffuse
- Pain moves to another area away from its origin;
- Constant or intermittent
- 0 - 10 pain scale (initial event and ongoing assessment)
- Duration

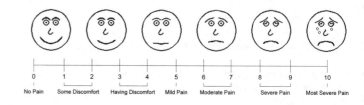

PATIENT ASSESSMENT & MANAGEMENT
Supplemental Information (Continued)

POISONING / OVERDOSE

- Type of substance
- Quantity and route of exposure (ingestion, inhalation, absorption, injection)
- Time of exposure
- Effect (altered level of consciousness, respiratory problems, abdominal pain/discomfort, nausea, vomiting, etc)
- Progression of symptoms
- Care rendered prior to EMS
- Response to treatment prior to EMS

RESPIRATORY DISTRESS

- When distress first began, gradual vs. sudden, and if acute or chronic
- Causative event (allergy, exertion, drugs, etc) and what makes it better or worse
- Effective ventilations, tidal volume, difficulty getting air in or air out, accessory muscle use, stridor, position, etc.
- Rate fast, slow, normal and respiratory pattern
- Initial or repeated episodes, time of last episode
- Rate the severity using mild, moderate, or severe and compare to previous episode or ongoing assessment
- Duration

Distress level considerations for chief complaint of shortness of breath (SOB)

Mild - tachypnea, normal position, answers in full sentences
Moderate - tachypnea, upright position if possible, answers in partial sentences
Severe - tachypnea, tripod position, answers in 2-3 words only

VAGINAL BLEEDING

- Precipitating event
- Time of onset
- Duration of event
- Last normal menstrual period (LNMP)
- Pregnant (how far along)
- Pain/cramping
- Amount of bleeding (number of saturated pads/hour)
- Passing blood clots/tissue
- Nausea, vomiting
- Dizziness

REFERENCES

- 502 - Patient Destination
- 506 - Trauma Triage
- 508 - Sexual Assault Patient Destination
- 510 - Pediatric Patient Destination
- 511 - Perinatal Patient Destination
- 512 - Burn Patient Destination
- 513 - ST Elevation Myocardial Infarction Patient Destination
- 515 - Air Ambulance Trauma Transport
- 518 - Decompression Emergencies/Patient Destination
- 519 - Management of Multiple Casualty Incidents
- 521 - Stroke Patient Destination
- 606 - Documentation of Prehospital Care
- 808 - Base Hospital Contact and Transport Criteria
- 834 - Patient Refusal of Treatment or Transport

Developed 11/99   Revised 12/01, 3/03, 10/08, 9/09,

RECEIVING FACILITIES

- Designated Stroke Center (DSC)
- Emergency Department Approved for Pediatrics (EDAP)
- Most Accessible Receiving (MAR)
- Pediatric Medical Center (PMC)
- Pediatric Trauma Center (PTC)
- Perinatal Center (N)
- Sexual Assault Center (SART)
- ST Elevation Myocardial Infarction Receiving Center (SRC)
- Trauma Center (TC)

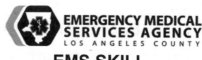

EMERGENCY MEDICAL
SERVICES AGENCY
LOS ANGELES COUNTY

EMS SKILL

PATIENT ASSESSMENT & MANAGEMENT

PERFORMANCE OBJECTIVES

Demonstrate competency in performing a complete medical or trauma assessment involving scene size-up, primary assessment, secondary assessment, physical examination, ongoing assessment, and perform life-threatening interventions as necessary.

CONDITION

Perform a medical or trauma assessment on a simulated patient and perform life-threatening interventions as necessary. Necessary equipment will be adjacent to the patient or brought to the field setting.

EQUIPMENT

Live model or manikin, oxygen tank with flow meter, oxygen tubing, BVM device, oxygen mask, nasal cannula, stethoscope, blood pressure cuff, pen light, timing device, clipboard, pen, goggles, various masks, gown, gloves.

PERFORMANCE CRITERIA

- Items designated by a diamond (♦) must be performed successfully to demonstrate skill competency.
- Items identified by double asterisks (**) indicate actions that are required if indicated.
- Items identified by (§) are not skill component items, but should be practiced.
- Patient assessment and management of life-threatening interventions must be completed within 10 minutes.

PREPARATION	
Skill Component	**Key Concepts**
♦ Take body substance isolation precautions	• Mandatory (minimal) personal protective equipment – gloves

SCENE SIZE-UP Critical Decisions	
Skill Component	**Key Concepts**
♦ Assess: • Personnel/patient safety • Environmental hazards • Number of patients • Mechanism of injury/Nature of illness	• The initial information obtained from the mechanism of injury or nature of illness assists in formulating the field impression.

♦ Determine need for:
• Additional resources
• Specialized equipment
• Extrication/spinal immobilization
  - Approach the patient from the front side
  - Direct patient not to move or turn head
  - Direct 2nd rescuer to stabilize the cervical spine
	• Assume that all trauma patients have the potential for a spinal injury.
	• Approaching the patient from the front side, minimizes the potential that the patient will turn his/her head to look at the EMS provider.
	• Manual spinal stabilization begins with manual control of the head. The C-collar is applied after the primary assessment is completed.

♦ Evaluate need for additional BSI precautions	• Situational - goggles, mask, gown

PRIMARY ASSESSMENT (Initial Assessment) Critical Management and Transport Decisions	
Skill Component	**Key Concepts**
♦ Consider: • General impression • Imminent Life-threatening condition • Observe for major disabilities **NOTE: The patient's condition may change at anytime. EMS providers must reassess and manage any changes in the patient's condition.**	• The general impression is determined by observing the appearance and hygiene, patient position, sounds, and smells. It establishes the overall condition of the patient and if immediate interventions are needed. Does the patient appear stable, potentially unstable, or unstable? • The primary assessment should be completed in 60 – 90 seconds. • Manage life-threatening situations when found.

such as bleeds big

Skill Component	Key Concepts
◆ Establish patient rapport: • Introduce yourself to the patient and/or caregiver • Ask the patient's name • Ask why EMS was called (preliminary C/C) • <u>Obtain permission to treat</u> • Respond with empathy • Use positive body language	• Situation and patient condition determines the level of rapport that is possible. • Establishing a positive rapport will decrease the patient's anxiety all will elicit a greater degree of cooperation. • Asking why EMS was called assists in determining the preliminary chief complaint and patient symptoms. • Responding with empathy develops trust and encourages essential patient communication. • All patients have the right to be treated with respect and should receive non-judgmental and impartial treatment. • Body language (non-verbal communication) refers to facial expressions, gestures and body movements that communicate a variety of messages to the patient regarding impressions of the healthcare provider; i.e. caring, helpful, dismissive, hostile, confident, incompetent, etc.
◆ Assess mental status/stimulus response (AVPU): • Alert • Verbal stimulus • Painful stimulus • Unresponsive	• The primary assessment only assesses the patient's response to environmental stimuli. This is <u>NOT</u> the time to obtain a comprehensive orientation level. • Use the lowest level of stimuli to determine mental status.
Airway ◆ Assess and manage airway: • Patent • Obstructed ** *Manage life-threatening situations:* • *Open and clear/suction airway - if indicated* • *Utilize basic airway adjuncts - if indicated* • *Initiate immediate transport – if unable to open the airway*	• Noisy respirations indicate an obstructed airway and airway positioning or maneuvers must be instituted to provide a patent airway. • Assess for foreign body such as food, gum, etc. • Use an NP airway for either responsive or unresponsive patients. • Use an OP airway for the unresponsive patient with no gag reflex. • Immediate transport should be initiated if unable to establish or maintain an adequate airway. • EMTs should transport prior to the arrival of ALS for life-threatening situations in which the ETA for ALS exceeds the ETA to the Most Accessible Receiving (MAR) hospital. See Reference No. 502.
Breathing ◆ Assess/Manage breathing: • Rate (fast, slow, normal or absent) • Rhythm (regular, irregular) • Quality (air movement, chest expansion) • Depth (tidal volume) • Rapid chest auscultation - *if difficulty breathing or shortness of breath* ** *Manage life-threatening situations:* • **Initiate appropriate delivery method for supplemental O$_2$** • **Use positive pressure ventilations - *if inadequate ventilation*** • **Initiate immediate transport - *if unable to manage ventilations***	• Visualize chest and signs of inadequate breathing. • The initial respiratory rate should not be counted at this time, but only observed if it is too fast, too slow or in the normal range. • Abnormal rates may not provide adequate ventilations or tidal volume. Use BVM to increase tidal volume or rate if necessary, especially if level of consciousness is decreased. • Administer O2 therapy if vital organs are at risk for hypoperfusion. • Rapid chest auscultation for presence and equality is performed in *2 locations only* (5th-6th intercostal space, mid-axillary line) bilaterally. • In life-threatening situations when the ETA for ALS exceeds the ETA to the MAR, EMTs should exercise their clinical judgment to transport prior to the arrival of ALS. See Reference No. 502.

Skill Component	Key Concepts

Circulation
 	
♦ Assess/Manage circulation:
  • Pulse – normal, too fast, too slow or absent
  • Skin - color, temperature, moisture
  • Uncontrolled external bleeding
  • Capillary refill - *if appropriate*
 	
** *Manage life-threatening situations:*
  • **Control *life-threatening external bleeding***
  • **Place in *shock position - if signs of hypoperfusion***
  • ***Place on cardiac monitor/AED - if indicated***
  • ***Consider venous access - if indicated***
  • ***Initiate immediate transport – if uncontrolled external bleeding***
	• Check the radial and carotid pulses at same time in critical situations. Check the femoral pulse if unable to obtain a carotid pulse. The radial pulse may be absent due to decreased blood pressure.
	
	• An irregular pulse is an indication for ECG monitoring.
	
	• Capillary refill is most accurate in pediatric patients. It is NOT always accurate in adults due to chronically poor peripheral circulation. It is not accurate in cold environments.
	
	• Capillary refill can be taken at any skin area such as: fingernail bed, palm of the hand, chest, forehead, etc. If using the ball of the foot in pediatric patients, the child must be in a supine position. The most accurate site to check capillary refill is a central site (chest wall) vs. a peripheral site.
	
	• In life-threatening situations when the ETA for ALS exceeds the ETA to the MAR, EMTs should exercise their clinical judgment to transport prior to the arrival of ALS. See Reference No. 502.
	
	• IV access should be started enroute in critical trauma patients.

Disability
 	
♦ Observe for abnormal body presentation:
  • Neurological deficits
  • Body position
	• Neurological deficits include: facial droop, slurred speech, drooling, paresthesia, and paralysis. Note GCS and pupils, prn.
	
	• Abnormal body presentation include tripod position, decerebrate or decorticate posturing, or contractures due to prolonged lack of use of the extremities, etc.

Expose ♦ Expose area associated with the preliminary chief complaint	• Preliminary chief complaint is the reason for summoning EMS to the scene. • Avoid inference of impropriety. Maintain patient modesty and dignity as much as possible.
Formulate ♦ Form a field impression ** *Manage life-threatening situations - if not already addressed* ** *Obtain blood glucose level - if altered level of consciousness*	• Field impression is determined by EMS personnel utilizing information gathered early in the assessment.

Identify
 	
♦ Identify priority patient and determine which secondary assessment and physical exam is needed:
  • Rapid medical or rapid trauma assessment
  • Comprehensive medical or trauma assessment
	• The primary assessment information determines which specific secondary assessment and physical exam is needed.
	
	• A rapid medical or rapid trauma assessment should be done when a patient is unresponsive or has sustained major trauma. It should take no longer than 60-90 seconds.

♦ Determine transport option:
  • Level of transport
  • Mode of transport
  • Destination
	• ALS or BLS transport is determined by designation of priority vs. non-priority patient.
	
	• Medical and minor trauma patients should be assessed and treated on scene before being transported.
	
	• Major trauma patients should receive a rapid trauma assessment and all life-threatening interventions performed on scene. All other assessment and treatment of injuries should be done enroute.
	
	• Mode of transport incorporates ground and air transport.
	
	• ALS and BLS providers should transport to the appropriate facility as indicated. See Reference No. 502, 506, 508, 510, 511, 512, 513, 515, 518 & 808.

SECONDARY ASSESSMENT
(Focused History and Physical Examination)

Skill Component	Key Concepts
◆ Perform a <u>rapid</u> medical or trauma assessment for all critical situations. <u>Briefly</u> assess and palpate: • head • pelvis • neck • lower extremities • chest • upper extremities • abdomen • back	• A rapid trauma assessment is a brief inspection and palpation of the body. It reveals life-threatening injuries which must be treated immediately and require rapid transport. The assessment should take only 60-90 seconds.

◆ Assess current complaint (illness or injury):
 	
<u>**SAMPLE History Assessment**</u>
 	
• **S**igns/**S**ymptoms
  - OPQRST for current complaint
 	
• **A**llergies
 	
• **M**edications
 	
• **P**ertinent history
  - <u>age</u>
  - weight
  - under physician's care/private medical doctor
  - pertinent medical/surgical history
 	
• **L**ast oral intake (last meal or when medication taken) - <u>*if pertinent*</u>
 	
• **E**vent leading to injury or illness
	• Evaluate if the current illness or injury reflects the chief complaint.
	• Assess pediatric patients starting at the feet then progress to their head (toe-to-head).
	• Use the pediatric emergency resuscitation tape to obtain an infant's or a child's weight.
	
	• OPQRST is a pneumonic to assist in asking questions to describe the signs/symptoms of the present complaint. Used primarily to asses pain and respiratory distress, but can be used to assess other conditions.
	
	  - **O**nset – activity at time the problem/pain started and did emotional or environmental factors contribute to problem
	  - **P**rovokes – what makes it worse, **P**alliative – what makes it better, **P**osition – in what position is the patient found
	  - **Q**uality – type of discomfort (burning stabbing crushing) and constant or intermittent
	  - **R**egion – area involved, **R**adiation – does the pain/discomfort spread from origin, **R**ecurrence – has this occurred before
	  - **S**everity – pain scale
	  - **T**ime – when did the problem/pain begin and what is the duration of time
	
	• Obtaining information such as under physician care, name of primary medical doctor or health plan assists in eliciting medical history and transport destination. *Obtain information from family or bystanders if patient is unable to provide the needed information.*
	
	• Pertinent history refers to past medical history that is pertinent to the chief complaint/problem such as: a heart condition, pulmonary problems, hypertension, diabetes, CVA, or recent surgery.
	
	• Last oral intake is important when there is a possibility the patient may require surgery or if there is a potential for aspiration.

◆ Assess vital signs:
• Cardiac status
 	
  - pulse - rate, rhythm, quality
  - ECG reading - <u>*if indicated and available*</u>
 	
• Respiratory status
  - respirations - rate, effort, tidal volume
  - breath sounds
  - oxygen saturation SpO$_2$% (Pulse oximetry - <u>*if available for patients at risk for hypoxemia*</u>)
 	
• Blood pressure
 	
• Skin signs
  - color
  - temperature
  - moisture
  - turgor
 	
• Pain
 	
** ***Re-evaluate the effectiveness of all primary assessment interventions performed - <u>if applicable</u>***
	• Pulse and respirations are actually counted at this time.
	• Oxygen saturation is not a vital sign, but some EMS providers utilize it to assess a patient's condition. Regardless of the reading, pulse oximetry SHOULD NOT prevent oxygen being administered to patients who require it, nor should it influence treatment without doing a thorough patient assessment.
	
	• The pulse oximetry device measures the level of hemoglobin that is saturated with oxygen or a chemical that displaces oxygen such as carbon monoxide.
	
	• Pulse oximetry is not reliable if a patient is exposed to carbon monoxide (includes tobacco and marijuana smokers), anemic patients, ingestion of certain kinds of poisons, hypoperfusion, cold or injured extremity, finger nail polishes or acrylic nails.
	
	• Both systolic and diastolic B/P should be auscultated. Palpate B/P <u>only</u> if unable to hear when auscultated.
	
	(Continued)

Skill Component	Key Concepts
	• Palpating blood pressure for convenience or saving time DOES <u>NOT</u> provide necessary cardiovascular information or evaluate changes in patients with cerebral edema, CHF, or other serious conditions.
	• It is important to document temperature information in suspected febrile seizures or environmental emergencies. This can be obtained by asking the caretaker for last temperature reading and by feeling the patient's trunk under the axillary region with the back of the hand.
	• Evaluation of skin condition involves assessment of moisture, color and skin turgor.
	• All patients must be assessed for presence of pain. Document what patient states the pain level is using the 0 - 10 scale. EMS providers must document what the patient states and not the provider's perception of the pain level.

♦ Examine neurological status
  • Comprehensive orientation level - person, place, time
  • Glasgow Coma Scale (GCS) - eyes, verbal, motor
  • Pupils – equal size, round, react to light (PERRL) and movement - *if indicated*
  • Extremities-circulation, movement, strength, sensation
 	
** *Perform glucose check – if indicated*
	• Comprehensive orientation level involves three (3) parameters of person, place, and time.
	
	• Glasgow Coma Scale (GCS) in Los Angeles County reverses the verbal and motor parameter assessments – *eyes, motor, verbal.*
	
	• Neuro symptoms described by the patient may include headache, blurred vision, photophobia, dizziness, paresthesia, etc.
	
	• Assess each extremity individually then compare findings.
	
	• The patient must be competent to refuse treatment or transport if indicated. See Reference No. 834.

♦ Expose and perform an examine specific to the painful area identified or injured ** *Render care based on assessment findings - <u>if not already addressed</u>*	• Avoid inference of impropriety. Maintain patient modesty and dignity as much as possible.
♦ Re-evaluate transport decision to appropriate facility	• See Reference No. 502, 506, 508, 510, 511, 512, 513, 515, 518, 521 & 808.

♦ Perform detailed physical examination:
  • Medical patient – <u>complete on scene</u>
  • Trauma patient – <u>complete enroute</u>
 	
** *Manage specific illness or injury on scene or enroute as indicated*
	• A detailed physical examination entails a complete body check on scene for a <u>medical patient</u>.
	
	EXCEPTION – if the patient is too unstable to remain in the field, EMS personnel should use their best judgment to transport immediately and attempt detailed examination enroute.
	
	• A detailed physical examination entails a complete body check for an unconscious patient and a major trauma patient.
	
	• Look for anything that is abnormal or does not fit the situation.

Patient Assessment & Management   © 1999, 2001, 2003, 2006, 2009 UCLA Skills Guide for EMT -1   Page 166   Page 5 of 12

DETAILED PHYSICAL EXAMINATION OR EXAMINATION OF AFFECTED AREA OR INJURY
(Assessment for Specific Illness or Injury)

Skill Component	Key Concepts

HEAD - Skull, Eyes, Ears, Nose, Mouth, Face
 	
◆ **Assess for DCAP/BTLS**:
• Deformity (visible and palpated)
• Contusions
• Abrasions
• Penetrations / Punctures
• Burns / Bruises
• Tenderness
• Lacerations
• Swelling / Scars
 	
◆ **Palpate for**:
• Tenderness
• Instability
• Crepitus
 	
◆ **Additional Assessment Elements**:
• Asymmetry of head and face
• Drainage
• Raccoon eyes
• Battle's sign
• Soot and singed nasal or facial hairs
• Coffee ground emesis
 	
◆ **Medical Devices**:
• Nasogastric Tube (NG)
 	
** *Maintain patent airway*
	• <u>Adults</u> - head-to-toe examination works best.
	
	• <u>Children</u> - toe-to-head examination works best to gain the child's confidence.
	
	• Asymmetry of head and face may due to trauma or medical problem such as stoke or Bell's Palsy (unilateral facial paralysis of sudden onset and unknown cause).
	
	• Battle's sign is bruising over the mastoid process and indicates a basilar skull fracture or fracture of the temporal bone.
	
	• Raccoon eyes is the bruising of one or both orbits and indicates fracture of the sphenoid sinus.
	
	• Battle's sign and raccoon eyes develop some time after the injury and generally are not seen upon EMS arrival, if noted, this may be due to a previous injury.
	
	• Fluid from the ear or nose also may indicate leakage of spinal fluid resulting from a basilar skull fracture.
	
	• Soot is fine black carbon particles from combustion.
	
	• Coffee ground emesis is partially digested blood found with upper GI bleeding.
	
	• <u>Definition of Crepitus</u>:
	  - grating of bone fragments
	  - crackling of joints
	  - air or gas in soft tissue (subcutaneous emphysema)

NECK/CERVICAL SPINE
 	
◆ **Assess for DCAP/BTLS**:
• Deformity (visible and palpated)
• Contusions
• Abrasions
• Penetrations / Punctures
• Burns/bruises
• Tenderness
• Lacerations
• Swelling / Scars
 	
◆ **Palpate for**:
• Tenderness
• Instability
• Crepitus
 	
◆ **Additional Assessment Elements**:
• Track marks and tattoos
• Medical alert tags
• Jugular vein distention (JVD)
• Tracheal deviation
• Accessory muscle use
• Carotid pulses
• Subcutaneous emphysema (crepitus)
• Stoma
 	
◆ **Medical Devices**:
• Tracheostomy
• Central venous catheters
 	
** *Maintain spinal immobilization - if indicated*
** *Apply occlusive dressing - if puncture wound to neck*
	• DO NOT simultaneously press on both carotid arteries.
	
	• <u>Paramedics</u> should consider spinal immobilization indications and <u>EMTs</u> shall perform spinal immobilization based on mechanism of injury.
	
	• Full face helmets should be removed to allow access to the patient's airway and provide in-line immobilization of the head and neck.
	
	• DO NOT REMOVE shoulder pads or custom fitted helmets such as football or hockey helmets unless respiratory distress is coupled with inability to access the airway. Remove face guard with rescue scissors or a screwdriver.
	
	• Leave infants and children in safety seats for assessment and for controlled spinal immobilization. Remove them only if the seat is damaged, child requires further assessment, or life-threatening treatment that cannot be performed in the safety seat.
	
	• Pad (shim) patients to maintain a neutral position and restrict movement on a long spine board:
	  - Adults - head and neck for comfort and to prevent hyper-extension
	  - Infant or child - immobilize in child safety seat, if possible, or - pad neck and shoulder area to maintain alignment if placed on long spine board.
	  - Elderly - head and neck to maintain comfort and prevent hyper-extension, airway obstruction, and skin breakdown
	  - Athletes - head and neck to prevent hyper-extension, if the shoulder pads are in place, and the helmet is removed
	• *Placing a cervical collar on patients who have a stoma is dangerous due to the possibility of the cervical collar shifting and occluding the airway.*

Skill Component	Key Concepts

CHEST – Clavicles, Sternum, Ribs
 	
♦ **Assess for DCAP/BTLS:**
• Deformity (visible and palpated)
• Contusions
• Abrasions
• Penetrations / Punctures
• Burns/bruises
• Tenderness
• Lacerations
• Swelling / Scars
♦ **Palpate for:**
• Tenderness
• Instability
• Crepitus
♦ **Additional Assessment Elements:**
• Paradoxical movement
• Accessory muscle use
• Sucking chest wound
• Subcutaneous emphysema (crepitus)
♦ **Auscultate:**
• Breath sounds in all lung fields
♦ **Percuss** - *if breath sounds are unequal*
♦ **Medical Devices:**
• Pacemaker
• Internal cardiac defibrillator (ICD)
• Central catheters
• Chest tubes
** Apply occlusive dressing to sucking chest wound - *if indicated*
** Splint flail segment - *if paradoxical motion is noted*
** Decompress chest - *if tension pneumothorax*
	• Maintain patient modesty and perform chest palpation in a manner as to avoid any inference of impropriety.
	
	• Complete breath sounds should be assessed in either anterior or posterior locations and auscultate for 2 breaths in all 3 fields.
	
	• Chest percussion assists in providing information if there is a hemothorax or a pneumothorax. Percussion on scene may be difficult due to environmental noise and patient condition – transport <u>should not be delayed</u> for this assessment.
	
	  - Hemothorax - dull sound
	  - Pneumothorax - hyperresonant sound
	
	• Paramedics must perform chest decompression once tension pneumothorax is suspected and to prevent irreversible shock.
	
	• Percussion is a paramedic skill and not performed by EMTs.

ABDOMEN ♦ **Assess for DCAP/BTLS:** • Deformity (visible and palpated) • Contusions • Abrasions • Penetrations / Punctures • Burns/bruises • Tenderness • Lacerations • Swelling / Scars ♦ **Palpate for:** • Tenderness ♦ **Additional Assessment Elements:** • Distention • Rigidity/guarding • Pulsating mass • Signs of pregnancy and/or complications • Subcutaneous emphysema (crepitus) ♦ **Auscultate:** ♦ **Medical Devices:** • Gastrostomy tube • Colostomy • Medication pumps	• DO NOT PALPATE pulsating masses – this may rupture an aneurysm. • EMS providers should palpate each of the 4 quadrants one time only to assess for rigidity and guarding. Further palpation does not add to examination findings and results in unnecessary pain. • Use finger pads of the first 3 fingers to palpate the abdomen. DO NOT use finger tips. • Assessing for rebound tenderness should not be performed. It causes severe pain and prehospital treatment will not change. - *This is a diagnostic test for peritoneal irritation caused by infection or internal bleeding and is rarely used by physicians due to the advancement of diagnostic technology.* • Guarding is a reflexive tightening of abdominal muscles as depth of palpation is increased. • Pregnancy related complications are; contractions, vaginal bleeding, rigid abdomen, back pain, etc. • The assessment element of instability is not pertinent in the abdomen since it is a soft cavity with malleable organs. • The assessment element of subcutaneous emphysema (crepitus) is only felt if the patient has developed gas gangrene (potentially deadly form of tissue death). It is caused by an anaerobic microorganism infection at the site of a recent surgical or traumatic wound. Gas gangrene develops rapidly and is often fatal.

Skill Component	Key Concepts

PELVIS
 	
♦ **Assess for DCAP/BTLS**:
  • Deformity (visible and palpated)
  • Contusions
  • Abrasions
  • Penetrations / Punctures
  • Burns/bruises
  • Tenderness
  • Lacerations
  • Swelling / Scars
♦ **Palpate for**:
  • Tenderness
  • Instability
  • Crepitus
♦ **Additional Assessment Elements**:
  • Femoral pulses
  • Incontinence
  • Priapism
  • Signs of pregnancy and/or complications
  • Vaginal bleeding
♦ **Medical Devices**:
  • Urinary catheter
	• Pelvic injuries are critical and have the potential for major blood loss. DO NOT palpate if there are obvious pelvic injuries or patient complains of pelvic pain, but transport immediately, if not already enroute.
	
	• Palpating femoral pulses is useful in the elderly if circulation to extremities is diminished. Maintain modesty and dignity and palpate in a manner as to avoid inference of impropriety.
	
	• Pregnancy related complications are; contractions, vaginal bleeding, rigid abdomen, back pain, etc.
	
	• Priapism is a prolonged painful penile erection not associated with sexual stimulation. It may be caused by:
	  - blood disorders such as Sickle cell anemia and leukemia
	  - prescription medications used for erectile dysfunction, antidepressants, psychiatric disorders, anti-anxiety and blood thinners
	  - illicit or recreational drugs
	  - spinal cord lesions
	  - spinal cord trauma
	  - enovation from the bite of a scorpion, black widow spider, and the Brazilian wandering spider

LOWER EXTREMITIES
 	
♦ **Assess for DCAP/BTLS**:
  • Deformity (visible and palpated)
  • Contusions
  • Abrasions
  • Penetrations / Punctures
  • Burns/bruises
  • Tenderness
  • Lacerations
  • Swelling / Scars
♦ **Palpate for**:
  • Tenderness
  • Instability
  • Crepitus
♦ **Additional Assessment Elements**:
  • Track marks and tattoos
  • Medical alert tags
  • Pedal pulses
  • Motor movement and function
  • Sensation
♦ **Medical Devices**:
  • IV catheters
	• Compare bilateral pulses, motor movement and sensation.
	
	• Midline calf tenderness may indicate deep vein thrombosis and should be assessed for in patients complaining of shortness of breath, chest pain, or signs of a stroke. Deep vein thrombosis may indicate migration of a clot to the lungs, coronary arteries or brain.
	
	• Abnormal sensations may be tingling, burning or numbness.

UPPER EXTREMITIES
 	
♦ **Assess for DCAP/BTLS**:
  • Deformity (visible and palpated)
  • Contusions
  • Abrasions
  • Penetrations / Punctures
  • Burns/bruises
  • Tenderness
  • Lacerations
  • Swelling / Scars
♦ **Palpate for**:
  • Tenderness
  • Instability
  • Crepitus   (Continued)
	• Compare bilateral pulses, motor movement and sensation.
	
	• Abnormal sensations may be tingling, burning or numbness.
	
	• Arteriovenous (AV) shunt or fistula connects an artery to a vein and is used for dialysis.

Skill Component	Key Concepts

UPPER EXTREMITIES (Continued)
 	
♦ **Additional Assessment Elements:**
  • Tract marks and tattoos
  • Medical alert tags
  • Brachial/radial pulses
  • Motor movement and function
  • Sensation
 	
♦ **Medical Devices**:
  • Arteriovenous (AV) shunt or fistula
  • IV catheters	

BACK - Posterior Thorax, Lumbar, Buttocks
♦ **Assess for DCAP/BTLS**:
  • Deformity (visible and palpated)
  • Contusions
  • Abrasions
  • Penetrations / Punctures
  • Burns/bruises
  • Tenderness
  • Lacerations
  • Swelling / Scars
♦ **Palpate for**:
  • Tenderness
  • Instability
  • Crepitus
♦ **Additional Assessment Elements:**
  • Tattoos
  • Brachial/radial pulses
  • Subcutaneous emphysema (crepitus)
  • Sacral edema
	• Log roll patient if suspected spinal injury.
	
	• Roll patient directly onto backboard once examination is complete.

REASSESSMENT
(Ongoing Assessment)

Skill Component	Key Concepts

♦ Reassess a patient at least every **5 minutes for priority** patients and every **15 minutes for stable** patients.
  • Primary assessment
  • Relevant portion of the secondary assessment
  • Vital signs
	• Priority patients are patients who have abnormal vital signs, S/S of poor perfusion, if there is a suspicion that the patient's condition may deteriorate, or when the patient's condition changes.

♦ Evaluate response to treatment	• Patients must be re-evaluated at least every 5 minutes if any treatment was initiated or medication administered.
♦ Evaluate results of reassessment and note any changes from patient's previous condition and vital signs ****Manage patient condition as indicated.**	• Evaluating and comparing results assists in recognizing if the patient is improving, responding to treatment or condition is deteriorating.
§ Explain the care being delivered and the transport destination to the patient/caregivers	• Communication is important when dealing with the patient, family or caregiver. This is a very critical and frightening time for all involved and providing information helps in decreasing the stress they are experiencing.
§ Give patient report to equal or higher level of care provider **Exception**: *Report may be given to a lower level of care provider when an ALS to BLS downgrade has occurred*	• Report should consist of all pertinent information regarding the assessment findings, treatment rendered and patients response to care provided.

Guide to Patient Assessment

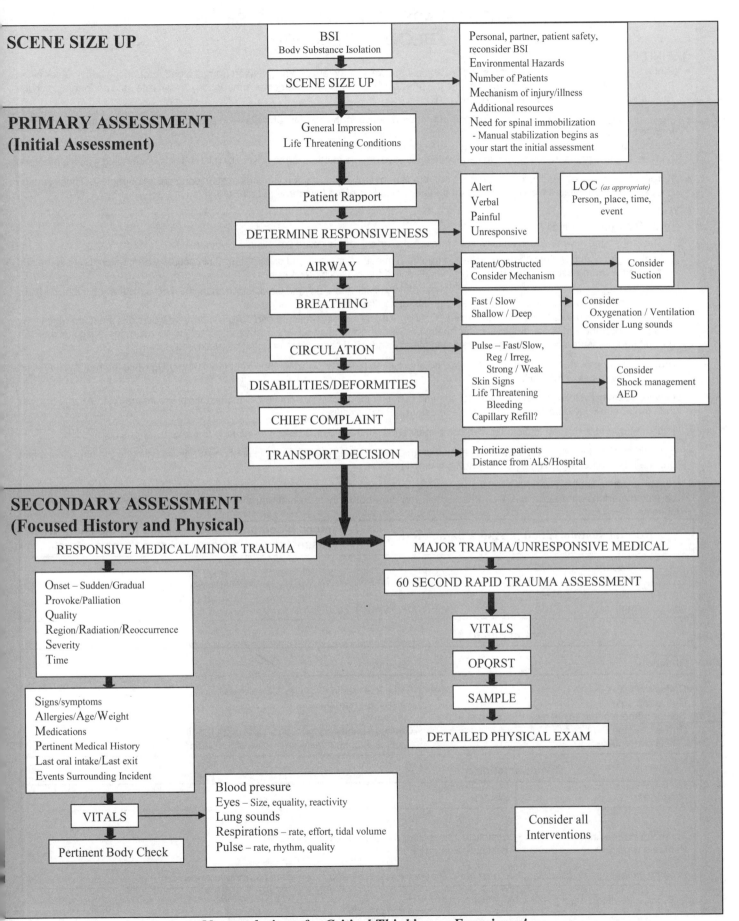

SCENE SIZE UP

BSI
Body Substance Isolation

SCENE SIZE UP

Personal, partner, patient safety, reconsider BSI
Environmental Hazards
Number of Patients
Mechanism of injury/illness
Additional resources
Need for spinal immobilization
 - Manual stabilization begins as your start the initial assessment

PRIMARY ASSESSMENT
(Initial Assessment)

General Impression
Life Threatening Conditions

Patient Rapport

DETERMINE RESPONSIVENESS

Alert
Verbal
Painful
Unresponsive

LOC *(as appropriate)*
Person, place, time, event

AIRWAY

Patent/Obstructed
Consider Mechanism

Consider Suction

BREATHING

Fast / Slow
Shallow / Deep

Consider
 Oxygenation / Ventilation
Consider Lung sounds

CIRCULATION

Pulse – Fast/Slow,
 Reg / Irreg,
 Strong / Weak
Skin Signs
Life Threatening
 Bleeding
Capillary Refill?

Consider
Shock management
AED

DISABILITIES/DEFORMITIES

CHIEF COMPLAINT

TRANSPORT DECISION

Prioritize patients
Distance from ALS/Hospital

SECONDARY ASSESSMENT
(Focused History and Physical)

RESPONSIVE MEDICAL/MINOR TRAUMA

MAJOR TRAUMA/UNRESPONSIVE MEDICAL

Onset – Sudden/Gradual
Provoke/Palliation
Quality
Region/Radiation/Reoccurrence
Severity
Time

60 SECOND RAPID TRAUMA ASSESSMENT

VITALS

OPQRST

SAMPLE

Signs/symptoms
Allergies/Age/Weight
Medications
Pertinent Medical History
Last oral intake/Last exit
Events Surrounding Incident

DETAILED PHYSICAL EXAM

VITALS

Blood pressure
Eyes – Size, equality, reactivity
Lung sounds
Respirations – rate, effort, tidal volume
Pulse – rate, rhythm, quality

Consider all Interventions

Pertinent Body Check

Not a substitute for Critical Thinking or Experience! UCLA Skills Guide Page 171

PATIENT ASSESSMENT / VITAL SIGNS
BLOOD PRESSURE

DEFINITIONS:

- <u>Blood pressure</u> - measurement of force applied against the walls of the arteries as the heart pumps blood through the body. Determined by stroke volume (amount of blood ejected into the arterial system with one ventricular contraction), heart rate, and peripheral vascular resistance (BP=combination of SV, HR, and PVR)

- <u>Pulse pressure</u> -is defined as the difference in pressure between the systolic and diastolic pressure. This diagnostic information is important in certain conditions:
  - widening pulse pressure may indicate increased intracranial pressure
  - narrowing pulse pressure may indicate cardiogenic, hypovolemic and other forms of shock which have a decreasing systolic pressure

- <u>Korotkoff's sounds</u> -   pulse sounds that are heard as sharp tapping or knocking sounds at each ventricular contraction. These sounds are caused by an inflated blood pressure cuff partially occluding blood flow through an artery.

NOTES:

- <u>Blood Pressure Readings</u>:
  - The <u>first sound</u> is when blood initially flows through the artery and is called the systolic pressure.
  - The <u>second sound</u> is when there is a change (muffled) in sound or the sound disappears. This occurs when the pressure in the cuff falls below the pressure in the artery. This is considered the diastolic pressure.
  - The <u>third sound</u> is when the sound disappears completely (if still heard beyond the diastolic change). This occurs when the blood flows freely through the artery and is considered the Aabsolute diastole@.

- **A palpated blood pressure is NOT preferred.** Only provides a systolic pressure and does not provide a diastolic pressure which may provide important additional diagnostic information. Should only be used when environmental noise overrides auscultation. An auscultated pressure should always be attempted initially and ASAP during the ongoing assessment.

- Brachial artery provides the most accurate reading and can be palpated down to approximately 70mmg/Hg while the radial artery is no longer palpable below 80mmHg.

- Lower extremity systolic pressure may be 10-40 mm/Hg higher than upper extremities. The diastolic pressure may be the same or lower than the arm. (Should be attempted if unable to use upper extremities.)

- If the first sound is missed, deflate the cuff completely and wait 30 seconds before re-inflation to prevent venous congestion.

- Sometimes the blood pressure should be taken in both arms, such as with the complaint of chest pain radiating to the back, this might provide information regarding a possible aortic dissection.

- Hypertension in adults is when the systolic pressure is sustained > 140mmHg **OR** diastolic pressure > 90mmHg. However, patients with chronic hypertension may be in shock when pressures drop below their normal and are considered adequate for non-hypertensive patients.

Normal systolic blood pressure parameters		Systolic blood pressures denoting hypotension when associated with signs and symptoms of shock	
Newborn	50-70	Males	< 90 Systolic
Infant	80-100	Females	< 80 Systolic
Child	80-110	Children	< 70 Systolic
Adult	90-140		

Common Pitfalls	
Situation	**Results**
Cuff is too large	False low reading
Cuff is too small	False high reading
Center of the bladder is not over the brachial artery	Inaccurate reading
Cuff is deflated too slowly	Causes venous congestion = false high reading
Cuff is over inflated	Causes vasospasms/pain = false high reading

Documentation	
Readings	**Written**
Two sound readings	Systolic/diastolic (120/72)
Three sound readings	Systolic/diastolic/final diastolic change (124/72/40).
Palpated reading	Systolic/palpated (90/P).
In <u>some situations</u> the diastolic sound may not disappear completely and is recorded as systolic/zero (72/0).	

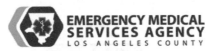

**EMERGENCY MEDICAL
SERVICES AGENCY**
LOS ANGELES COUNTY

EMS SKILL

PATIENT ASSESSMENT / VITAL SIGNS
BLOOD PRESSURE

PERFORMANCE OBJECTIVES

Demonstrate proficiency in obtaining an accurate auscultated and palpated blood pressure reading.

CONDITION

Auscultate a systolic and diastolic blood pressure and palpate a systolic blood pressure on a live model. Necessary equipment will be adjacent to the patient or brought to the field setting.

EQUIPMENT

Live model, large/medium/pediatric sphygmomanometer, stethoscope/dual teaching stethoscope, goggles, mask, gown, gloves.

PERFORMANCE CRITERIA

- Items designated by a diamond (♦) must be performed successfully to demonstrate skill competency.
- Items identified by double asterisks (**) indicate actions that are required if indicated.
- Items identified by (§) are not skill component items, but should be practiced.
- Reading must be within +/- 6 mmHg (systolic and diastolic) of examiner's determination.

PREPARATION	
Skill Component	**Key Concepts**
♦ Take body substance isolation precautions	• Mandatory personal protective equipment - gloves • Situational - goggles, mask, gown

♦ Select appropriate size blood pressure cuff	• Each EMS unit should carry a large, adult, and pediatric cuff.
	• Appropriate cuff size must be selected or an inaccurate reading will be obtained.
	  - Cuff width should cover 2/3 of the upper portion of the limb.
	  - Cuff bladder should encircle 2/3 the circumference of the limb.

♦ Select an appropriate site: • Upper extremity • Lower extremity	• Blood pressure measurements should not be taken on an extremity that is injured, paralyzed, edematous or has an IV, central catheter, arteriovenous fistula or shunt, or in an arm on the same side as a mastectomy. • Constriction of the arm or limb held in a tense position may result in inaccurate readings, discomfort, blood clots, injury to the vein or damage to the device.

♦ Position the extremity at appropriate level	• The extremity should be at the level of the heart and in a relaxed position or readings will be inaccurate:
	  - above heart level — false low reading
	  - below heart level — false high reading

UPPER EXTREMITY AUSCULTATED BLOOD PRESSURE PROCEDURE	
Skill Component	**Key Concepts**
♦ Place cuff snugly around arm: • Approximately 1" above antecubital space • Center the bladder over the brachial artery • Ensure bulb and tubing are at bottom of cuff - *if possible*	• Arm should be approximately at the level of the heart for the best sound to be heard. • Center of the bladder must be placed over brachial artery in order to register sounds clearly. • Bulb and tubing should be at the bottom of the cuff unless limb contractures or other positioning problems prevent this.
♦ Locate the brachial artery and palpate pulse	• Purpose for locating brachial artery is to find the best site for sound reproduction. • Use the fingertips to palpate and NOT the thumb.

Skill Component	Key Concepts
◆ Insert the stethoscope earpieces into ears	• Make sure earpieces are facing forward. This allows for better sound conduction.
◆ Place the diaphragm/bell over the brachial artery	• Radial artery does not allow for the placement of a stethoscope. • If stethoscope has a dual head, use the bell for better sound conduction.
◆ Inflate cuff rapidly 20-30mmHg above the level where the pulse sound is obliterated	• Over inflation of the cuff causes vasospasms or pain and results in a false high reading.
◆ Deflate cuff 2-4 mmHg/second and note where the first sound is heard *(systolic pressure)*	• Slow cuff deflation causes venous congestion and results in a false high reading. • The first sound heard is when blood initially flows through the artery (ventricular contraction ejecting blood into the arterial system). • If the first sound is missed, deflate the cuff completely and wait 30 seconds before re-inflation to prevent venous congestion.
◆ Continue to deflate cuff 2-4 mmHg/second and note where the first change in tone is heard *(diastolic pressure)*	• The sounds may disappear completely at this point or they may change in tone (muffled). This change occurs because the pressure in the cuff falls below the pressure in the artery. This is considered the diastolic pressure (ventricles in diastole - resting phase). This is recorded as the 2nd or last sound (120/80).
◆ Continue to deflate cuff 2-4 mmHg/second and note where the sound disappears entirely *(absolute diastole)* - *if sound continues to be heard*	• This is considered the "absolute diastole" (not routinely heard). The sound disappears when the blood flows freely through the artery. This is recorded as the 3rd sound (120/80/40).

LOWER EXTREMITY AUSCULTATED BLOOD PRESSURE PROCEDURE

Skill Component	Key Concepts

◆ Place cuff snugly around thigh:
  • Approximately 1" above knee
  • Center the bladder over the popliteal artery
  • Ensure bulb and tubing are at bottom of cuff - *if possible*
	• Lower extremity blood pressure should be attempted when unable to use upper extremities.
	• Patient should be in a supine position and limb relaxed for an accurate reading
	• Center of the bladder must be placed over popliteal artery in order to register sounds clearly.
	• Lower extremity systolic pressure may be 10-40 mmHg higher than upper extremities. The diastolic pressure may be the same or lower than the arm.

◆ Locate the popliteal artery and palpate pulse	• Purpose for locating popliteal artery is to find the proper site to place the stethoscope. • Use the fingertips to palpate and NOT the thumb.
◆ Insert the stethoscope earpieces into ears	• Make sure earpieces are facing forward. This allows for better sound conduction.
◆ Place the diaphragm/bell of the stethoscope over the popliteal artery	• If stethoscope has a duel head, use the bell for better sound conduction.
◆ Inflate cuff rapidly 20-30 mmHg above the level where the auscultated pulse sound was obliterated	
◆ Deflate cuff 2-4 mmHg/second and note where the first sound is heard *(systolic pressure)*	
◆ Continue to deflate cuff 2-4 mmHg/second and note where the last distinct sound is heard *(diastolic pressure)*	

PALPATED BLOOD PRESSURE
PROCEDURE

Skill Component	Key Concepts

◆ Place cuff snugly around arm:
  • Approximately 1" above antecubital space
  • Center the bladder over the brachial artery
  • Ensure bulb and tubing are at bottom of cuff - _if possible_
	• **_Palpated blood pressure is NOT preferred._** Only provides a systolic pressure and does not provide a diastolic pressure which may provide important additional diagnostic information. Should only be used when environmental noise overrides auscultation. An auscultated pressure should always be attempted initially and ASAP during the ongoing assessment.
	• The arm should be approximately at level of the heart for best measurement.
	• Center of the bladder must be placed over brachial artery in order to obtain an accurate measurement.
	• Palpated pressure readings are lower than auscultated readings.

◆ Locate and palpate pulse at the brachial or radial artery	• Brachial artery provides the most accurate reading and can be palpated down to approximately 70mmg/Hg while the radial artery is no longer palpable below 80mmHg.
◆ Inflate cuff rapidly to 20-30mmHg above the level where the palpated pulse is obliterated	
◆ Deflate cuff 2-4 mmHg/second and note where the first beat is felt	

REASSESSMENT
(Ongoing Assessment)

Skill Component	Key Concepts

§ Reassess auscultated or palpated blood pressure as required:
  • Priority patients every 5 minutes
  • Stable patients every 15 minutes
	• If palpated blood pressure obtained initially, attempt an auscultated blood pressure ASAP. This allows for a more accurate pressure and obtaining a systolic and diastolic pressure provides a better assessment picture.
	• Take bilateral extremity pressures if pressure obtained does not correlate with clinical picture, pressure is high, bilateral pulses are unequal, or when there is suspicion of aortic dissection.

PATIENT REPORT AND DOCUMENTATION

Skill Component	Key Concepts

§ Verbalize/Document:
  • Blood pressure reading
  • Site used
  • Patient's position
	• If blood pressure is palpated or a lower extremity is used to obtain a blood pressure, document the rationale for using this method or site.
	• The site used may provide different pressure values which are specific to the upper or lower extremity.
	• Important to document patient's position as to standing, sitting or lying down.
	• Documentation must be on either the Los Angeles County EMS Report form or departmental Patient Care Record form.

Developed 3/02   Revised 9/02, 1/10

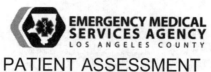

PATIENT ASSESSMENT
CHEST AUSCULTATION
Supplemental Information

DEFINITIONS:

- <u>Adventitious</u> - abnormal sounds. Result from obstruction of either the large or small airways and are most commonly heard on inspiration - crackles, wheezes and rhonchi.

- <u>Atelectasis</u> - a collapse or airless condition of the lungs. May be caused by obstruction, hypoventilation, mucus plugs or excessive secretions.

- <u>Bronchial</u> -sounds heard over a major bronchus; harsh, high-pitched with an equal inspiratory and expiratory phase.

- <u>Death Rattle</u> - "audible rales" heard without a stethoscope. Usually heard as patient is dying.

- <u>Lobectomy</u> - The surgical removal of a lobe of the lung or any organ.

- <u>Tracheal</u> - sounds heard over the trachea; loud and high-pitched with a pause between inspiratory and expiratory phase (expiratory phase slightly longer).

- <u>Vesicular</u> - normal breath sounds heard all over the chest distal to the central airways; soft sound and is primarily an inspiratory sound. May be diminished in older, obese, or very muscular patients. Harsher sounds heard if ventilations are rapid and deep or in children due to their thin, elastic chest walls.

BREATH SOUNDS	OTHER TERMS	DESCRIPTION
Normal	Clear	Clear and quiet breath sounds heard during inspiration and expiration - louder during inspiration.
Rales	Crackles Crepitation Wet	Crackling, popping sound produced by air passing over airway secretions/fluid or the sudden opening of collapsed airways. May be coarse or fine and heard usually on inspiration but can be heard on expiration - louder during inspiration.
Rhonchi	Sonorous rales Congested	Low- pitched continuous rumbling, snoring sound produced by narrowing of the larger airways due to thick secretions or muscle spasms. Sonorous wheezing sound may be heard on inspiration or expiration (usually expiration). This often clears or changes with coughing.
Wheezes	Musical rales	High-pitched continuous sound produced by narrowing of the smaller airways. Whistling sound may be heard on inspiration or expiration - louder during expiration. More severe if heard on inspiration.
Stridor	Crowing	Brassy, crowing sound produced by obstruction in the upper airways. May be caused by epiglottitis, viral croup, or foreign body - most prominent on inspiration. Heard best over the larynx or trachea.

NOTES:

- Firm pressure is necessary to eliminate friction sounds of chest hairs rubbing against stethoscope.

- Breath sounds are heard more prominently at the mid-lung field because the lungs are smaller at the apices and bases.

- Compare sounds heard bilaterally and listen to both the inspiratory and expiratory phase.

- DO NOT listen to breath sounds over clothing. This results in <u>significant</u> alteration of sounds heard.

- If rales are suspected, but difficult to hear, have patient cough to clear secretions.

- As patients become more severe breath sounds may cross over and a combination of sounds may be heard or one sound obliterated by another.

Auscultation Sites

Anterior	Posterior
<u>Apices</u> - 1 inch below the clavicle at mid-clavicular line	<u>Apices</u> - vertebral border at the level of T-3 (3rd rib)
<u>Mid-lung fields</u> - 3rd-4th ICS at mid-clavicular line	<u>Mid-lung fields</u> - inferior angle of the scapula
<u>Bases</u> - 6th intercostal space at mid- axillary line	<u>Bases</u> - 3 finger breadths below the inferior angle of the scapula at the level of the diaphragm (approx. 10th rib)

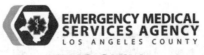

EMERGENCY MEDICAL SERVICES AGENCY
LOS ANGELES COUNTY

EMS SKILL

PATIENT ASSESSMENT
CHEST AUSCULTATION

PERFORMANCE OBJECTIVES
Demonstrate proficiency in performing rapid and/or comprehensive auscultation of the anterior and posterior breath sounds.

CONDITION
Auscultate anterior and posterior breath sounds and perform rapid chest auscultation in critical situations using a live model or respiration simulator. Necessary equipment will be adjacent to the patient or brought to the field setting.

EQUIPMENT
Live model or respiration simulator, stethoscope/dual teaching stethoscope, goggles, mask, gown, gloves.

PERFORMANCE CRITERIA
- Items designated by a diamond (♦) must be performed successfully to demonstrate skill competency.
- Items identified by double asterisks (**) indicate actions that are required if indicated.
- Items identified by (§) are not skill component items, but should be practiced.

PREPARATION	
Skill Component	**Key Concepts**
♦ Take body substance isolation precautions	• Mandatory personal protective equipment - gloves
♦ Direct patient to breathe <u>deeply</u> in and out through open mouth when ready to listen at specific areas	• Breathing with an open mouth increases air velocity resulting in more accurate sounds. • Having patient cough if breaths are congested will clear secretions result in hearing clearer sounds such as crackles (rales).
♦ Place diaphragm of stethoscope directly on patient's skin over auscultation site	• Hold the stethoscope head between index and middle fingers and press firmly against the chest; allows better transmission of breath sounds and eliminates external noises. • Maintaining patient modesty, diaphragm of the stethoscope may be slipped into place under clothing without exposing patient.

RAPID AUSCULTATION PROCEDURE	
Skill Component	**Key Concepts**
♦ Listen for <u>presence</u> and <u>equality</u> of bilateral breath sounds only: • Instruct patient to take a deep breath - *if responsive* • Listen at 5th - 6th intercostal space mid-axillary line	• Rapid auscultation should be done in emergency situations and after endotracheal tube/esophageal tracheal combitube intubation. • Assess only 1-2 breaths to confirm presence and equality of breath sounds. • Determining the type of breath sounds present requires further evaluation which is not appropriate at this time.

ANTERIOR CHEST AUSCULTATION PROCEDURE	
Skill Component	**Key Concepts**
♦ Listen to a minimum of 3 bilateral anterior fields: • Apices - 1" below the clavicle at mid-clavicular line • Mid-lung fields - 3rd - 4th ICS at mid-clavicular line • Bases - 6th intercostal space at mid-axillary line	• <u>Apices</u> - sound is more bronchial (air movement) and quieter • <u>Mid-lung fields</u> - usually heard the loudest • <u>Bases</u> - sounds more vesicular (alveolar exchange) and quieter • In <u>infants and small children</u>, breath sounds may be heard over the entire chest and abdomen due to the small size of the chest.

POSTERIOR CHEST AUSCULTATION
PROCEDURE

Skill Component	Key Concepts
◆ Listen to a minimum of 3 bilateral posterior fields: • Apices - vertebral border at the level of T-3 (3rd rib) • Mid-lung fields - inferior angle of the scapula • Bases - 3 finger breadths below the inferior angle of the scapula at the level of the diaphragm (approx. 10th rib)	• Flex shoulders anteriorly to spread scapulae in order to hear breath sounds more accurately. • In pediatric patients breath sounds may be heard throughout torso. • *Auscultation of the posterior chest is preferred because sounds can be heard better in this location.*

REASSESSMENT
(Ongoing Assessment

Skill Component	Key Concepts
§ Auscultate anterior or posterior breath sounds as required:	• Rapid chest auscultation may be appropriate in situations where only breath sounds confirmation is needed. • Full assessment of all 6 fields either anteriorly or posteriorly may be needed to assess changes in patient's pulmonary status.

PATIENT REPORT AND DOCUMENTATION

Skill Component	Key Concepts

§ Verbalize/Document:
• Initial and ongoing breath sounds:
  - type of sounds heard
  - absent sounds
• Location of auscultation (anterior or posterior)
• Site of sounds heard - *if abnormal*
	• Documentation must be on either the Los Angeles County EMS Report form or departmental Patient Care Record form.
	• If absent breath sounds or unable to obtain, document reason sounds could not be heard/obtained.
	  - If absent - may be due to lobectomy, atelectasis, tight airways, bronchospasms, or an unknown reason.
	  - If unable to obtain, may be due to environment too noisy or dangerous, patient refuses, etc.

Developed 3/02   Revised 1/10

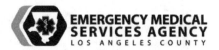

PATIENT ASSESSMENT / VITAL SIGNS
ORTHOSTATIC
Supplemental Information

PURPOSE:

- To assess potential for hidden blood loss or decrease in circulating blood volume.

INDICATION:

- Suspicion of possible hypovolemia in patients who have a normal blood pressure and pulse rate.

CONTRAINDICATIONS:

- Hemorrhage/hypovolemia
- Altered level of consciousness
- Possible spinal injury
- Signs of inadequate perfusion - weakness, dizziness, syncope
- Signs of decreased circulating volume
- Patients with irregular pulse or bradycardia

NOTES:

- Orthostatic vital signs are also known as postural vital signs or tilt test. This is a diagnostic procedure and not pertinent for field assessment.
- Orthostatic vital signs are normally performed in 3 steps: lying → sitting → standing.
- A decrease of 10-20mm/Hg in either the systolic or diastolic pressure, or an increase of 10-20 beats/minute in the pulse rate represents positive orthostatic changes. Physicians and text sources vary as to what values are considered positive; therefore 10-20 range is given.
- Only one factor, a decrease of the systolic or diastolic blood pressure or an increase in the pulse, is required to determine a positive orthostatic change.
- Patients with positive orthostatic changes should be suspected of having hidden blood loss and transported to the hospital for further evaluation.
- Important to obtain a medical history as to medications because patients on calcium channel or beta blockers may not have the ability to raise their pulse rate.

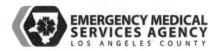

EMERGENCY MEDICAL SERVICES AGENCY
LOS ANGELES COUNTY

EMS SKILL

PATIENT ASSESSMENT / VITAL SIGNS
ORTHOSTATIC

PERFORMANCE OBJECTIVES

Demonstrate competency in obtaining accurate orthostatic vital signs.

CONDITION

Demonstrate competency in taking an accurate blood pressure and pulse to determine orthostatic vital signs on a live model with the patient lying supine, sitting and standing. Necessary equipment will be adjacent to the patient or brought to the field setting.

EQUIPMENT

Live model, large/medium sphygmomanometer, stethoscope/dual teaching stethoscope, timing device, gloves.

PERFORMANCE CRITERIA

- Items designated by a diamond (♦) must be performed successfully to demonstrate skill competency.
- Items identified by double asterisks (**) indicate actions that are required if indicated.
- Items identified by (§) are not skill component items, but should be practiced.
- Reading must be within +/- 6 mm/Hg for blood pressure and +/- 4 beats/minute for pulse of examiner's determination.

PREPARATION	
Skill Component	**Key Concepts**
♦ Take body substance isolation precautions	• Mandatory (minimal) personal protective equipment – gloves

PROCEDURE	
Skill Component	**Key Concepts**
♦ Have patient lie supine for full 1 minute: • Auscultate blood pressure • Assess pulse for rate, quality, and regularity	• Appropriate cuff size must be selected or inaccurate readings will be obtained. • The supine position for 1 minute allows patient to equilibrate to the highest pressure reading. • If hypovolemia is suspected, treat as orthostatic positive. DO NOT sit or stand patient up.
♦ Have patient sit for 1 full minute: • Auscultate blood pressure • Assess pulse for rate, quality, and regularity	• If signs of dizziness or syncope occur, place patient in supine position and discontinue test.
♦ Have patient stand for 1 full minute: • Auscultate blood pressure • Assess pulse for rate, quality, and regularity	• Decrease of 10-20 points in either the systolic or diastolic pressure indicates positive orthostatic change. • Increase of 10-20 beats per minute in pulse rate indicates positive orthostatic change.

REASSESSMENT	
(Ongoing Assessment)	
Skill Component	**Teaching Points**
♦ Repeat assessment at least every **5 minutes for priority** patients and every **15 minutes for stable** patients. • Primary assessment • Relevant portion of the secondary assessment • Vital signs	• Priority patients are patients who have abnormal vital signs, S/S of poor perfusion, if there is a suspicion that the patient's condition may deteriorate, or when the patient's condition changes.

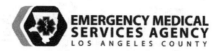

PATIENT ASSESSMENT / VITAL SIGNS
PULSE
Supplemental Information

DEFINITIONS:

- Rate - number of heart beats per minute:

  - Initial assessment - determine if fast or slow, rate is not counted during the initial assessment

  - Focused/Ongoing assessment - rate can be calculated by counting for 30 seconds and multiplying by 2
  - A 6 second pulse count is NOT acceptable due to inaccuracy of the count and mathematical errors
  - A 15 second pulse count should not be used due to missing an irregular rhythm that may be present

- Rhythm (regularity) - heart rhythm may be either regular or irregular. The rhythm may be either regularly-irregular or irregularly-irregular.

  - Regular rhythm - consistent interval between beats

  - Irregular rhythm - a beat may be early, late or missed. An irregular pulse should be counted for 1 full minute.

  * *All irregular rhythms are considered abnormal rhythms until proven otherwise.* The young and athletes have commonly regularly-irregular pulses as a normal event called sinus arrhythmia. Pulse accelerates with inspiration and slows with expiration.

- Quality (strength) - determines the feel of the pulse and described as: strong, full or bounding, weak or thready

Normal Pulse Rate		Pulse Quality/Strength		Palpated Pulse in Relation to Blood Pressure
Adult	60-100	Strong	normal	Adult blood pressures
Adolescent 11-14 years	60-105	Full/bounding	stronger than normal	Radial approximately ≥ 80 Systolic
School Age 6-10 years	70-110	Weak/thready	difficult to feel	Brachial approximately ≥ 70 Systolic
Preschool 3-5 years	80-120			Femoral approximately ≥ 70 Systolic
Toddler 1-3 years	80-130			Carotid approximately ≥ 60 Systolic
Infant 6-12 months	80-140			
Infant 0-5 months	90-140			*(pressure is lost in the order indicated -- from radial to the carotid pulse)*
Newborn (Neonate) 0-28 days	120-140			

COMMON CAUSES OF ABNORMAL PULSE RATE OR RHYTHM		
Tachycardia	**Bradycardia**	**Irregular Rhythm**
Exercise Hypoxia Fever Infection Hypovolemia Hyperthyroidism Emotional upset Stimulating drugs/medications Myocardial infarction Pain Hyperthermia	Heart disease Organophosphates Calcium channel or beta blocking agents Vagal response Myocardial infarction Pain Intracranial pressure CNS depressing drugs/medications Athletic conditioning Hypothermia	Electrolyte imbalance Conduction defects Cardiac damage (MI) Drug/Chemical ingestion or exposure Medications Hypoxia Abnormal body temperature

Note:
- 10-15% of pedal pulses are difficult to find. Check other signs of circulation. Mark pulses with an "X" if located.

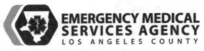

PATIENT ASSESSMENT / VITAL SIGNS
PULSE

PERFORMANCE OBJECTIVES
Demonstrate competency in performing an accurate pulse assessment.

CONDITION
Perform an accurate pulse assessment for the primary and secondary assessment. The examiner assesses the opposite radial or brachial pulse to determine the accuracy of the assessment. Necessary equipment will be adjacent to the patient or brought to the field setting.

EQUIPMENT
Live model, timing device, stethoscope, goggles, mask, gown, gloves.

PERFORMANCE CRITERIA
- Items designated by a diamond (♦) must be performed successfully to demonstrate skill competency.
- Items identified by double asterisks (**) indicate actions that are required if indicated.
- Items identified by (§) are not skill component items, but should be practiced.
- Reading must be within +/- 4 beats/minute of examiner's determination.

PREPARATION	
Skill Component	**Key Concepts**
♦ Take body substance isolation precautions	• Mandatory (minimal) personal protective equipment – gloves

§ Locate the most common arterial points:
 	
• Peripheral
  - brachial
  - radial
  - ulnar
  - popliteal
  - tibial (posterior tibial)
  - pedal (dorsalis pedis)
• Central
  - carotid
  - femoral
  - apical
	• Students should be able to locate and palpate all major arterial points.
	• An auscultated apical pulse should be taken on pediatric patients, trauma patients with no detectable pulse, and on patients who are to be pronounced dead in the field.
	• Central pulses should be palpated if unable to palpate peripheral pulses.
	• If patient is critical, peripheral and central pulses should be palpated simultaneously.
	• Palpate pulse with 2 fingers. DO NOT use thumb to palpate due to the possibility of feeling one's own pulse.
	• Femoral pulses are palpated in the inguinal fold - avoid inference of impropriety.
	• Pedal pulses (10-15%) are often difficult to find. Check other signs of circulation. Mark pulses with an "X" if located.

PRIMARY ASSESSMENT	
Skill Component	**Key Concepts**

♦ Assess pulse:
• Rate (normal, fast, slow)
• Rhythm (regularity)
• Quality (strength)
 	
** *Consider cardiac monitor - if pulse is irregular*
	• Rate - determine if fast or slow. The actual beats per minute are not counted during the primary assessment.
	• Rhythm (regularity) - heart rhythm may be either regular or irregular.
	  - regular rhythm - consistent interval between beats
	  - irregular rhythm - a beat may be early, late or missed. The rhythm may be either regularly-irregular or irregularly-irregular.
	  * *All irregular rhythms are abnormal rhythms.*
	• Quality (strength) - determines the feel of the pulse and described as: strong (normal), full or bounding (stronger than normal), weak or thready (difficult to feel).

SECONDARY ASSESSMENT

Skill Component	Key Concepts

◆ Assess pulse:
  • Rate (beats/minute)
  • Rhythm (regularity)
  • Quality (strength)
 	
** *Consider cardiac monitor - if pulse is irregular*
	• Rate can be calculated by counting for 30 seconds and multiplying by 2.
	  - A 15 second count may be inaccurate and irregular rhythms may be missed.
	  - A 6 second pulse count is NOT acceptable due to inaccuracy of the count, missing irregular rhythms and mathematical errors.
	• An irregular pulse should be counted for 1 full minute.
	• DO NOT rely on monitor rate indicator. The monitor may pick up various wave forms and count as a pulse if the gain is too high or may not pick up the pulse if the gain is too low.

REASSESSMENT
(Ongoing Assessment)

Skill Component	Key Concepts

§ Repeat pulse assessment:
 	
  • Every 5 minutes for priority patients
  • Every 15 minutes for stable patients	

§ Re-assess pulse:
  • Rate (beats/minute)
  • Rhythm (regularity)
  • Quality (strength)
 	
** *Consider cardiac monitor - if pulse is irregular*	

PATIENT REPORT AND DOCUMENTATION

Skill Component	Key Concepts

§ Verbalize/Document:
 	
  • Rate (beats/minute)
  • Rhythm (regularity)
  • Quality (strength)
  • ECG reading - *if applicable*
	• If patient is placed on a monitor, run at least two (2) 6 second strips and attach one strip to the provider copy and one strip to the receiving copy of the EMS form.
	• If the monitor is applied, document the palpated pulse and the pulse rate on the monitor. DO NOT rely just on the monitor read out .
	• Documentation must be on either the Los Angeles County EMS Report form or departmental Patient Care Record form.

Developed: 3/02 Revised 12/09

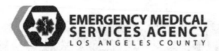

PATIENT ASSESSMENT / VITAL SIGNS
RESPIRATIONS / BREATHING
Supplemental Information

DEFINITIONS:

- Accessory muscles - muscles used when a patient has difficulty breathing. They include the shoulder muscle (trapezius), neck muscles (sternocleidomastoid and scalenus), chest muscles (pectoralis and intercostals), and abdominal muscles.

- Dyspnea - subjective feeling of shortness of breath - usually associated with heart or lung disease, but occurs normally with intense physical activity or in high altitudes.

- Inspiratory-Expiratory ratio (I:E ratio) - this ratio is time of inspiration to time of expiration. The active inhalation phase lasts 1/3 the time of the passive exhalation phase. It takes longer to exhale than to inhale. If the rate of breathing increases, the ratio may change to 1:2 or 1:1 depending on the rate. In patients with COPD and asthma, air trapping occurs and to exhale completely the ratio may increase to 1:4.

- Respiration (ventilations) - in normal breathing each breath includes 2 phases; inspiration and expiration

- Tripod position - abnormal position to keep airway open. The patient is in a sitting position leaning forward on both arms and demonstrates a conscious effort to breathe

NOTES:

- The amount of air exchange that occurs is dependent on the rate and the tidal volume.

- Respiratory rate can be calculated by counting for 30 seconds and multiplied by 2. Abnormal pattern should be counted for 1 full minute.

- Respiratory rate > 40 or < 10 may not provide adequate tidal volume. Be prepared to assist with bag-valve-mask ventilation if level of consciousness is decreased.

- An adult patient breathing slower than 10 breaths/minute or faster than 24 breaths/minute should be evaluated for inadequate breathing.

- Signs of respiratory distress:

  - Respiratory rate slower than 10 breaths/minute or greater than 24 breaths/minute
  - Accessory muscle use
  - Intercostal and sternal retractions
  - Pale, cyanotic, or cool (clammy) skin
  - Abnormal I:E ratio
  - Abnormal respiratory pattern
  - Decreased, unequal or abnormal lung sounds
  - labored breathing
  - Shallow or uneven chest rise and fall
  - Unable to speak in complete sentences between breaths (only 2-3 words at a time)

Type of Respirations	Characteristics	Possible Cause
Normal/Adequate	Breathing is ordinary - neither deep or shallow	Normal respirations
Shallow	Slight movement of the chest or abdomen	Respiratory depression, chest wall injury, pleuritic pain
Labored	Increased effort of breathing, use of accessory muscles, *nasal flaring, *intercostal retractions, * sternal retraction * mostly seen in infants and children	Respiratory insufficiency and failure *(In infants and children, cardiac arrest is most commonly caused by respiratory arrest)*
Noisy	Snoring, wheezing, gurgling, crowing and stridor	Partial airway obstruction from a foreign object, swelling, neck position, fluid in the lungs, or constriction of the airways

PATIENT ASSESSMENT / VITAL SIGNS
RESPIRATIONS / BREATHING
(Continued)

Tidal Volume	Normal Respiratory Rates	Accessory Muscles
Normal/Adequate Increased Shallow (decreased)	Adults 12-20 Child 15-30 Infants 25-50 Newborn 30-60	**Adults** • Trapezius (shoulder) *[assist with inspiration]* • Sternocleidomastoid (neck) *[assist with inspiration]* • Scalenus (neck) *[assist with inspiration]* • Abdominal *[assist with expiration]* **Pediatric** • Intercostal retractions • Sternal retractions **"Children retract in severity from the bottom up"**

Respiratory Patterns

Graph obtained from Saunders, Paramedic Textbook 2nd ed. Fig. 11-13

Respirations	Definition
Eupnea	Normal breathing
Bradypnea	Slower than normal rate
Apnea	No breathing
Tachypnea	Faster than normal rate
Hyperventilation (hyperpnea)	Increased rate and/or depth (faster and/or deeper than normal respirations)
Ataxic	Irregularly - irregular
Biot's	Irregular with periods of apnea (similar to but not as regular as Cheyne Stokes)
Cheyne-Stokes	Regular increase and decrease in depth followed by a period of apnea
Kussmaul	Rapid, regular deep respirations caused by diabetic ketoacidosis or other metabolic acidosis
Central Neurogenic Hyperventilation	Pattern similar to Kussmaul but caused by increased intracranial pressure (head injury)
Air trapping	Prolonged but inefficient expiratory effort, commonly seen in COPD or asthma
Sighing	An occasional deep, audible inspiration that is insignificant

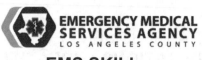

PATIENT ASSESSMENT / VITAL SIGNS
RESPIRATIONS / BREATHING

PERFORMANCE OBJECTIVES
Demonstrate proficiency in performing an accurate respiratory assessment.

CONDITION
Perform an accurate respiratory assessment for the primary and secondary assessment. The examiner will assess respirations with the examinee to determine the accuracy of the assessment. Necessary equipment will be adjacent to the patient.

EQUIPMENT
Live model, timing device, goggles, mask, gown, gloves.

PERFORMANCE CRITERIA
- Items designated by a diamond (♦) must be performed successfully to demonstrate skill competency.
- Items identified by double asterisks (**) indicate actions that are required if indicated.
- Items identified by (§) are not skill component items, but should be practiced.
- Reading must be within +/- 2 breaths/minute of examiner's determination.

PREPARATION	
Skill Component	**Key Concepts**
♦ Take body substance isolation precautions ** ***Place a mask on the patient - if suspected airborne disease*** ** ***Place mask on patient and a HEPA respirator on rescuer - if suspected tuberculosis***	• Mandatory personal protective equipment - gloves • Situational - goggles, mask, gown

PRIMARY ASSESSMENT	
Skill Component	**Key Concepts**
♦ Observe or feel for rise and fall of chest or abdomen	• Evaluate patient's respirations as subtly as possible. Patients have a tendency to increase their respirations if they know they are being assessed. • The rescuer may have to feel the patient's chest or abdomen to check for rise and fall if tidal volume is decreased or patient is dressed in a large jacket or many layers of clothing. Lay patient's arm over chest or abdomen, watch movement of shoulders, etc. • Infants are "abdominal breathers" which causes the abdomen to protrude and the chest wall to retract.
♦ Assess respirations/Manage breathing: • Rate (normal, fast, slow) • Effort/Quality • Tidal volume ** ***Consider O₂ therapy*** ** ***Consider BVM - if inadequate ventilation***	• <u>Rate</u> - determine if fast or slow. Rate is not counted during the initial assessment. • <u>Effort/Quality</u> - evaluated by the use of accessory muscles, patient position (tripod, reclined, etc.) sounds clear or diminished, are equal, labored, noisy, absent and the ability to speak in words, sentences or unable due to being short of breath. • <u>Tidal volume</u> - determine if normal, adequate, shallow, increased or decreased. • Determine if tidal volume and rate are adequate to assure effective ventilation - use BVM to increase tidal volume or rate if necessary. • Administer O2 whenever vital organs are at risk for hypoperfusion and/or hypoxia.
♦ Assess breath sounds (rapid chest auscultation) - *if difficulty breathing or shortness of breath*	• Assess only 1-2 breaths to confirm presence and equality of breath sounds at 5th - 6th intercostal space mid-axillary line.

SECONDARY ASSESSMENT

Skill Component	Key Concepts
♦ Observe or feel for rise and fall of chest or abdomen	
♦ Assess/Manage breathing: • Rate (respirations/minute) • Effort/Quality • Tidal volume • Rhythm/Pattern (regular/irregular) ** *Consider O₂ therapy* ** *Consider BVM - if inadequate ventilation* ** *Place a mask on the patient - if suspected airborne disease and not already done* ** *Place mask on patient and a HEPA respirator on rescuer - if suspected tuberculosis and not already done*	• Rate can be calculated by counting for 30 seconds and multiplying by 2. Abnormal pattern should be counted for 1 full minute. • Respiratory rate >40 or <10 may not provide adequate tidal volume. Be prepared to assist with bag-valve-mask ventilation if level of consciousness is decreased. • Respiratory rhythm assessed is either regular or irregular. • Respiratory pattern is determined after complete assessment and may include any of the following: 　- normal　　　- sighing　　　- Biot's 　- bradypnea　- Cheyne-Stokes　- ataxic 　- tachypnea　- Kussmaul　　- air-trapping 　- agonal　　　- hyperventilation (hyperpnea)
♦ Assess breath sounds (3 bilateral anterior or posterior fields) - *if difficulty breathing or shortness of breath*	• Breath sounds are assessed in three (3) bilateral anterior or posterior fields; apices, mid-lung, and bases.

REASSESSMENT
(Ongoing Assessment)

Skill Component	Key Concepts
§ Repeat respiratory assessment: • Every 5 minutes for priority patients • Every 15 minutes for stable patients	• Priority patients are patients who have abnormal vital signs, S/S of poor perfusion, if there is a suspicion that the patient's condition may deteriorate, or when the patient's condition changes.
§ Observe or feel for rise and fall of chest or abdomen	
§ Re-assess/Manage breathing: • Rate (respirations/minute) • Effort/Quality • Tidal volume • Rhythm/Pattern (regular or irregular) ** *Consider O₂ therapy* ** *Consider BVM - if inadequate ventilation*	
§ Re-assess breath sounds (3 bilateral anterior or posterior fields) - *if difficulty breathing or shortness of breath*	• Re-assess full breath sounds whenever there is a change in patient's condition or respiratory pattern.
§ Give patient report to equal or higher level of care provider **Exception**: *Report may be given to a lower level of care provider when an ALS to BLS downgrade has occurred*	• Report should consist of all pertinent information regarding the assessment findings, treatment rendered and patients response to care provided.

PATIENT REPORT AND DOCUMENTATION

Skill Component	Key Concepts
§ Verbalize/Document: • Respiratory assessment: 　- rate (respirations/minute) 　- effort/quality 　- tidal volume 　- rhythm/pattern (regular or irregular) • Breath sounds • Oxygen administration: 　- airway adjunct/ventilatory devices used 　- oxygen liter flow 　- ventilation rate	• Respiratory rate, tidal volume, rhythm/pattern and breath sounds should be reported and documented. • Airway adjuncts and ventilatory devices are mechanical aids that assist in maintaining a patent airway, ventilating or delivering oxygen. These adjuncts/devices include: oxygen mask, nasal cannula, oropharyngeal and nasopharyngeal airway, bag-valve-mask, a tracheostomy, endotracheal or esophageal combitube, etc. • Documentation must be on either the Los Angeles County EMS Report or departmental Patient Care Record form.

SOFT TISSUE INJURY / BANDAGING
ABDOMINAL EVISCERATION

NOTES:

- The exposed organs must be covered with a moist dressing and kept warm because an open abdominal cavity radiates body heat and exposed organs lose fluid rapidly.

- Sterile or tap water should never be used to wet dressings because the water is hypotonic and will draw water into cells resulting in cell destruction.

- Flexing the patient's legs and knees relieves pressure on the abdominal wall musculature.

- Dry dressings adhere and dry out normally moist tissues which causes further destruction and necrosis of the exposed organs.

- DO NOT touch or try to replace any eviscerated organ.

- DO NOT delay transport to apply an occlusive dressing, this is only necessary if there is a possibility of long field or transport time. The healthcare provider should frequently check to see that dressings remain moist and if necessary wet them as needed.

- DO NOT use any material that is adhering or loses substance when wet.

- DO NOT use aluminum foil, this may cause laceration of the eviscerated organ. Occlusive dressings consist of clear plastic wrap.

Developed: 1/02

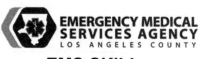

EMERGENCY MEDICAL SERVICES AGENCY
LOS ANGELES COUNTY

EMS SKILL

SOFT TISSUE INJURY / BANDAGING
ABDOMINAL EVISCERATION

PERFORMANCE OBJECTIVES

Demonstrate competency in applying a dressing to an open abdominal injury with an evisceration of the intestines.

CONDITION

Assess and dress an open abdominal injury with an evisceration of the intestines. Necessary equipment will be adjacent to the patient or brought to the field setting.

EQUIPMENT

Manikin or live model, bag-valve-mask device, O_2 connecting tubing, oxygen source with flow regulator, 4"x4" dressings, large lap or multitrauma dressings, clear plastic wrap, tape, goggles, masks, gown, gloves.

PERFORMANCE CRITERIA

*   Items designated by a diamond (♦) must be performed successfully to demonstrate skill competency.
*   Items identified by double asterisks (**) indicate actions that are required if indicated.
*   Items identified by (§) are not skill component items, but should be practiced.

PREPARATION	
Skill Component	**Key Concepts**
♦ Take body substance isolation precautions	• Mandatory (minimal) personal protective equipment – gloves
♦ Assess scene safety/scene size-up ** ***Consider spinal immobilization - if indicated***	• Spinal immobilization should be initiated when spinal trauma is suspected by taking bystander information and mechanism of injury into consideration.
♦ Evaluate need for additional BSI precautions	• Situational - goggles, mask, gown
♦ Assess severity of bleeding: • Arterial • Venous • Capillary	
♦ Remove enough clothing to expose the entire wound	

PROCEDURE	
Skill Component	**Key Concepts**
♦ Soak a large sterile dressing with sterile saline	• DO NOT use water (sterile or tap) to wet dressings; water is hypotonic and may draw water from the cells resulting in cell dehydration.
♦ Place several (2-3 layers) sterile moist dressings over wound	• Scoop up the eviscerated organ using a moist saline dressing and DO NOT directly handle the eviscerated parts with hands or unsterile objects. • DO NOT attempt to replace eviscerated organs but cover them with a moist sterile dressing or an air tight non-adhering dressing to prevent organ dehydration. *Dry dressings adhere to and dry out moist tissues resulting in further destruction and necrosis of abdominal organs.* • DO NOT use petroleum gauze, adhering material, or any material that may lose substance when wet.

Skill Component	Key Concepts
♦ Apply a dry abdominal dressing or an occlusive dressing over the moist dressing ** ***Prepare for rapid transport***	• Occlusive dressings consist of plastic wrap or sheeting or additional dry dressings over the moist dressing. DO NOT use aluminum foil, this may cause laceration of the eviscerated organ. • DO NOT delay transport to apply an occlusive dressing over the moist dressing. • Secure dressings by taping around all sides or tying cravats above and below the position of the exposed eviscerated organ • Cravats are ties used to keep dressings secured; especially if patients are allergic to tape or have excoriated skin.
♦ Flex patient's hips and knees – *if uninjured and spinal immobilization is not required*	• Flexing the patient's hips and knees decreases tension on abdominal muscles. • Place a pillow or other padding material under knees to keep the knees flexed.
♦ Keep eviscerated organs moist and warm ** ***Re-saturate dressings as needed to prevent dressings from becoming dry***	• Organ dehydration and heat loss occurs rapidly with an open abdominal cavity. Place towels or occlusive dressings over the dressings already applied. • The EMS provider should frequently check to see that dressings remain moist and wet them as needed.
♦ Transport patient supine with hips and knees flexed	• When hips and knees are flexed it decreases discomfort/pain and relaxes the abdominal muscles.
§ Explain the care being delivered and transport destination to the patient/caregiver	• Communication is important when dealing with the patient, family or caregiver. This is a very critical and frightening time for all involved and providing information helps in decreasing the stress they are experiencing.

REASSESSMENT
(Ongoing Assessment)

Skill Component	Key Concepts
♦ Repeat assessment at least every **5 minutes for priority** patients and every **15 minutes for stable** patients. • Primary assessment • Relevant portion of the secondary assessment • Vital signs	• Priority patients are patients who have abnormal vital signs, S/S of poor perfusion, if there is a suspicion that the patient's condition may deteriorate, or when the patient's condition changes.
♦ Evaluate response to treatment	• Patients must be re-evaluated at least every 5 minutes if any treatment was initiated, medication administered or unless a change in the patient's condition is anticipated.
♦ Evaluate results of reassessment and note any changes from patient's previous condition and vital signs ** ***Manage patient condition as indicated.***	• Evaluating and comparing results assists in recognizing if the patient is improving, responding to treatment or condition is deteriorating.

PATIENT REPORT AND DOCUMENTATION

Skill Component	Key Concepts
§ Verbalize/Document: • Mechanism of injury • Description of injury • Treatment rendered	• Documentation must be on either the Los Angeles County EMS Report or departmental Patient Care Record form. • Documenting reassessment information provides a comprehensive picture of patient's response to treatment. • Last reassessment information (before patient care is transferred) should be documented in the section of the EMS form that is called "Reassessment after Therapies and/or Condition on Transfer".

Developed: 1/02   Revised: 9/09

SOFT TISSUE INJURY / BANDAGING
IMPALED OBJECT

INDICATIONS:

• Any impaled object.

CONTRAINDICATIONS

• Impaled objects in the cheek may be removed if the airway is compromised. Impaled objects directly interfering with CPR may also be removed.

COMPLICATIONS:

• Improper stabilization my further aggravate existing trauma

NOTES:

• The use of an occlusive dressing should be considered in treating impaled object in chest and neck.

Developed 7/07

SOFT TISSUE INJURY / BANDAGING
IMPALED OBJECT

PERFORMANCE OBJECTIVES

The examinee will demonstrate proficiency in stabilizing an impaled object.

CONDITION

The examinee will be requested to properly stabilize from a patient with an impaled object located in the chest.

EQUIPMENT

Adult CPR/trauma manikin or live model, all necessary sterile and occlusive dressings, bandages, 1 inch tape, gloves, stethoscope.

PERFORMANCE CRITERIA

- 100% accuracy required on all items designated by a diamond (♦) for skills testing and must manage successfully all items indicated by double asterisks (**).
- Documentation, identified by the symbol (§), must be practiced, but is not a required test item.
- Appropriate body substance isolation precautions must be instituted.

SPECIFIC SKILL PREPARATION	
Skill Component	**Teaching Points**
♦ Take body substance isolation precautions	• Mandatory personal protective equipment - gloves • Situational - long sleeves, goggles, masks, gown
♦ Explain Procedure to patient	• Maintain patient rapport
♦ **Hold impaled object to stabilize**	• Ensure that assistant is in proper position

PROCEDURE	
Skill Component	**Teaching Points**
♦ Expose site, if signs of sucking chest wound are present place an occlusive dressing around object, directly on patients skin	
♦ Place several layers of a bulky dressing around the object and secure in place while maintaining stabilization	

ONGOING ASSESSMENT	
Skill Component	**Teaching Points**
§ Continue to reassess patient	• Emphasize the possible indications of tension pneumothorax when stabilizing a penetrating chest injury

DOCUMENTATION	
Skill Component	**Teaching Points**
§ Verbalize/Document: • Mechanism of injury • Description of injury • Treatment provided	

Developed 7/07

SOFT TISSUE INJURY / BANDAGING
OCCLUSIVE DRESSING

INDICATIONS:

- Penetrating trauma to the thorax, upper abdomen (bandage to be taped on three sides)
- Penetrating trauma to the neck (bandage to be taped on four sides)

CONTRAINDICATIONS

- Do **NOT** allow Vaseline near an abdominal evisceration.

COMPLICATIONS:

- Tension pneumothorax
- Inadequate flutter valve effect due to blood building up under dressing

NOTES:

- Oxygen therapy should always be initiated as soon as possible.
- After applying an occlusive dressing to the thorax or upper abdomen, the EMT should be alert for signs and symptoms suggesting a tension pneumothorax. These include increasing dyspnea, shock, jugular venous distension, and rarely tracheal deviation; should this occur, the dressing should be immediately removed to relieve the tension pneumothorax.
- All chest wounds you believe entered the thoracic cavity should be sealed regardless of whether or not they are bubbling.

Developed 7/07

SOFT TISSUE INJURY / BANDAGING
OCCLUSIVE DRESSING

PERFORMANCE OBJECTIVES

The examinee will demonstrate proficiency in applying an occlusive dressing.

CONDITION

The examinee will be requested to properly apply an occlusive dressing to either the head or neck.

EQUIPMENT

Adult CPR/trauma manikin or live model, all necessary sterile and occlusive dressings, bandages, 1 inch tape, gloves, stethoscope.

PERFORMANCE CRITERIA

- 100% accuracy required on all items designated by a diamond (♦) for skills testing and must manage successfully all items indicated by double asterisks (**).
- Documentation, identified by the symbol (§), must be practiced, but is not a required test item.
- Appropriate body substance isolation precautions must be instituted.

APPLICATION OF OCCLUSIVE DRESSING PREPARATION	
Skill Component	**Teaching Points**
♦ Take body substance isolation precautions	• Mandatory personal protective equipment - gloves • Situational - long sleeves, goggles, masks, gown
♦ Explain Procedure to patient	• Maintain patient rapport
♦ Remove any clothing in affected body area	
♦ Shave area if needed	
♦ Remove any blood from the area of penetrating trauma	

PROCEDURE	
Skill Component	**Teaching Points**
♦ Place occlusive dressing to area	• If the patient is responsive, ask the patient to cough. Place the dressing on the wound after the cough.
♦ Seal three sides of the occlusive dressing with tape if in thoracic area, seal all four sides if in the neck	• Insure that dressing extends past margin of wound.

ONGOING ASSESSMENT	
Skill Component	**Teaching Points**
§ Observe and assess patient (watch for signs and symptoms of tension pneumothorax)	• If applied to thoracic area and condition deteriorates, remove occlusive dressing and reapply as indicated. Tension pneumothorax should be considered if condition worsens, shock occurs, tracheal deviation is present or patient develops jugular venous distension (JVD). • If blood builds up under the dressing and prevents air from escaping, consider removing the dressing, clean the injury site, and reapply the dressing.

Skill Component	Teaching Points
§ Verbalize/Document: • Mechanism of injury • Description of injury • Treatment provided	

Developed 7/07

UCLA CENTER FOR PREHOSPITAL CARE

Los Angeles County Department of Health Services Prehospital Policies

REFERENCE	TITLE
815.2	State EMS Authority Approved (DNR) Medallion
816	Phyician at Scene
819	Organ Donor Identification
821	Physicians Orders for Life Sustaining Treatment (POLST)
821.1	Physicians Orders for Life Sustaining Treatment (POLST) Form
822	Suspected Child Abuse / Neglect Reporting Guidelines
822.2	Suspected Child Abuse Report
823	Elder Abuse and Dependent Adult Abuse Reporting Guidelines
832	Treatment / Transport of Minors
834	Patient Refusal of Treatment or Transport
836	Communicable Disease and Exposure Testing
838	Application of Patient Restraints
1014	EMT Certification

| SUBJECT: | **PRIVATE AMBULANCE PROVIDER** | (EMT-I/PARAMEDIC) |
| | **NON 9-1-1 MEDICAL DISPATCH** | REFERENCE NO. 226 |

PURPOSE: To establish minimum standards for private ambulance medical dispatch.

AUTHORITY: Health and Safety Code, Division 2.5, Sections 1797.220 and 1798 (a), California Code of Regulations, Sections 100172, 100173 and 100175, Ambulance Ordinance 07.16.010 E, G, H,

DEFINITIONS:

ALS Ambulance: Ambulance transport of a patient who requires, or may require, skills or treatment modalities that do not exceed the paramedic scope of practice. An ALS transport may be required for either a non-emergency or emergency transport.

BLS Ambulance: Ambulance transport of a patient who requires skills or treatment modalities that do not exceed the EMT-I scope of practice or expanded scope of practice. A BLS transport may be sufficient to meet the needs of the patient requiring either a non-emergency or emergency transport.

Continuing Dispatch Education: Development and implementation of educational experiences designed to enhance knowledge and skill in the application of medical dispatch.

Emergency call: A request for an ambulance where an individual has a need for immediate medical attention, or where the potential for such need is perceived by the emergency medical personnel or a public safety agency.

Dispatch Medical Director: A physician licensed in California, board certified or qualified in emergency medicine, who possesses knowledge of emergency medical systems in California and the local jurisdiction, and who provides medical dispatch medical direction and oversees medical dispatch.

Non 9-1-1 Medical Dispatcher/Call taker: A person employed by an agency providing medical dispatch services, who has completed an EMS Agency approved medical dispatch program.

Level II Dispatch: A level of service in which a dispatcher is responsible for determining, through key medical questions, whether the call is a life-threatening or non-life-threatening emergency or non-emergency.

Non-emergency call: A request for the transport of a stretcher patient to or from a medical facility in a licensed ambulance and which is neither an emergency call nor a critical care transport.

EFFECTIVE: 10-15-06
REVISED: 10-15-09
SUPERSEDES: 10-15-06

APPROVED: _____
Director, EMS Agency

_____
Medical Director, EMS Agency

Nurse-Staffed Critical Transport (CCT): Ambulance interfacility transport of a patient who requires, or may require, skills or treatment modalities that exceed the paramedic scope of practice. A critical care transport may be required for either a non-emergency or emergency interfacility transport.

PRINCIPLE:

All callers requesting emergent or non-emergent prehospital care shall have direct access to qualified private provider medical dispatch personnel for the provision of dispatch services.

POLICY:

I.   Non 9-1-1 Medical Dispatching

      A.   The dispatcher is responsible for determining, through key medical questions, whether the call is emergent or non-emergent and the level of service required. The dispatcher takes action on the request using pre-established guidelines, determining the level and type of response. In all cases, a medical response is dispatched.

II.   Private Provider Medical Dispatch Standards

      A.   All private ambulance providers shall have written policies approved by the EMS Agency which, at minimum, address all the following requirements:

            1.   Basic Medical Dispatcher Training

            2.   Quality Improvement (QI) Program

            3.   Policies and Procedures

            4.   Staffing

            5.   Medical Direction and Oversight

III.   Basic Medical Dispatcher Program Training

      A.   Medical Dispatcher duties include:

            1.   Receiving and processing calls for non 9-1-1 and/or emergency medical assistance

            2.   Determining the nature and urgency of a medical incident

            3.   Prioritizing the dispatch response

            4.   Dispatching appropriate level of resources and mode of response

            5.   Giving corresponding information to responding personnel

            6.   Coordinating with public safety and EMS providers

B.   Minimum qualifications for medical dispatcher:

1.   Current First Responder BLS Cardiopulmonary Resuscitation (CPR) certification according to the standards of the American Heart Association or equivalent

2.   Current certification of Emergency Medical Dispatcher (EMD) or Emergency Telecommunicator (ETC) meeting the standards of the National Academies of Emergency Medical Dispatch

3.   Completion of provider specific in-service program on response and documentation of emergency calls

IV.   Quality Improvement Program:

A.   Be established according to the California EMS Authority's Emergency Medical Services Dispatch Program Guidelines and Los Angeles County's EMS Quality Improvement Program.

B.   Include indicators specific to Emergency Medical Dispatch to foster continuous improvement in performance and quality patient care.

V.   Policies and Procedures shall:

A.   Ensure the medical dispatch call is completed and call back number is obtained.

B.   Provide systematized caller interview questions.

C.   Establish protocols that determine vehicle response mode and configuration based on the medical dispatcher's evaluation of injury or illness severity.

D.   Establish a call classification coding system, for quality assurance and statistical analysis.

E.   Establish a written description of the communications system configuration for the service area including telephone and radio service resources.

F.   Establish a record-keeping system, including report forms or a computer data management system to permit evaluation of patient care records.

VI.   Staffing

A.   The dispatch center shall be staffed with sufficient personnel to accomplish all dispatch operations and management which include:

1.   A readily accessible dispatch supervisor or designee

2.   Medical dispatchers who have met minimum requirements

3.   Medical dispatch staffing on a continuous 24 hour basis

VII.   Medical Direction and Oversight

   A.   Dispatch centers shall appoint a medical director who will provide medical oversight of the dispatch center by review and approval of:

   1.   Policies and procedures related to program approval

   2.   Continuing education processes

   3.   Dispatch guidelines

   B.   Oversee quality improvement, risk management programs and compliance standards.

VIII.   Records Management

   A.   The provider shall retain records of each medical dispatcher training and course completion records in individual emergency medical dispatcher's training file:

   1.   Copy of current CPR certification

   2.   Proof of current EMD or ETC certification

   3.   Continuing Dispatch Education (CDE) including course title, course dates, locations, and number of CDE hours completed

IX.   Continuous Evaluation of Medical Dispatch Centers

   A.   Upon request of the EMS Agency, the following data shall be submitted for continuous evaluation of Medical Dispatch Centers:

   1.   Data Collection

          Such information will include, at minimum, the date and time (hours, minutes, and seconds) for the:

          a.   Initial call

          b.   Dispatch of ambulance

          c.   Ambulance enroute to call

          d.   Ambulance on scene of incident

          e.   Ambulance enroute to facility

          f.   Ambulance arrival at hospital

          g.   Ambulance available

          h.   Canceled, if applicable

i.   Documentation of all calls that have been referred to 9-1-1

2.   Site surveys

The EMS Agency will conduct annual site surveys to audit compliance with medical dispatch standards, agreement obligations, policy and procedure, and any other regulations applicable to the operations of medical dispatch.

CROSS REFERENCES:

Prehospital Care Policy Manual:
Reference No. 517,   **Private Provider Agency Transport/Response Guidelines**
Reference No. 620,   **EMS Quality Improvement Program (EQIP)**
Reference No. 620.1, **EMS Quality Improvement Program (EQIP) Plan**

California Emergency Medical Services Authority Emergency Medical Service Dispatch Program Guidelines #132

DEPARTMENT OF HEALTH SERVICES
COUNTY OF LOS ANGELES

SUBJECT: **PATIENT DESTINATION**

PURPOSE: To ensure that 9-1-1 patients are transported to the most appropriate facility that is staffed, equipped, and prepared to administer emergency and/or definitive care appropriate to the needs of the patient.

AUTHORITY: Health and Safety Code, Division 2.5, Section 1797.220
California Code of Regulations, Title 13, Section 1105 (c)

PRINCIPLES:

1.   9-1-1 patients shall ordinarily be transported to general acute care hospitals with a basic emergency department permit. Transport to other medical facilities (hospitals with a stand-by permit, clinics and other medical facilities approved by the EMS Agency) shall be performed only in accordance with this policy.

2.   In the absence of decisive factors to the contrary 9-1-1 patients shall be transported to the most accessible medical facility equipped, staffed, and prepared to receive emergency cases and administer emergency care appropriate to the needs of the patient.

3.   The most accessible receiving (MAR) facility may or may not be the closest facility geographically. Transport personnel shall take into consideration traffic, weather conditions or other similar factors, which may influence transport time when identifying which hospital is most accessible.

4.   The most appropriate health facility for a patient may be that health facility which is affiliated with the patient's health plan. Depending upon the patient's chief complaint and medical history, it may be advantageous for the patient to be transported to a facility where they can be treated by a personal physician and/or the individual's personal health plan and where medical records are available.

5.   ALS units utilizing Standing Field Treatment Protocols (SFTPs) shall transport patients in accordance with this policy.

6.   Patients shall not be transported to a medical facility that has requested diversion due to internal disaster.

7.   Notwithstanding any other provision of this reference and in accordance with Reference No. 503, Guidelines for Hospitals Requesting Diversion of ALS Patients, final authority for patient destination rests with the base hospital handling the call. Whether diversion requests will be honored depends on available system resources.

EFFECTIVE: 7-20-84
REVISED: 4-01-09
SUPERSEDES: 12-18-06

PAGE 1 OF 5

APPROVED: _____
Director, EMS Agency

_____
Medical Director, EMS Agency

POLICY:

I.   Transport of Patients by EMT-I Personnel

    A.   EMT-I personnel shall transport 9-1-1 patients deemed stable and requiring only basic life support (BLS) to the MAR regardless of its diversion status (exception: internal disaster). For pediatric patients, the MAR is considered to be the most accessible Emergency Department Approved for Pediatrics (EDAP). For perinatal patients, the MAR is considered to be the most accessible perinatal center.

    B.   EMT-I personnel may honor patient requests to be transported to other than the MAR provided that the patient is deemed stable and requires basic life support measures only and the ambulance is not unreasonably removed from its primary area of response.

    C.   In life-threatening situations (e.g., unmanageable airway or uncontrollable hemorrhage) in which the estimated time of arrival (ETA) of the paramedics exceeds the ETA to the MAR, EMT-Is should exercise their clinical judgement as to whether it is in the patient's best interest to be transported prior to the arrival of paramedics.

    D.   EMT-I personnel may transfer care of a patient to another EMT-I team if necessary.

II.   Transport of Patients by Paramedic Personnel

    A.   Patients should be transported to the MAR unless:

        1.   The base hospital determines that a more distant hospital is more appropriate to meet the needs of the patient; or

        2.   The patient meets criteria or guidelines for transport to a specialty care center (i.e., Trauma, Pediatric Trauma, ST-Elevation Myocardial Infarction Receiving Center, EDAP, Pediatric Medical Center, Perinatal, Stroke); or

        3.   The patient requests a specific hospital; and

            a.   The patient's condition is considered sufficiently stable to tolerate additional transport time; and

            b.   The EMS provider has determined that such a transport would not unreasonably remove the unit from its primary area of response. If requests cannot be honored, the provider should attempt to arrange for alternate transportation, i.e., private ambulance, to accommodate the patient's request; and

            c.   The requested hospital does not have a defined service area. (For hospitals with a defined service area, refer to Section V of this policy.)

4. The medical facility has requested diversion to 9-1-1 patients requiring advanced life support (ALS) as specified in Ref. No. 503. ALS patients may be directed to an alternate open facility provided:

   a. The patient does not exhibit an uncontrollable problem in the field as defined by unmanageable airway or uncontrolled hemorrhage.

   b. The involved ALS unit estimates that it can reach an alternate facility within fifteen (15) minutes, Code 3, from the incident location. If there are no open facilities within this time frame, ALS patients shall be directed to the MAR, regardless of its diversion status (exception: Internal Disaster).

B. Paramedic personnel may transfer care of a patient to another paramedic team if necessary. If base hospital contact has been made, the initial paramedic team shall advise the base hospital that another paramedic team has assumed responsibility for the patient.

NOTE: On an "as needed" basis, the EMS Agency may extend the maximum transport time.

III. Destination of Restrained Patients

A. Restrained patients shall be transported to the most accessible basic emergency department facility within the guidelines of this policy. Allowable exceptions:

   1. Patients without a medical complaint, with a 5150 order written by a designated Department of Mental Health Team, when transport to a psychiatric facility has been arranged.

   2. A law enforcement request for transport to medical facilities other than the closest may be honored with base hospital concurrence.

IV. Transport to Health Facilities without a Basic Emergency Department Permit

A. <u>Hospitals with a Stand-by Emergency Department Permit</u>: Patient requests for transport to hospitals with a Stand-by Emergency Department Permit may be honored by EMT-I or paramedic personnel if base hospital contact is made; and

   1. The base hospital concurs that the patient's condition is sufficiently stable to permit the estimated transport time; and

   2. The base hospital contacts the requested hospital and ensures that a physician is on duty and willing to accept the patient.

B. <u>Other medical facilities approved on an individual basis by the EMS Agency</u>: 9-1-1 patients may be transported to medical facilities other than hospitals (i.e., clinics) only when approved in advance by the EMS Agency.

V.   Transport to Health Facilities with a Designated Service Area (Service Area Hospitals)

   A.   Patients shall be transported by EMT-I or paramedic personnel to hospitals with a designated service area whenever the incident location is within the hospital's defined service area (exception: diversion to Internal Disaster). In most instances, the service area hospital is also the MAR.

   B.   If a patient within the defined service area meets criteria or guidelines for a specialty care center not provided by the service area hospital, this patient shall be transported to the appropriate specialty care center.

   C.   Patient requests for transport to: 1) a service area hospital when the incident location is outside the hospital's defined service area or inside the service area of another hospital or; 2) a hospital without a service area when the incident location is within another hospital's defined service area, may be honored by:

      1.   EMT-I personnel if it is a BLS patient, the receiving hospital is contacted and agrees to accept the patient, and the transporting unit is not unreasonably removed from its primary response area.

      2.   Paramedic personnel if the base hospital is contacted and concurs that the patient's condition is sufficiently stable to permit the estimated transport time, the requested hospital agrees to accept the patient, and the transporting unit is not unreasonably removed from its primary response area. The receiving hospital may be contacted directly if the ALS unit is transporting a BLS patient.

VI.   Transport to Specialty Care Centers

   A.   Trauma Center and Pediatric Trauma Center: Transport of trauma patients shall be in accordance with Ref. Nos. 504, 506 and 510. Requests for diversions due to trauma care may be honored as outlined in Ref. No. 503.

   B.   Pediatric Medical Center (PMC): Transport of pediatric patients shall be in accordance with Ref. Nos. 504, 506 and 510. The MAR for the pediatric patient is the most accessible EDAP.

   C.   Perinatal Center: Patients meeting Perinatal Center criteria shall be transported in accordance with Ref. No. 511. The MAR for the perinatal patient is the most accessible Perinatal Center.

   D.   STEMI Receiving Center (SRC): Patients who are experiencing an ST-elevation myocardial infarction (STEMI) as determined by a field 12-lead EKG should be transported to an approved STEMI Receiving Center, regardless of service agreement rules and/or considerations.

   E.   Approved Stroke Center (ASC): Patients who have met the Modified Los Angeles Prehospital Stroke Screen (mLAPSS) criteria and are suspected of experiencing a stroke should be transported to an ASC in accordance with Ref.

No. 521, regardless of service agreement rules and/or considerations.

CROSS REFERENCE:

DEPARTMENT OF HEALTH SERVICES
COUNTY OF LOS ANGELES

SUBJECT: **TRAUMA PATIENT DESTINATION**

(EMT-I, PARAMEDIC, MICN)
REFERENCE NO. 504

PURPOSE: To determine the appropriate trauma patient destination with regards to the trauma center's catchment area.

AUTHORITY: California Administrative Code, Title 22, Chapter 7

DEFINITIONS:

Trauma Catchment Area: A geographical area surrounding a trauma center which may be defined by streets or by transport time.

Secure Trauma Catchment Area: A geographical area surrounding a trauma center strictly defined by streets/freeways or other physical landmarks.

Open Trauma Catchment Area: A geographical area surrounding a trauma center defined by a 30-minute, Code-3 transport time. Open trauma catchment areas may vary due to variations in weather and traffic patterns.

Undesignated Trauma Area (Antelope Valley): Geographical area of Los Angeles County that does not fall within a trauma catchment area.

PRINCIPLES:

A. Trauma patients should be transported to the designated trauma center or the designated pediatric trauma center.

B. Only the Department of Health Services may alter trauma catchment areas.

C. Only patients from incident locations within the strictly defined area shall be transported to those trauma centers with secure trauma catchment areas.

D. To facilitate appropriate trauma team activation, direct contact with the anticipated receiving trauma center should be made whenever possible.

POLICY:

I. Responsibilities of the Paramedic:

A. Maintain current knowledge of trauma centers with secure trauma catchment areas, open trauma catchment areas, pediatric trauma centers, and undesignated trauma areas within their assigned area.

B. Establish direct base contact with the receiving trauma center on all trauma center criteria, trauma guideline patients, or if in the paramedic's judgement it is in the patient's best interest to be transported to the designated trauma center.

EFFECTIVE: 4-15-95
REVISED: 3-20-09
SUPERSEDES: 5-1-06

PAGE 1 OF 3

APPROVED: _____
Director, EMS Agency

_____
Medical Director, EMS Agency

II.   The following table identifies trauma centers, pediatric trauma centers, and trauma centers with **secure** trauma catchment areas:

Trauma Centers	Pediatric Trauma Centers	Secure Trauma Catchment Areas
California Hospital Medical Center		X
Cedars Sinai Medical Center	X	X
Childrens Hospital of Los Angeles	X	
Henry Mayo Newhall Memorial Hospital		X
Huntington Memorial Hospital		X
LAC Harbor/UCLA Medical Center	X	
LAC + USC Medical Center	X	
Long Beach Memorial Medical Center	X	X
Northridge Hospital Medical Center – Roscoe Campus		X
Providence Holy Cross Medical Center		
St. Francis Medical Center		X
St. Mary Medical Center		
Ronald Reagan UCLA Medical Center	X	X

All Pediatric Trauma Centers have an OPEN trauma catchment area for pediatric trauma patients.

III.   When the designated trauma center requests diversion to trauma, a trauma patient may be transported to:

A.   The closest open trauma center with an open trauma catchment area within the 30-minute transport guideline; or

B.   The closest open County-operated trauma center within the 30-minute transport guideline; or

C.   The designated trauma center, when the base hospital determines it is in the patient's best interest, despite the temporary request for trauma diversion.

IV.   For multiple casualty incidents, secure trauma catchment areas shall be adhered to. However, it is understood that during a multiple casualty incident, as a result of normal triage procedures, injured patients may ultimately be transported to a trauma center as the next closest receiving hospital (crossing trauma catchment areas), as receiving hospitals in the surrounding geographical area are utilized to their maximum capacity.

CROSS REFERENCES:

<u>Prehospital Care Policy Manual</u>:
Reference No. 501,   **Hospital Directory**
Reference No. 502,   **Patient Destination**
Reference No. 503,   **Guidelines for Hospitals Requesting Diversion of ALS Units**
Reference No. 506,   **Trauma Triage**
Reference No. 510,   **Pediatric Patient Destination**
Reference No. 515,   **Air Ambulance Trauma Transport**
Reference No. 515.2, **Antelope Valley Air Ambulance Trauma Transport**
Reference No. 519,   **Management of Multiple Casualty Incidents**

PURPOSE: To establish criteria and standards which ensure that patients requiring the care
of a trauma center are appropriately triaged and transported.

AUTHORITY: California Code of Regulations, Title 13, Section 1105(c) California Code of
Regulations, Title 22, Section 100236 et seq. Health and Safety Code, Div. 2.5,
Section 1797 et seq., and 1317.

PRINCIPLES:

1.   Trauma patients should be secured and transported from the scene as quickly as
possible, consistent with optimal trauma care.

2.   An emergency patient should be transported to the most accessible medical facility
appropriate to their needs. The base hospital physician's determination in this regard is
controlling.

3.   Paramedics shall make base hospital contact with the area's trauma center, when it is
also a base hospital, on all injured patients who meet Base Contact and Transport
Criteria (Prehospital Care Policy, Ref. No. 808), trauma triage criteria and/or guidelines,
or if in the paramedic's judgment it is in the patient's best interest to be transported to a
trauma hospital. Contact shall be accomplished in such a way as not to delay transport.

POLICY:

I.   Trauma Criteria - Requires immediate transport to a designated trauma center.

Patients who fall into one or more of the following categories are to be transported
directly to the area's designated trauma center, if transport time does not exceed 20
minutes; patients can be transported an additional 10 minutes to a maximum of 30
minutes, if the provider based resources at the time of transport allow.

A.   Adults with blood pressure < 90 systolic or children with blood pressure
< 70 systolic

B.   Penetrating cranial injury

C.   Penetrating thoracic injury between the midclavicular lines

D.   Gunshot wound to trunk

E.   Blunt injury to chest with unstable chest wall (flail chest)

F.   Penetrating injury to neck

EFFECTIVE DATE: 6-15-87
REVISED: 11-15-09
SUPERSEDES: 12-28-06

PAGE 1 OF 3

APPROVED: _____
Director, EMS Agency

_____
Medical Director, EMS Agency

UCLA Skills Guide Page 212

G.   Diffuse abdominal tenderness

H.   Patients surviving falls from heights > 15 feet

I.   Intrusion of the motor vehicle into passenger space

J.   Patients in cardiopulmonary arrest with penetrating torso trauma

K.   Blunt head injury associated with altered consciousness (GCS equal to or less than 14, excluding patients less than 1 year old), seizures, unequal pupils, or focal neurological deficit

L.   Open or closed injury to the spinal column associated with sensory deficit or weakness of one or more extremities

M.   Extremity injuries with neurological and/or vascular compromise, excluding isolated hand or foot injuries.

II.   Triage Guidelines - At the discretion of the base hospital, a patient who falls into one of the following categories may be directed to a trauma center.

Mechanism of injury is the most effective method of selecting critically injured patients before unstable vital signs develop. Paramedics and base hospital personnel should consider mechanism of injury when determining patient destination. Transportation to a trauma center is advisable for patients such as:

A.   Surviving victims of vehicular accidents in which fatalities occurred and who complain of injury

B.   Pedestrians struck by automobiles

C.   Patients ejected from vehicles

D.   Patients requiring extrication

E.   Very young and very old patients and those with precarious previous medical histories

III.   Extremis Patients - Requires immediate transportation to the most accessible receiving facility:

A.   Patients with an obstructed airway

B.   Other patients, as determined by the base hospital personnel, whose lives would be jeopardized by transportation to any but the most accessible receiving facility

IV.   When for whatever reason base hospital contact cannot be made, the destination of injured patients will be made by paramedics using the guidelines set forth.

V.   Basic life support personnel shall transport patients to the most accessible receiving facility or service area hospital when applicable.

CROSS REFERENCE:

Prehospital Care Manual:
Ref. No. 501, **Hospital Directory**
Ref. No. 502, **Patient Destination**
Ref. No. 503, **Guidelines for Hospitals Requesting Diversion of ALS Units**
Ref. No. 504, **Trauma Patient Destination**
Ref. No. 808, **Base Hospital Contact and Transport Criteria**

SUBJECT: **SEXUAL ASSAULT PATIENT DESTINATION**

(EMT-I, PARAMEDIC, MICN)
REFERENCE NO. 508

PURPOSE: To provide guidelines for transporting patients who are alleged victims of sexual assault to the most accessible medical facility appropriate to their needs.

DEFINITION:

Sexual Assault Patient: A person who states they were sexually assaulted or a person suspected by the 9-1-1 personnel to have been the victim of a sexual assault.

SART: Sexual Assault Response Team - a coordinated interdisciplinary intervention model between law enforcement, crime laboratory, District Attorney's Office, medical and advocacy experts to meet the forensic need of the criminal justice system and the medical and emotional needs of the sexual assault patient.

SART Center: A licensed general acute care hospital, a licensed basic or comprehensive emergency department or a hospital sponsored program clinic that has met the specific requirements approved by the County of Los Angeles to receive patients who are victims of sexual assault.

PRINCIPLE:

1. When considering which facility is most appropriate to the needs of the sexual assault patient, the importance of evidence collection for legal proceedings should be one of the factors considered. However, in all cases, the health and well-being of the patient is the overriding consideration in determining hospital destination.

POLICY:

I. Sexual assault patients who deny physical injuries and who do not meet base hospital contact and transport criteria may be released at the scene to the local law enforcement agency for appropriate follow-up. Law enforcement personnel are highly encouraged to transport these patients to a designated SART Center. EMS personnel shall document on the EMS Report Form to whom the patient was released.

II. Every effort should be made to transport sexual assault patients who meet base hospital contact and transport criteria to the most accessible receiving (MAR) facility that has an affiliated designated SART Center. If EMS personnel determine that such a transport would unreasonably remove the transport unit from its primary response area, the patient should be transported to the MAR facility.

III. EMS personnel shall notify the local law enforcement agency of sexual assault patients regardless of whether the patient complains of physical injuries. EMS personnel shall document on the EMS Report Form to whom the incident was reported.

EFFECTIVE: 3-31-97
REVISED: 3-1-05
SUPERSEDES: 3-31-97

PAGE 1 OF 2

APPROVED:

Director, EMS Agency

Medical Director, EMS Agency

UCLA Skills Guide Page 215

CROSS REFERENCES:

Prehospital Care Policy Manual:

Ref. No. 501,	Hospital Directory
Ref. No. 502,	Patient Destination
Ref. No. 503,	Guidelines for Hospitals Requesting Diversion of ALS Units
Ref. No. 506,	Trauma Triage
Ref. No. 508.1	SART Center Roster
Ref. No. 510,	Pediatric Patient Destination
Ref. No. 511,	Perinatal Patient Destination
Ref. No. 808,	Base Hospital Contact and Transport Criteria

PURPOSE: To identify designated service area hospitals and define service area policies and boundaries.

AUTHORITY: California Administrative Code, Title 22, Chapter 7
Health and Safety Code, Division 2.5, Section 1797.220
California Code of Regulations, Title 13, Section 1105 (c)

DEFINITION:

Service Area: A defined geographic area assigned to a hospital from which 9-1-1 patients are transported.

Service Area Hospital: A hospital designated by the Emergency Medical Services (EMS) Agency to have a service area for 9-1-1 transports. This hospital has agreed to ensure that it will meet all requirements for Basic Emergency Department licensure to include Emergency Department Approved for Pediatrics (EDAP) designation unless sharing a service area with an EDAP approved hospital.

Shared Service Area: A defined geographic area with boundaries that are shared between two service area hospitals from which 9-1-1 patients are transported.

PRINCIPLES:

1. Patients shall be transported by EMS personnel to a service area hospital with a designated service area whenever the incident location is within the defined service area.

2. For a shared service area, patients shall be transported by EMS personnel to either service area hospital whenever the incident location is within the defined shared service area.

3. Service area hospitals have agreed not to request diversion for any categories other than internal disaster except for those with a shared service area (these hospitals may divert to each other).

4. Hospitals within a service area are bound by the same patient destination policies and boundaries of the hospital with the service area. Since these hospitals may not meet all of the service area requirements, these hospitals may divert 9-1-1 patients to the service area hospital only.

5. Only the EMS Agency may alter or lift service area boundaries.

EFFECTIVE: 1-1-05
REVISED: 8-01-08
SUPERSEDES: 12-20-06

PAGE 1 OF 4

APPROVED: _____
Director, EMS Agency

_____
Medical Director, EMS Agency

6.   Patients who meet criteria or guidelines for a specialty care center (e.g. Pediatric Medical Center, Pediatric Trauma Center, Perinatal or Trauma Centers) not provided by the service area hospital will be transported to the appropriate specialty care center.

7.   Patients exhibiting unmanageable airway or uncontrollable external bleeding will be transported to the most accessible receiving (MAR) facility regardless of incident location.

8.   Patients from multiple casualty incidents may be transported across service area boundaries.

9.   Patient request should be honored whenever possible in accordance with Section VI of this policy.

POLICY:

I.   Role of the Paramedic

A.   Maintain current knowledge of service area rules and boundaries within their assigned area.

B.   Advise the base hospital of the receiving service area hospital based on the incident location. For paramedic personnel authorized to utilize Standing Field Treatment Protocols (SFTP), patient destination shall be determined according to service area rules and boundaries.

II.   Role of the Base Hospital

A.   Provide online medical direction as needed.

B.   Assist as needed with patient destination.

C.   Notify receiving facilities of incoming patients.

III.   Role of the Service Area Hospital

A.   Receive 9-1-1 transports from within their defined service area.

B.   Ensure that hospital meets all requirements for a basic Emergency Department licensure and EDAP designation.

C.   In unusual circumstances that overwhelm ED resources, service area hospitals may contact the Medical Alert Center (MAC) and request for their service area to be lifted temporarily.

1.   If all hospitals surrounding the requesting facility are on diversion to ED saturation, the request will be denied. If at least one facility is open, the request will be granted on a case-by-case basis.

2.   The service area will be lifted for a two hour period only, during which the ReddiNet will reflect that the hospital is on ED diversion.

3.   If the unusual circumstances persist beyond two hours, the hospital may recontact the MAC and request to speak to the Administrator on Duty (AOD) regarding additional time on diversion.

4.   During the two-hour period when the service area is lifted, the hospital shall continue to receive basic life support (BLS) traffic from calls originating inside of their service area boundaries.

IV.   Hospitals with Designated Service Areas in Los Angeles County

A.   Shared: California Hospital Medical Center (CAL) and Good Samaritan Hospital (GSH)

B.   Centinela Hospital Medical Center (CNT)

C.   White Memorial Medical Center (WMH)

D.   Memorial Hospital of Gardena (MHG)

V.   Hospital within a Service Area

A.   East Los Angeles Doctor's Hospital is located within White Memorial Medical Center's service area.

VI.   Transport of patients from outside of the service area boundaries: Patient requests for transport to a service area hospital when the incident location is outside the hospital's defined service area or inside the service area of another hospital may be honored by:

A.   BLS personnel: if it is a BLS patient, the receiving hospital is contacted (via the HEAR or dispatch center) and agrees to accept the patient, and the transporting unit is not unreasonably removed from its primary response area.

B.   Advance Life Support (ALS) personnel: if the base hospital is contacted and concurs that the patient's condition is sufficiently stable to permit the estimated transport time, the requested hospital agrees to accept the patient, and the transporting unit is not unreasonably removed from its primary transport response area. The receiving hospital may be contacted directly if the ALS unit is utilizing SFTPs or transporting a BLS patient.

CROSS REFERENCES:

Prehospital Care Policy Manual:
Ref. No. 501,   **Hospital Directory**
Ref. No. 502,   **Patient Destination**
Ref. No. 503,   **Guidelines for Hospitals Requesting Diversion of ALS Patients**
Ref. No. 506,   **Trauma Triage**
Ref. No. 509.1, **Service Area for Centinela Hospital Medical Center**
Ref. No. 509.2, **Shared Service Area for California Hospital Medical Center and Good Samaritan Hospital**
Ref. No. 509.3, **Service Area for Memorial Hospital of Gardena**
Ref. No. 509.4, **Service Area for White Memorial Medical Center**
Ref. No. 510,   **Pediatric Patient Destination**
Ref. No. 511,   **Perinatal Patient Destination**
Ref. No. 519,   **Management of Multiple Casualty Incidents**

DEPARTMENT OF HEALTH SERVICES
COUNTY OF LOS ANGELES

SUBJECT: **PEDIATRIC PATIENT DESTINATION**

PURPOSE: To ensure that 9-1-1 pediatric patients are transported to the most appropriate facility that is staffed, equipped and prepared to administer emergency and/or definitive care appropriate to the needs of the pediatric patient.

AUTHORITY: Health and Safety Code, Division 2.5, Section 1797.220
California Code of Regulations, Title 13, Section 1105 C

DEFINITIONS:

Pediatric patient: Children 14 years of age or younger.

Emergency Department Approved for Pediatrics (EDAP): A licensed basic emergency department that is approved by the County of Los Angeles EMS Agency to receive 9-1-1 pediatric patients. These emergency departments provide care to pediatric patients by meeting specific requirements for professional staff, quality improvement, education, support services, equipment, supplies, medications, and established policies, procedures, and protocols.

Pediatric Medical Center (PMC): A licensed acute care hospital that is approved by the County of Los Angeles EMS Agency to receive critically ill 9-1-1 pediatric patients based on guidelines outlined in this policy. These centers provide referral centers for critically ill pediatric patients.

Pediatric Trauma Center (PTC): A licensed acute care hospital that is approved by the County of Los Angeles EMS Agency to receive injured 9-1-1 pediatric patients based on guidelines outlined in this policy. These centers provide tertiary-level pediatric care and serve as referral centers for critically injured pediatric patients.

PRINCIPLES:

1.   In all cases, the health and well being of the patient is the overriding consideration in determining patient destination. Factors to be considered include severity and stability of the patient's illness or injury; current status of the pediatric receiving facility; anticipated transport time; and request by the patient, family, guardian or physician.

2.   For purposes of this policy, the most accessible receiving hospital is the most accessible EDAP.

POLICY:

I.   Guidelines for transporting pediatric patients to an EDAP, PMC, PTC or Trauma Center:

    A.   Patients who require transport and do not meet guidelines for transport to a PMC and PTC shall be transported to the most accessible EDAP.

EFFECTIVE: 5-1-85
REVISED: 3-15-09
SUPERSEDES: 2-1-06

APPROVED: _____
Director, EMS Agency

_____
Medical Director, EMS Agency

PAGE 1 OF 3

B.   BLS units shall call for an ALS unit or transport pediatric patients to the most accessible EDAP as outlined in Ref. No. 808, Base Hospital Contact and Transport Criteria.

C.   Patients meeting <u>medical guidelines</u> for transport to a PMC:

   1.   Shall be transported to the most accessible PMC if ground transport is 20 minutes or less.

   2.   If ground transport time to a PMC is greater than 20 minutes, the patient may be transported to the most accessible EDAP.

D.   Patients meeting <u>trauma criteria/guidelines</u> for transport to a PTC:

   1.   Shall be transported to the most accessible PTC, if the transport time does not exceed 20 minutes. Patients can be transported an additional 10 minutes, to a maximum of 30 minutes, if the provider based resources at the time of transport allow.

   2.   Childrens Hospital Los Angeles shall be the primary receiving pediatric trauma center for pediatric trauma patients transported by air ambulance from the Antelope Valley and the East San Gabriel Valley.

   3.   If a PTC cannot be accessed but a trauma center can be accessed under the parameter in (D.1), the patient may be transported to the trauma center.

   4.   If a PTC or trauma center cannot be accessed as specified above, the patient may be transported to the most accessible EDAP.

E.   Pediatric patients who have an uncontrollable, life-threatening situation (e.g., unmanageable airway or uncontrollable hemorrhage) shall be transported to the most accessible EDAP.

F.   Pediatric patients may be transported to a non-EDAP provided all of the following are met:

   1.   The patient, family, or private physician requests transport to a non-EDAP facility.

   2.   The patient, family, or private physician is made aware that the receiving facility is not an EDAP and may not meet current EDAP standards.

   3.   The base hospital concurs and contacts the requested facility and ensures that the facility has agreed to accept the patient. This includes those providers functioning under SFTPs.

   4.   All of the above shall be documented on the EMS Report Form.

II.   Guidelines for identifying critically **ill** pediatric patients who require transport to a PMC:

   A.   Cardiac dysrhythmia

   B.   Severe respiratory distress

   C.   Cyanosis

   D.   Persistent altered mental status

   E.   Status epilepticus

   F.   ALTE (Apparent Life Threatening Event) $\leq$ 12 months of age

III.   Guidelines for identifying critically **injured** pediatric patients who require transport to a PTC:

   Trauma triage criteria and/or guidelines identified in Ref. No. 506, Trauma Triage

CROSS REFERENCE:

Prehospital Care Policy Manual:
Ref. No. 502, **Patient Destination**
Ref. No. 504, **Trauma Patient Destination**
Ref. No. 506, **Trauma Triage**
Ref. No. 512, **Burn Patient Destination**
Ref. No. 519, **Management of Multiple Casualty Incidents**
Ref. No. 808, **Base Hospital Contact and Transport Criteria**
Ref. No. 816, **Physician at Scene**
Ref. No. 832, **Treatment/Transport of Minors**
Ref. No. 834, **Patient Refusal of Treatment or Transport**

Los Angeles County EDAP Standards
Los Angeles County PMC Standards
State of California Emergency Medical Services Authority Guidelines for Children (EMSC)

PURPOSE: To provide guidelines for transporting perinatal patients to the most accessible facility appropriate to their needs.

DEFINITIONS:

1.   Perinatal – For the purpose of this policy, "perinatal" refers to patients who are at least 20 weeks pregnant.

2   Perinatal Center – For the purpose of this policy, "perinatal center" refers to a general acute care hospital with a basic emergency department permit <u>and</u> obstetrical service. This terminology is not intended to indicate the absence or presence of a neonatal intensive care unit (NICU).

3.   EDAP – Emergency Department Approved for Pediatrics.

4.   PMC – Pediatric Medical Center.
     PTC – Pediatric Trauma Center

PRINCIPLES.

1.   Perinatal patients should be transported to the most accessible facility appropriate to their needs. This determination will be made by the base hospital physician or Mobile Intensive Care Nurse (MICN) after consideration of the guidelines established in this policy. Final authority for patient destination rests with the base hospital handling the call.

2.   If delivery occurs prior to arrival at a hospital, the mother and the newborn should be transported to the same facility.

3.   BLS units shall call for an ALS unit or transport perinatal patients to the most accessible perinatal center as outlined in Reference No. 808, Base Hospital Contact and Transport Criteria.

4.   In all cases, the health and well being of the patient is the overriding consideration in determining patient destination. Factors to be considered include: severity and stability of the patient's illness or injury; current status of the pediatric receiving facility; anticipated transport time; and request by the patient, family, guardian or physician.

POLICY:

I.   The following perinatal patients should be transported to the most accessible perinatal center:

EFFECTIVE DATE: 6-15-87
REVISED: 10-01-08
SUPERSEDES: 12-23-05

PAGE 1 OF 2

APPROVED: _____   _____
          Director, EMS Agency   Medical Director, EMS Agency

A.   Patients who appear to be in active labor, whether or not delivery appears imminent.

B.   Patients whose chief complaint appears to be related to the pregnancy. Patients who appear to be having perinatal complications.

C.   Injured patients who do not meet trauma criteria or guidelines.

II.   Perinatal patients who have delivered prior to arriving at a health facility should be transported to the most accessible perinatal center which is also an EDAP (consider a perinatal center with a NICU).

III.   Perinatal patients meeting trauma criteria and/or guidelines should be transported to a trauma center.

IV.   Perinatal patients for whom transportation to a perinatal center would exceed 20 minutes should be transported to a receiving facility which is also an EDAP.

V.   The following perinatal patients should be transported to the most accessible receiving facility:

A.   Patients in acute respiratory distress.

B.   Patients in full arrest.

C.   Patients whose chief complaint is clearly not related to the pregnancy.

VI   Consideration may be given by the base hospital to:

A.   Direct patients who are equal to or less than 34 weeks pregnant, whose chief complaint appears to be related to the pregnancy, to a perinatal receiving facility with a NICU, regardless of service area considerations/rules.

B.   Honor patient destination requests for those patients who have made previous arrangement for obstetrical care at a given hospital. This consideration should be based on the following:

1.   If the condition of the patient permits such transport.

2.   Transportation to the requested obstetrical facility would not exceed 20 minutes and would not unreasonably remove the ALS unit from its area of primary response.

CROSS REFERENCES:

Prehospital Care Policy Manual:
       Reference No. 502, **Patient Destination**
       Reference No. 506, **Trauma Triage**
       Reference No. 510, **Pediatric Patient Destination**
       Reference No. 808, **Base Hospital Contact and Transport Criteria**

DEPARTMENT OF HEALTH SERVICES
COUNTY OF LOS ANGELES

SUBJECT: BURN PATIENT DESTINATION

(EMT-I, PARAMEDIC, MICN)
REFERENCE NO. 512

PURPOSE: To ensure the appropriate destination for Los Angeles County patients who sustain burn injuries.

POLICY:

I. Paramedics should make base contact whenever any patient sustaining burn injuries meets the guidelines established in the Prehospital Care Policy Reference No. 808, Base Hospital Contact and Transport Criteria.

II. The base hospital should initiate appropriate orders as outlined in the Base Hospital Treatment Guidelines.

III. Destination of patients sustaining burn injuries will be determined as follows:

    A. Patients who meet trauma or Pediatric Medical Center (PMC) criteria and/or guidelines should be transported to the appropriate trauma center or PMC.

    B. Patients who do not meet trauma or PMC criteria and/or guidelines should be transported to the closest, most accessible medical receiving facility appropriate for their age.

IV. The receiving hospital should:

    A. Provide appropriate stabilization of the patient

    B. Arrange, in conjunction with the Medical Alert Center (MAC), for transfer to an appropriate burn facility if necessary. Provide MAC with the following information:

        1. Status of airway control

        2. Percentage, degree, and location of the burns

        3. Type of burn (electrical, thermal, chemical, radiation)

        4. Level of care the patient requires (ICU, med/surg)

        5. Circulatory status (vital signs and perfusion of burned extremity if applicable)

        6. Level of consciousness

EFFECTIVE: 6-5-79
REVISED: 8-15-08
SUPERSEDES: 12-1-05

PAGE 1 OF 2

APPROVED:

Director, EMS Agency

Medical Director, EMS Agency

UCLA Skills Guide Page 226

7.   Other injuries

8.   Past medical history, pre-existing major systemic disease and current medications

9.   Treatment(s) already rendered and in progress

CROSS REFERENCES:

Prehospital Care Policy Manual:
Ref. No. 502, Patient Destination
Ref. No. 506, Trauma Triage
Ref. No. 510, Pediatric Patient Destination
Ref. No. 808, Base Hospital Contact and Transport Criteria

Los Angeles County Base Hospital Treatment Guidelines

SUBJECT: **PRIVATE PROVIDER AGENCY** (EMT-I/PARAMEDIC/MICN)
TRANSPORT/RESPONSE GUIDELINES REFERENCE NO. 517

PURPOSE: To provide guidelines for private ambulance providers handling requests for emergency, urgent and non-emergency transports.

AUTHORITY: Ambulance Ordinance, Section 7.16.005 E, H, M,
Health & Safety Code, Division 2.5, Sections 1250, 1797.52 - 1797.84,
California Code of Regulations Section 1104.

DEFINITIONS:

Advanced Life Support (ALS) Transport: A ground or air ambulance transport of a patient who requires, or may require, skills or treatment modalities that do not exceed the paramedic scope of practice. An ALS transport may be required for either a non-emergency or emergency transport.

NOTE: Both Nurse-Staffed and ALS (paramedic-staffed) transports are considered CCTs, but are differentiated by level of staffing.

Base Hospital Contact Criteria: Those signs, symptoms, chief complaints, or special circumstances of patients for which paramedics are required to contact a base hospital for medical direction and/or patient destination as outlined in Ref. No. 808, Base Hospital Contact and Transport Criteria.

Basic Life Support (BLS) Transport: A ground or air ambulance transport of a patient who requires skills or treatment modalities that do not exceed the EMT-I scope of practice or expanded scope of practice. A BLS transport may be sufficient to meet the needs of the patient requiring either a non-emergency or emergency transport.

Life-Threatening Medical Condition: An acute medical condition that, without immediate medical attention, could reasonably be expected to result in serious jeopardy to the health of an individual (or, in the case of a pregnant woman, the health of the woman or her unborn child) or serious impairment or dysfunction of any bodily organ or part.

Health Facility: For purposes of this policy, a health care facility may include any of the following:

> General Acute Care Hospitals
> Skilled Nursing Facilities
> Clinics/Urgent Care Centers
> Physicians Offices
> Dialysis Centers
> Intermediate Care Facilities
> Acute Psychiatric Facilities

Interfacility Transport (IFT): The transport of a patient from one health facility to another health facility as defined above.

EFFECTIVE: 1-5-88
REVISED: 10-15-09
SUPERSEDES: 5-01-06

APPROVED: _____
Director, EMS Agency

PAGE 1 OF 7

_____
Medical Director, EMS Agency

Nurse-Staffed Critical Care Transport (CCT): An ambulance or air ambulance interfacility transport of a patient who requires or may require skills or treatment modalities that exceed the paramedic scope of practice. A critical care transport may be required for either a non-emergency or emergency interfacility transport.

Respiratory Care Practitioner (RCP) Specialty Transport: An ambulance or air ambulance interfacility transport of a patient who requires skill or treatment modalities that do not exceed the EMT-I scope of practice or expanded scope-of-practice or the RCP scope of practice. A RCP transport team (minimum of two EMT-Is and one RCP) may be sufficient to meet the needs of the patient requiring non-emergency transport.

Stable for Transfer: The treating physician attending to the patient has determined, with reasonable clinical confidence, that the patient is expected to leave the health facility and be received at the second facility with no material deterioration in medical condition. However, patients requiring a higher level of care and who may generally not satisfy the definition of stable for transfer may be transported when the benefits of transfer outweigh the risk of not being transferred.

9-1-1 Response: An emergency response by the primary emergency transportation provider or its designee for that geographic area in which the response is requested.
9-1-1 requests are generally made by the public, but may include requests from acute and non-acute care health facilities.

PRINCIPLES:

1. Private ambulance providers are prohibited from dispatching to any call that would normally be considered an emergency 9-1-1 call for the authorized emergency transportation operator for that geographical area, unless the call is from either a public entity or such authorized emergency transportation operator requesting backup services.

2. Any ambulance personnel observing the scene of a traffic collision or other emergency should:

   a. Contact their respective communications center and request that the jurisdictional 9-1-1 provider agency be notified.

   b. Follow the internal policy developed by their employer in regard to stopping at the scene of an observed emergency.

3. Privately owned or operated ambulances may not be equipped and operated as emergency vehicles nor respond to an emergency call unless the operating provider agency has been licensed to do so by the Commissioner of the California Highway Patrol.

4. It is the responsibility of the requested transport provider, in consultation with the facility requesting the transport, to provide the appropriate level of transport (ALS, BLS, Critical Care and/or Respiratory Care Practitioner) based on the transferring physician's determination of the medical needs of the patient.

5. Health facilities shall provide the transport provider agency with appropriate transfer documents in compliance with COBRA/EMTALA principles and Centers for Medicaid and Medicare Services Requirements.

6. Personnel providing interfacility transports shall be legally qualified to provide appropriate medical measures needed by the patient enroute and to operate any special equipment required for the patient.

7. General acute care hospitals with basic or comprehensive emergency departments have staffing and equipment resources available to assess, treat and monitor a patient awaiting an interfacility transport. Other types of health care facilities may not have the staffing and equipment available to assess, treat and/or monitor a patient for extended time frames. Therefore, 9-1-1 emergency responses may be necessary for those patients whose condition may deteriorate while waiting for a private provider response.

POLICY:

I. Transport Modalities

   A. BLS Transport

      1. Unit is staffed with two EMT-Is.

      2. Requests may be for emergency, urgent, or non-emergency response.

      3. Patient does not require care, which exceeds the EMT-I basic or expanded scope of practice.

      4. Patient does not meet Base Hospital Contact Criteria at time of transport.

      5. The receiving hospital, if applicable, has accepted transfer from the sending facility.

      6. Patient destination requested by the sending facility will be honored. However, if the patient's condition deteriorates enroute, the patient shall be diverted to the most accessible facility appropriate to the needs of the patient.

         EXCEPTION: Patients with a valid Do-Not-Resuscitate (DNR) form or order shall be transported as outlined in Reference No. 815, Honoring Prehospital Do-Not-Resuscitate Orders.

   B. ALS Transport

      1. Unit is staffed with two paramedics unless the ambulance provider has been given approval by the EMS Agency to staff ALS IFT units with one paramedic and one EMT-I.

      2. Request may be for emergency, urgent or non-emergency response.

      3. Patient does not require skills or treatment modalities, which exceed the paramedic scope of practice.

      4. Base hospital contact is <u>not</u> required for routine IFTs unless the patient's condition deteriorates enroute. In these circumstances, Procedures Prior to Base Contact (Ref. No. 806) may be initiated and base hospital contact

made. The base hospital will determine if the patient should be diverted to the most accessible receiving facility appropriate to the needs of the patient or if the patient may be transported to the original destination requested by the sending facility.

EXCEPTION: For patients with a valid DNR form or order:

a.   **Base hospital contact is only required to obtain orders for ALS supportive measures as outlined in Ref. No. 815.**

b.   **Transport shall be performed as outlined in Ref. No. 815.**

5.   Paramedics are not required to make base hospital contact to monitor therapies established by the sending facility prior to transport if such therapies fall within the paramedic scope of practice.

6.   With the exception of patients with a valid Do-Not-Resuscitate form or order, paramedics may not accept standing orders or medical orders from the transferring physician or provider medical advisor. Should a patient's condition change enroute, paramedics must contact a base hospital for medical orders.

C.   Nurse-Staffed Critical Care Transport

1.   Unit is staffed by a qualified registered nurse and two EMT-Is or paramedics. Other medical personnel (e.g., physician, respiratory care practitioner) may be added to meet the needs of the patient.

2.   Request may be for emergency, urgent or non-emergency response.

3.   Patient requires, or may require, skills or treatment modalities that exceed the paramedic scope-of-practice.

4.   Registered nurses, who function under the provisions of the California Nurse Practice Act, are not required to make base hospital contact. Nurses may follow medical orders of the transferring physician and/or orders approved by the Critical Care Transport Medical Director for patient care enroute. However, CCT nurses may not give medical orders to paramedics who may be part of the transport team.

5.   The receiving hospital, if applicable, has accepted transfer from the sending hospital.

6.   Patient destination requested by the sending facility will be honored;

7.   Patient destination requested by the sending facility will be honored. However, if the patient's condition deteriorates enroute, the patient shall be diverted to the most accessible facility appropriate to the needs of the patient.

      EXCEPTION: Patients with a valid Do-Not-Resuscitate form or order shall be transported as outlined in Reference No. 815, Honoring Prehospital Do-Not-Resuscitate (DNR) Orders.

D. Respiratory Care Practitioner (RCP) Specialty Transport

1. Unit is staffed by a qualified respiratory care practitioner and two EMT-Is or paramedics.

2. RCP staffed ambulances are not approved for 9-1-1 responses.

3. Requests may be for urgent or non-emergency response.

4. The specialty care needs of the patient do not require skills or treatment modalities that exceed the RCP scope of practice.

5. The RCP will practice under the license and guidelines/protocols approved by the program medical advisor.

6. The receiving hospital, if applicable, has accepted transfer from the sending hospital.

7. Patient destination requested by the sending facility will be honored; however, if the patient's condition deteriorates enroute, the patient shall be diverted to the most accessible facility appropriate to the need of the patient.

    EXCEPTION: Patients with a valid Do-Not-Resuscitate form or order shall be transported as outlined in Reference No. 815, Honoring Prehospital Do-Not-Resuscitate (DNR) Orders.

II. Levels of Responses/Requests

A. Emergency (Code 3) Response Requests

1. Request by a 9-1-1 Provider Agency

    Ambulance providers shall dispatch an ambulance within a reasonable time in response to an emergency call from a public agency or authorized emergency transportation operator for that geographical area, unless the caller is immediately advised of a delay in responding to the call.

2. Request by a Health Facility

    a. If a physician has evaluated and stabilized the patient to the best extent possible and arranged an interfacility transfer, a private ground (or air) ambulance transport may be arranged and the 9-1-1 provider is not ordinarily contacted.

        NOTE: A 9-1-1 provider may be contacted if the ETA of the private provider is too long and the condition of the patient warrants a rapid response and transport. Patient destination will then be determined as outlined in Ref. No. 502, Patient Destination.

b.   If a patient at a health facility has an emergency medical condition which has not been evaluated or stabilized by a physician prior to the facility requesting an emergency response, the dispatcher for the private ambulance provider should refer the call to the 9-1-1 provider.

c.   If upon arrival EMT-Is or paramedics find that the patient has a life-threatening medical condition, the private ambulance provider shall determine whether it is in the best interest of the patient to request the primary 9-1-1 provider to respond or to provide rapid transport to the most accessible receiving facility. If on-scene personnel determine that immediate transport is indicated, the 9-1-1 provider shall be notified and justification shall be documented on the EMS Report Form.

3.   Request by a Private Citizen

a.   If information obtained from the calling party indicates that the patient has an emergency medical condition or meets Base Hospital Contact Criteria, the call shall immediately be referred to the jurisdictional 9-1-1 provider. A private ambulance provider which is not designated as the primary 9-1-1 provider for a geographic area shall not respond Code 3 to a private call from the public unless requested or authorized to do so by the primary 9-1-1 provider for that jurisdiction.

b.   If upon arrival EMT-Is or paramedics find that the patient has a life-threatening medical condition, the private ambulance provider shall determine whether it is in the best interest of the patient to request the primary 9-1-1 provider to respond or to provide rapid transport to the most accessible receiving facility. If on-scene personnel determine that immediate transport is indicated, the 9-1-1 provider shall be notified and justification shall be documented on the EMS Report Form.

B.   Urgent (Code 2) Response Requests

1.   A request from a health facility for transport of a patient who has, or is perceived to have, a stabilized medical condition which is urgent, but not an emergency.

2.   Transports may be handled by BLS, ALS, CCT or RCP Specialty Units depending upon the medical requirements of the patient.

C.   Non-Emergency Response Requests

1.   A request for transport of a patient who does not have, or is not perceived to have, an emergency or urgent medical condition.

2.   Transports are handled by a private ambulance provider with BLS, ALS, CCT or RCP Specialty Units, depending upon the medical requirements of the patient and the associated scope of practice of the prehospital personnel.

III. Role of the Base Hospital in Interfacility Transports

A. To provide immediate medical direction to paramedics if the patient's condition deteriorates during transport from one health facility to another.

B. To determine if a patient should be diverted to the most accessible 9-1-1 receiving facility or be allowed to continue to the pre-designated receiving facility if the patient's condition changes while enroute to a designated facility. If diverted, the base hospital shall:

1. Contact the new receiving hospital and communicate all appropriate patient information.

2. Advise the original receiving hospital that a diversion has occurred.

C. To clarify the scope of practice of EMS personnel when requested to do so by a sending facility.

NOTE: It is not the responsibility of the base hospital or the transport personnel to determine whether the transfer is appropriate. The transferring physician, in consultation with the receiving physician, assumes this responsibility.

CROSS REFERENCE:

Prehospital Care Policy Manual:

Ref. No. 304, Role of the Base Hospital
Ref. No. 414, Registered Nurse/Respiratory Specialty Care Transport Provider
Ref. No. 502, Patient Destination
Ref. No. 514, Prehospital EMS Aircraft Operations
Ref. No. 802, EMT-I Scope of Practice
Ref. No. 802.1 EMT-I Scope of Practice
Ref. No. 803, Paramedic Scope of Practice
Ref. No. 806, Procedures Prior to Base Contact
Ref. No. 808, Base Hospital Contact and Transport
Ref. No. 815, Honoring Prehospital Do-Not-Resuscitate (DNR) Orders

SUBJECT: **DECOMPRESSION EMERGENCIES/**   (EMT-I, PARAMEDIC, MICN)
                 PATIENT DESTINATION   REFERENCE NO. 518

PURPOSE: To provide a procedure for transporting patients with potential decompression emergencies to the most appropriate and accessible medical facility.

POLICY:

I.   Responsibilities of the Provider Agency:

       A.   Contact assigned base hospital for any patient suspected of having a decompression emergency.

       B.   Obtain dive incident history of the patient and dive partner, if possible.

            This includes:

            1. Maximum dive depth
            2. Time spent at depth
            3. Rate of ascent
            4. Number of dives
            5. Surface interval
            6. Gas(ses) used

       C.   Coordinate patient transportation to the appropriate receiving facility.

            NOTE: Transportation of patients with potential decompression emergencies may involve the United States Coast Guard (USCG) helicopter which does not include paramedic level staffing. In some circumstances, the USCG helicopter may be able to accommodate a Los Angeles County paramedic to accompany the patient to the receiving facility. If this is not possible and rapid transport is in the best interest of the patient, care may be transferred from the paramedics handling the call to the USCG medical personnel.

       D.   Retrieve patient's dive equipment (e.g., dive computer, regulator, tank, buoyancy compensator, gauges and weight belt) and transport with patient. If the transporting unit cannot accommodate the equipment, the provider agency shall take custody of it and notify the receiving facility of the dive equipment location.

            NOTE: As a general rule, the integrity of the dive equipment should be maintained and not tampered with except by investigating authorities.

APPROVED: _____   _____
                Director, EMS Agency   Medical Director, EMS Agency

II.   Responsibilities of the Base Hospital Physician or Mobile Intensive Care Nurse (MICN):

A.   Contact the Medical Alert Center (MAC) by dialing the general number (866) 940-4401 and choose option 8 for "hyperbaric treatment". The MAC will coordinate the transport of hyperbaric chamber personnel to the chamber.

B.   Provide medical orders for patient care.

C.   In consultation with the hyperbaric chamber physician on call (arranged through the MAC), determine if the patient should be transported directly from the incident location to a hyperbaric chamber or to the most accessible receiving facility (MAR). The following guidelines should be considered for any patient with a history of recent underwater compressed gas use:

1.   Transport to a MAC-listed hyperbaric chamber (Immediate)

a.   Unconscious, or
b.   Apneic, or
c.   Pulseless

2.   Transport to a MAC-listed hyperbaric chamber and/or the MAR after consultation with the hyperbaric chamber physician (Emergent)

a.   Any neurological symptoms, or
b.   Severe dyspnea, or
c.   Chest discomfort
d.   Premature ascent with reported failure to complete any required underwater decompression stop(s) (omitted decompression) with or without symptoms

3.   Transport to the MAR with potential secondary transfer to a hyperbaric chamber after consultation with the hyperbaric chamber physician (Non-Emergent)

a.   Delayed symptoms after flying, or
b.   Delayed minor symptoms after 24 hours

NOTE: Patient destination for patients with decompression emergencies shall be determined by the hyperbaric chamber physician on call.

III.   Responsibilities of the Medical Alert Center

A.   Contact the hyperbaric chamber physician on call at LAC+USC Medical Center and arrange communication between the physician and the base hospital directing the call.

B.   Following consultation with the hyperbaric physician on call, determine which hyperbaric chamber is most appropriate to the needs of the patient. Factors to be considered include distance; altitude; weather; ETA of available transportation; the limitations of various aircraft and the condition of the patient.

C.   Inform the appropriate receiving facility of the patient's condition and ETA.

D.   Coordinate transportation to the hyperbaric chamber for the hyperbaric chamber personnel.

E.   Coordinate secondary transfers from the receiving facility as needed.

CROSS REFERENCES:

Prehospital Care Policy Manual:
Ref. No. 502, **Patient Destination**
Ref. No. 506, **Trauma Triage**
Ref. No. 808, **Base Hospital Contact and Transport Criteria**
Ref. No. 814, **Determination/Pronouncement of Death in the Field**

| SUBJECT: | **MANAGEMENT OF MULTIPLE** | (EMT, PARAMEDIC, MICN) |
| | **CASUALTY INCIDENTS** | REFERENCE NO. 519 |

PURPOSE: To provide guidelines for the efficient management of multiple casualty incidents (MCI) through coordination between prehospital care personnel, receiving facilities and the Medical Alert Center (MAC) to allow for maximum resource allocation, patient distribution and to prevent unnecessary delays in patient care and transport.

To provide guidelines for transition from a MCI response to a Mass Casualty Incident Management Response.

This policy defines the roles of the provider agency, MAC, base hospital and receiving facilities during an MCI.

DEFINITIONS : Refer to Reference No. 519.1, MCI – Definitions.

PRINCIPLES:

1. The Incident Command System (ICS) should be utilized at all MCI's.

2. Terminology is standardized.

3. Expedient and accurate documentation is essential.

4. The MAC is equipped to communicate with multiple receiving facilities simultaneously and can rapidly assess system wide emergency department bed status, hospital and ambulance resources.

5. Request for hospital diversion status should be considered when determining patient destination; however, if appropriate, patients may be directed to hospitals requesting diversion (Exception: Internal Disaster).

6. Patients requiring Advanced Life Support (ALS) treatment or procedures should be transported by paramedics whenever possible; however, these patients may be transported by Basic Life Support (BLS) units based on available resources during the MCI. BLS units may transport to other than the Most Accessible Receiving (MAR) facility if the patient meets specialty care center criteria and based on available system resources.

7. The EMS Agency will facilitate a post-incident debriefing of large scale incidents to include all affected agencies.

8. To maintain system readiness, provider agencies, hospitals, MAC and other disaster response teams should carry out regularly schedule MCI, disaster drills and monthly HEAR radio checks.

EFFECTIVE: 5-1-92
REVISED: 12-1-09
SUPERSEDES: 5-1-05

APPROVED: _____   _____
            Director, EMS Agency   Medical Director, EMS Agency

PAGE 1 OF 5

UCLA Skills Guide Page 238

9.   On any MCI in which the need for air transport is identified, early notification to air operations providers is essential in order to ensure rapid access to medical care and preserve life.

POLICY:

I.   Role of the Provider Agency

   A.   Institute ICS as necessary.

   B.   Implement MCI Triage Guidelines (modified START & Jump START) as necessary (see Ref. No. 519.2).

   C.   Establish early communication with either the:

      1.   MAC for 10 or more patients (via HEAR when possible) for hospital bed availability, authorization of Procedures Prior to Base Contact (Ref. No. 806.1), lifting of trauma catchment and service areas; or

      2.   Base hospital for the purpose of patient destination and/or medical direction.

   D.   If the need for additional BLS transport units exceeds the jurisdictional provider agency's capability, additional transport resources may be requested by the jurisdictional dispatch center or the Fire Operational Area Coordinator (FOAC) as per Ref. No. 1126, Multiple Casualty Incident Transportation Management.

   E.   Request hospital based medical resources from the MAC as outlined in Ref. No. 817, Hospital Emergency Response Team (HERT) if necessary.

   F.   Provide the following scene information to the MAC or base hospital:

      1.   Nature of incident

      2.   Location of incident

      3.   Medical Communications Coordinator (Med Com) provider unit and agency

      4.   Agency in charge of incident

      5.   Total number of estimated immediate, delayed, minor and deceased patients. If indicated, include total number and category of pediatric patients

      6.   Nearest receiving facilities including trauma centers, PMCs, PTCs and EDAPs

      7.   Transporting provider, unit number and destination

8. Type of hazardous material, contamination, level of decontamination completed, if indicated

G. Document the following patient information on the appropriate EMS Report Form:

1. Patient name

2. Chief complaint

3. Mechanism of injury

4. Age

5. Sex

6. Brief patient assessment

7. Brief description of treatment provided

8. Sequence number

9. Transporting provider, unit number and destination

H. Reassess situational status to identify available resources and resource needs. If the anticipated resource needs exceed available local and mutual aid resources, contact the FOAC. Additional resources beyond the operational area shall be requested through the Regional Disaster Medical and Health Coordinator (RDMHC).

I. Whenever departmental resources allow, the paramedic provider should consider assigning a provider agency representative to report to the MAC to assist with communications and coordination of patient destination.

II. Role of the Medical Alert Center

A. Provide prehospital care personnel with emergency department bed availability and diversion status as indicated by the ReddiNet poll.

B. Assist prehospital care personnel as necessary with patient destinations.

C. Arrange for additional ambulance transport units as requested by the FOAC or RDMHC.

D. Coordinate activation of HERT as requested.

E. Notify receiving facilities of incoming patients immediately via the ReddiNet.

F. Document, under the authority of the MAC Medical Officer on Duty (MOD) the implementation of Procedures Prior to Base Contact (Ref. No. 806.1). Lifting of trauma catchment and service areas is an EMS Administrator on Duty (AOD) function.

G.   Maintain an "open MCI victim list" via the ReddiNet for 72 hours.

H.   Complete a written report to include a summary of the incident and final disposition of all patients involved as indicated.

I.   Notify the EMS AOD per MAC policies and procedures.

J.   The EMS Agency, as the Medical and Health Operational Area Coordinator (MHOAC) for the County of Los Angeles, will assess the situational status and evaluate available resources and resource needs. If the anticipated resource needs exceed the available resources the EMS Agency, via its role as the RDMHC, will request resources from surrounding counties.

K.   Maintain a paramedic provider agency Medical/Health Resource Directory and assist paramedic providers with MCI resource management when requested.

III.   Role of the Base Hospital

A.   Notify the MAC of the MCI as soon as possible, especially for newsworthy events, HAZMAT, multi-jurisdictional response and potential terrorism incidents.

B.   Provide prehospital care personnel with emergency department bed availability and diversion status.

C.   Assist prehospital care personnel as needed with patient destination.

D.   Provide medical direction as needed.

E.   Notify receiving facilities of incoming patients.

IV.   Role of the Receiving Facility

A.   Provide the MAC or base hospital with emergency department bed availability upon request.

B.   Level I Trauma Centers are automatically designated to accept 6 Immediate patients from MCIs that involve 20 victims or more.

C.   Level II Trauma Centers are automatically designated to accept 3 Immediate patients from MCIs that involve 20 victims or more

D.   When activated by the EMS Agency, Burn Resource Centers (BRC) can accept up to 12 critically burned patients.

E.   Accept MCI patients with minimal patient information.

F.   Monitor the HEAR and ReddiNet.

G. Provide the MAC or base hospital with patient disposition information, sequence numbers and/or triage tags when requested and enter information into the ReddiNet.

H. Maintain the "Receiving Facility" copy of the EMS Report Form and/or triage tag as part of the patient's medical record.

I. Ensure that requested patient information is entered as soon as possible into the ReddiNet "MCI victim list" for all patients received from the MCI. The "MCI victim list" will remain open for 72 hours after the incident.

J. Notify the MAC if resource needs exceed available resources.

CROSS REFERENCE:

Prehospital Care Policy Manual:
Ref. No. 201,   **Medical Direction of Prehospital Care**
Ref. No. 502,   **Patient Destination**
Ref. No. 503,   **Guidelines for Hospitals Requesting Diversion of ALS Units**
Ref. No. 506,   **Trauma Triage**
Ref. No. 510   **Pediatric Patient Destination**
Ref. No. 511,   **Perinatal Patient Destination**
Ref. No. 519.1, **MCI Definitions**
Ref. No. 519.2, **MCI Triage Guidelines**
Ref. No. 519.3, **MCI Transport Priority Guidelines**
Ref. No. 519.4, **MCI Field Decontamination Guidelines**
Ref. No. 519.5, **Regional MCI Maps and Bed Availability Worksheets**
Ref. No. 803,   **Paramedic Scope of Practice**
Ref. No. 806.1, **Procedures Prior to Base Contact**
Ref. No. 807,   **Medical Control During Hazardous Material Exposure**
Ref. No. 808,   **Base Hospital Contact and Transport Criteria**
Ref. No. 814,   **Determination/Pronouncement of Death**
Ref. No. 817,   **Hospital Emergency Response Team (HERT)**
Ref. No. 1126, **Multiple Casualty Incident Transportation Management**

FIRESCOPE's Field Operations Guide ICS 420-1.

Decontamination (Decon): The physical and/or chemical process of removing or reducing contamination from personnel or equipment, or in some other way preventing the spread of contamination by persons and equipment.

Fire Operational Area Coordinator (FOAC): Los Angeles County Fire District, which is contacted through its Dispatch Center.

Hazardous Material: Any solid, liquid, gas, or mixture thereof that can potentially cause harm to the human body through respiration, ingestion, skin absorption or contact and may pose a substantial threat to life, the environment, or to property.

Hospital Emergency Administrative Radio (HEAR): The HEAR radio frequency is the designated MCI communication system for paramedic providers to contact the MAC.

Hospital Emergency Response Team (HERT): An organized group of health care providers from a designated Level I Trauma Center, with Emergency Medical Services (EMS) Agency approval as a HERT provider, who are available 24 hours/day to respond and provide a higher level of on-scene surgical expertise.

Incident Command Post (ICP): Location at which the primary command functions are executed and usually coordinated with the incident base.

Incident Command System (ICS): A management system utilized to rapidly and efficiently manage the scene of any type of a large incident. This includes a combination of facilities, equipment, personnel, procedures, and communications operating within a common organizational structure with responsibility for the management of assigned resources to effectively accomplish stated objectives pertaining to an incident.

ICS Components (five major management functions):

1. **Incident Command:** Sets the incident objectives, strategies, and priorities and has overall responsibility at the incident or event.

2. **Operations Section:** Conducts tactical operations to carry out the plan. Develops tactical objectives and organization, and directs all tactical resources.

3. **Planning Section:** Prepares and documents the Incident Action Plan to accomplish the objectives, collects and evaluates information, maintains resource status, and maintains documentation for incident records.

4. **Logistics Section:** Provides support, resources, and all other services needed to meet the operational objectives.

5. **Finance/Administration Section:** Monitors costs related to the incident. Provides accounting, procurement, time recording, and cost analysis.

Jump START: A pediatric MCI field triage tool developed to parallel the START triage system, which adequately addresses the unique anatomy and physiology of children.

Medical Alert Center (MAC): Assists provider agencies and base hospitals with patient destination decisions and multiple casualty incidents. It serves as the control point for the HEAR and ReddiNet systems.

Medical and Health Operational Area Coordinator (MHOAC): Responsible for all medical and health operations for the operational area. The EMS Agency administrator is the designated MHOAC and is contacted through the MAC.

Medical Officer on Duty (MOD): Designated medical officer on duty for the MAC.

Multiple Casualty Incident (MCI): The combination of numbers of ill/injured patients and the type of injuries going beyond the capability of an entity's normal first response.

National Incident Management System (NIMS): A comprehensive, national approach to incident management that is applicable at all jurisdictional levels and across functional disciplines. The intent of NIMS is to be applicable across a full spectrum of potential incidents and hazard scenarios, regardless of size or complexity. The management system serves to improve coordination and cooperation between public and private entities in a variety of domestic incident management activities.

Rapid Emergency Digital Data Information Network (ReddiNet): An emergency medical communications network linking hospitals, regional EMS agencies, paramedics, dispatch centers, law enforcement, public health officials and other healthcare systems. The system provides participants with tools for managing MCIs, determining hospital bed availability, assessing available healthcare system resources, communicating emergency department diversion status, participating in syndromic surveillance, and sending the network messages.

Simple Triage and Rapid Transport (START): A triage system that provides guidelines for prehospital care personnel to rapidly classify victims so that patient treatment and transport are not delayed. Patients are triaged into the following categories:

Deceased: Patients who do not have spontaneous respirations after repositioning the airway.

Immediate: Patients who exhibit severe respiratory, circulatory, or neurological symptoms. Patients who require rapid assessment and medical intervention for survival.

Delayed: Patients who are neither immediate nor minor but will require a gurney upon arrival at the hospital. Delayed patients are the second priority in patient treatment. These patients require aid but injuries are less severe.

Minor: Patients who are ambulatory with injuries requiring simple, rudimentary first-aid.

Standardized Emergency Management System (SEMS): A system required by Government Code 806 (a), for managing responses to multi-agency and multi-jurisdictional emergencies in California. SEMS consists of five organizational levels which are activated as necessary: (1) field response; (2) local government; (3) operational area; (4) regional; and (5) state.

Staging Area: The location where incident personnel and equipment are assigned on a three-minute available status.

Triage: A system that provides guidelines for prehospital care personnel to rapidly classify victims so that patient treatment and transport are not delayed (see Ref. Nos. 519.2, 519.3 and 519.4).

Triage Tag: A tag used by triage personnel to identify and document the patient's triage category.

Unified Command: A team effort that allows all agencies with jurisdictional responsibility for the incident, either geographical or functional, to manage an incident by establishing a common set of incident objectives and strategies. This is accomplished without losing or abdicating agency authority, responsibility or accountability.

Key Incident Command System Positions:

Air Ambulance Coordinator: Located on the ground, reports to the Patient Transportation Unit Leader. Essential functions include maintaining communications with the Air Operations Branch Director regarding air ambulance transportation assignments. The Air Ambulance Coordinator is to establish and maintain communications with the Medical Communications Coordinator, the Treatment Dispatch Manager and to provide air ambulances upon request from the Medical Communications Coordinator. The position is responsible to assure that necessary equipment is available in the air ambulance for patient needs during transportation. The Coordinator is responsible to maintain records as required and Unit/Activity Log (ICS Form 214).

Air Operations Branch Coordinator: Is ground based and is primarily responsible for preparing the air operations portion of the Incident Action Plan and providing logistical support to helicopters operating on the incident.

Delayed Treatment Area Manager: Responsible for the treatment and re-triage of patients assigned to the Delayed Treatment Area and requesting Medical Teams as necessary. This position assigns treatment personnel to patients received in the Delayed Treatment Area, ensures treatment of patients triaged to the Delayed Treatment Area, ensures that patients are prioritized for transportation and coordinates transportation of patients with Treatment Dispatch Manager.

Ground Ambulance Coordinator: Reports to the Patient Transportation Unit Leader with responsibility to manage the ambulance staging area(s) and to dispatch additional ambulances/transportation resources as needed. Essential duties include establishment of appropriate staging area for ambulances; identify routes of travel for ambulances; and maintain communications with the Air Operations Branch Director regarding air ambulance transportation assignments. The position is to maintain communications with the Medical Communications Coordinator and Treatment Dispatch Manager and to provide ambulances upon request. The Ground Ambulance Coordinator is to assure that necessary equipment is available in the ambulance for patient needs during transportation, provide an inventory of medical supplies available at ambulance staging area for use at the scene, and maintain records as required and Unit/Activity Log (ICS Form 214).

Helicopter Coordinator (Helco): Is often the senior provider agency pilot on scene who is responsible for the overall air traffic control of the incident. This position is responsible for maintaining a position in the air that allows direct visual and radio communications with all helicopters both public and private. Essential duties include establishing arrival and departure routes, communicating with Fire, Law Enforcement and News Media helicopters and coordinating traffic with the Air Ambulance Coordinator.

Immediate Treatment Area Manager: Responsible for treatment and re-triage of patients assigned to the Immediate Treatment Area. This position requests medical teams as necessary, assigns treatment personnel to patients, assures that patients are prioritized for transportation and coordinates transportation of patients with the Treatment Dispatch Manager. This position is responsible for identifying immediate patients who exhibit severe respiratory, circulatory or neurological symptoms and who meet one or more categories of Trauma Center Criteria. These patients require rapid assessment, medical intervention and transport to a 9-1-1 receiving, Trauma Center or other specialty center whenever system resources allow.

Litter Bearer: Personnel assigned by the Triage Unit Leader who are responsible for the transport of patients to the appropriate treatment areas.

Litter Bearer Manager: Position assigned by Triage Unit Leader, the Litter Bearer Manager is responsible for the management of personnel assigned to transport triaged patients to the appropriate treatment areas.

Medical Communications Coordinator (Med Com): Establishes communications with the Medical Alert Center or designated base hospital to obtain status of available hospital beds. The Med Com assigns appropriate patient destinations based on available resources. This position receives basic patient information and condition from Treatment Dispatch Manager and provides the Medical Alert Center or base hospital with information on the assigned patient destinations and transporting ambulance unit.

Medical Group/Division Supervisor: Supervises the Triage Unit Leader, Treatment Unit Leader, Patient Transportation Unit Leader and Medical Supply Coordinator and establishes command and control within a medical group. This position determines the amount and types of additional medical resources and supplies needed to handle the incident (medical caches, backboards, litters, and cots), ensures activation or notification of hospital alert system, local EMS/health agencies and maintains Unit/Activity Log.

Minor Treatment Area Manager: Responsible for the treatment and re-triage of patients assigned to the Minor Treatment Area and requests medical teams as necessary. This position assigns treatment personnel to patients received in the Minor Treatment Area, ensures treatment of patients triaged to the Minor Treatment Area, ensures that patients are prioritized for transportation and coordinates transportation of patients with Treatment Dispatch Manager.

Patient Transportation Group Supervisor: Supervises the Medical Communications Coordinator and the Ground Ambulance Coordinator. The Patient Transportation Group Supervisor is responsible for the coordination of patient transportation and maintenance of records relating to the patient's identification, condition, and destination. This position designates the Ambulance Staging Area(s), ensures that patient information and destination are recorded, notifies Ambulance Ground Coordinator of ambulance requests, and coordinates requests for air ambulance transportation through the Air Operations Branch Director.

Triage Personnel: Reports to the Triage Unit Leader, triage patients, tag patients, and assign them to appropriate treatment areas. Triage personnel direct the movement of patients to proper treatment areas and provide appropriate medical treatment to patients prior to movement as incident conditions allow.

Triage Unit Leader: Supervises Triage Personnel, Litter Bearers, Litter Bearer Manager and the Morgue Manager. The Triage Unit Leader assumes responsibility for providing triage management and movement of patients from the triage area. This position implements the triage process, coordinates movement of patients from the triage area to the appropriate treatment area and maintains security and control of the triage area.

Treatment Dispatch Manager: Responsible for coordinating with the Patient Transportation Unit Leader (or Group Supervisor if established) the transportation of patients out of the Treatment Areas. This position establishes communications with the Immediate, Delayed, Minor Treatment Area Managers and the Patient Transportation Unit Leader. The position verifies that patients are prioritized for transportation and advises Medical Communications Coordinator of patient readiness and priority for transport. This position coordinates transportation of patients with Medical Communications Coordinator and coordinates ambulance loading with the Treatment Managers and ambulance personnel.

Treatment Unit Leader: Assumes responsibility for treatment, preparation for patient transport, and directs movement of patients to loading location(s). This position establishes communications and coordination with Patient Transportation Unit Leader and ensures continual triage of patients throughout Treatment Areas. This position directs movement of patients to ambulance loading area(s) and gives periodic status reports to Medical Group Supervisor.

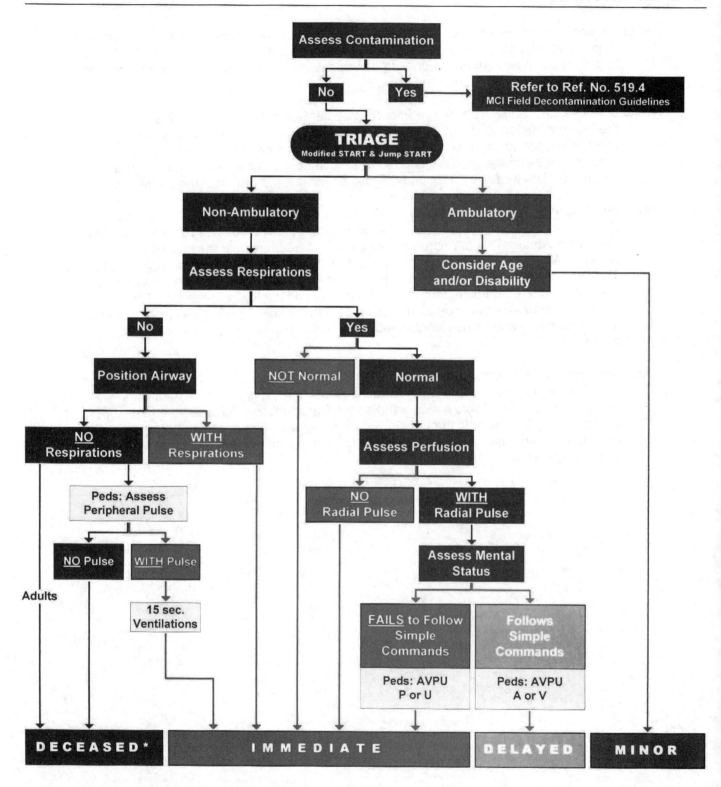

* Coordinate with Law Enforcement / Coroner

DEPARTMENT OF HEALTH SERVICES
COUNTY OF LOS ANGELES

SUBJECT: **MCI TRANSPORT PRIORITY GUIDELINES**

(EMT-I, PARAMEDIC, MICN)
REFERENCE NO. 519.3

PURPOSE: To provide guidelines for the Treatment Unit Leader, Treatment Area Manager and Patient Transportation Unit Leader for transport decisions that provide the maximum utilization of hospital resources during a Multiple Casualty Incident (MCI).

PRINCIPLES:

1. The Transport Priority Guidelines were developed to assist EMS personnel in determining which of the "Immediate" patients have the most life threatening injuries/illness requiring priority transport and would receive the greatest benefit from time critical medical interventions and definitive care.

2. Patients that meet Trauma Center Criteria (Ref. No. 506) should be transported to designated Trauma Centers whenever possible.

3. Pediatric patients should be transported to designated Pediatric Trauma Centers (PTC), Pediatric Medical Centers (PMC) or Emergency Department Approved for Pediatrics (EDAP) as appropriate to their condition.

TRANSPORT PRIORITY GUIDELINES:

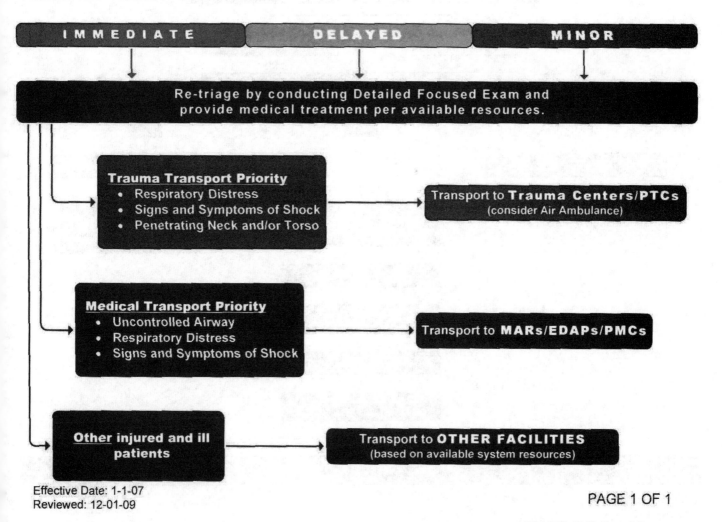

Effective Date: 1-1-07
Reviewed: 12-01-09

PAGE 1 OF 1

PRINCIPLES:

1. The need for decontamination should not delay the provision of time critical medication and treatment (i.e., Mark 1 antidote).

2. Patients shall not be transported to the receiving facility unless decontamination has been completed.

3. If incident involves chemical contamination and treatment is required, provider shall contact the base hospital or Medical Alert Center. Treatment should be based on the Hazardous Chemical Agent Emergency E3 guideline of the Base Hospital Treatment Guideline or Communication Failure Protocol.

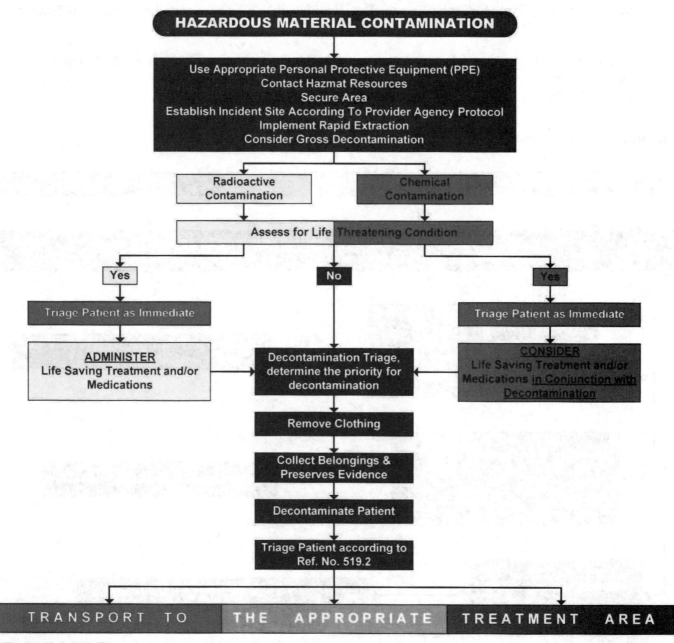

DEPARTMENT OF HEALTH SERVICES
COUNTY OF LOS ANGELES

SUBJECT: **CONFIDENTIALITY OF PATIENT**   (EMT-I, PARAMEDIC, MICN, BASE PHYSICIAN)
             INFORMATION   REFERENCE NO. 602

PURPOSE: To delineate local EMS Agency policy on disclosure of patient identity or medical
           information.

AUTHORITY: Health Insurance Portability and Accountability Act of 1996
           California Code of Regulations Title 22
           California Civil Code 56 & 1714, 1798
           California Health and Safety Code, 1797.98a – 1797.98g, 103885
           Welfare and Institutions Code Section 5325-5337

DEFINITIONS:

Medical information: Any Protected Health Information (PHI) possessed by a health care provider
           regarding a patient's medical history, mental or physical condition, or treatment, or the
           specific circumstances surrounding a specific patient identifiable incident (e.g. suspected
           child/elder abuse).

Protected Health Information (PHI): Individually identifiable health information that is maintained or
           transmitted in any form or medium, including paper, which can be linked to an individual
           (includes but is not limited to name, address, date, phone number, social security
           numbers, medical record numbers, certificate/license numbers, and any other unique
           identifying number, characteristic or code). Information can be shared for training
           purposes if personal information specific to a patient is redacted.

Prehospital Care Records: Prehospital records exist in various formats and include those on which
           written, spoken, printed, or digital information is recorded or preserved.

POLICY:

I.   Persons receiving health care services have a right to expect that the confidentiality of PHI
       obtained by health care providers is reasonably preserved. Therefore:

       A.   No provider of prehospital care shall disclose medical information regarding a patient of
              the provider without first obtaining an authorization from the patient or the patient's
              legally authorized representative except when such disclosure is permitted or required
              by law.

       B.   Paramedic communication shall be limited to that information that is relevant to the field
              care of the patient. If the patient's name is necessary, base hospitals shall request
              paramedics to landline the hospital if at all possible.

II.   Prehospital care providers transporting patients to hospitals shall disclose all relevant
       information only to health care professionals assuming care of the patient at the receiving
       hospital as required by applicable prehospital care policies.

EFFECTIVE: 3-24-75   PAGE 1 OF 2
REVISED: 4-01-09
SUPERSEDES: 5-15-06

APPROVED: _____   _____
          Director, EMS Agency   Medical Director, EMS Agency
                                             UCLA Skills Guide Page 251

DEPARTMENT OF HEALTH SERVICES
COUNTY OF LOS ANGELES

SUBJECT: **DOCUMENTATION OF PREHOSPITAL CARE**   (EMT-I, PARAMEDIC, MICN)
REFERENCE NO. 606

PURPOSE: To identify the hospital and Emergency Medical Services (EMS) provider procedures for documentation of Prehospital Care.

AUTHORITY: California Code of Regulations, Title 22, Article 9, Section 100176

DEFINITIONS:

Patient: A person who seeks or appears to require medical assessment and/or medical treatment.

EMS Response: The physical response of an EMS provider due to activation of the EMS system with a request for medical evaluation.

Patient Response: An EMS response that results in an actual patient or patients.

Multiple Casualty Incident (MCI): An incident involving multiple patients who might require transport.

PRINCIPLES:

1.   The EMS Report/Base Hospital Form is a:
   a.   Patient care record
   b.   Legal document
   c.   QI instrument
   d.   Billing resource
   e.   Record of cancelled calls and no patient found (EMS Report Form only)

2.   Any assessment or treatment provided to and medical history obtained from the patient shall be accurately and thoroughly documented on the EMS Report Form.

3.   Any person who alters or modifies the medical record of any person, with fraudulent intent, or who, with fraudulent intent, creates any false medical record, is guilty of a misdemeanor (section 471.5 of the California Penal Code).

4.   An EMS Report Form must be completed for every EMS response if a provider agency is unable to submit a quarterly volume report to the EMS Agency for the following types of calls:

   a.   Canceled calls
   b.   No patient(s) found
   c.   False alarms

POLICY:

I.   Form Completion

   A.   Paramedic/EMT-I Personnel

EFFECTIVE: 06-25-1974
REVISED: 04-11-06
SUPERSEDES: 10-15-2004

APPROVED: _____   _____
Director, EMS Agency   Medical Director, EMS Agency

PAGE 1 OF 4

1.   EMS providers shall document prehospital care according to procedures identified in the EMS Report Form Training Manual.

2.   Manual EMS Report Form Completion:

    a.   Paramedic/EMT personnel from the first responding agency shall complete one local EMS Agency approved EMS Report Form (one for each patient) for every 911 patient response which includes the following:
        i.   Regular runs
        ii.   DOA (dead on arrival; patients determined or pronounced dead per Reference No. 814, Determination/Pronouncement of Death in the Field
        iii.   ALS interfacility transfer patients

        Note: In the event of an automatic or mutual aid incident when two first responding providers have responded and have each completed an EMS Report Form, each provider agency shall legibly handwrite the Sequence Number from the other provider's form just above the imprinted Sequence Number (or in the space designated by their provider agency). Do not cross out or line through the imprinted Sequence Number. If care of the patient is transferred from one ALS provider agency to another, each provider agency shall complete an EMS Report Form and legibly handwrite the Sequence Number from the other provider's form just above the imprinted Sequence Number (or in the space designated by their provider agency). Do not cross out or line through the imprinted Sequence Number.

3.   Electronic EMS Report Form Completion

    a.   Paramedic/EMT-I personnel may document and submit prehospital care data electronically in lieu of the standard EMS Report Form provided that their department has received prior authorization from the EMS Agency.

    b.   Paramedic/EMT-I personnel shall complete one EMS Agency approved electronic EMS Report Form (one for each patient) for every patient response and one for each ALS interfacility transferred patient.

4.   Multiple Casualty Incident (MCI)

    a.   One standard EMS Report Form or one EMS Agency approved MCI EMS Report Form must be initiated for each patient transported in a multiple casualty incident. The MCI EMS Form may be initiated for incidents involving three (3) or more patients based on patient acuity and availability of resources.

    b.   Critical or unstable patients should have a standard EMS Report Form initiated whenever possible.

    c.   Non-transported patients may be included on a standard EMS Report Form, an EMS Agency approved MCI Report Form, or a patient log.

5.   Completion of EMS Report Form Prior to Distribution

    a.   EMT-Is and paramedics responsible for documenting prehospital care on EMS Reports shall ensure that, whenever possible, the EMS Report Form is completed in its entirety, prior to dissemination of copies. In most instances, this means that the form is completed at the scene or upon arrival at the receiving facility.

    b.   An exception to this is when a first responding agency is giving the receiving hospital (red/pink) copy to a transporting agency. In the interest of expediting the transfer of care, it is recognized that information such as the unit times may not be documented on the receiving hospital (red/pink) copy of the EMS Report Form.

6.   Completion of Page 2/Field Transfer of Patient Care Form

    a.   When the care of a patient has been transferred from the first responding ALS or BLS provider agency to a BLS provider agency for transport to a receiving facility, the provider agency receiving the patient should complete a Page 2/Field Transfer of Patient Care Form and not a standard EMS Report Form.

    b.   The provider agency completing the Page 2/Field Transfer of Patient Care Form must ensure that the Sequence Number from the EMS Report Form completed by the first responding provider agency is legibly and accurately transcribed onto the Page 2/Field Transfer of Patient Care Form.

    c.   The Receiving Hospital (red/pink) copy of the EMS Report Form, as well as the Page 2/Field Transfer of Patient Care Form (red/pink copy), must accompany the patient to the receiving facility where it becomes part of the patient's medical record.

B.   Base Hospital MICN and/or Physicians

1.   Base hospital personnel (MICNs and Physicians) shall document prehospital care according to procedures identified in the Base Hospital Form Training Manual.

2.   Base Hospital Form Completion

    a.   MICNs and/or physicians shall complete at least one EMS Agency approved Base Hospital Form (one for each patient in which medical direction is given) for every base hospital paramedic radio/telephone contact.

    b.   MICNs and/or physicians may document and submit base hospital data electronically in lieu of the standard Base Hospital Form provided that the base hospital has received prior authorization from the EMS Agency.

3.   Multiple Casualty Incidents (MCI)

    a.   ALS patients: Compete one standard Base Hospital Form or one EMS Agency approved MCI Base Hospital Form for each ALS patient.

b.   BLS patients: If the incident involves only BLS patients on whom no medical direction is given, only one form (for one patient) needs to be initiated in order to document the Sequence Number for the incident.

c.   ALS and BLS patients: One standard Base Hospital Form or one EMS Agency approved MCI Base Hospital Form must be completed for each ALS patient. BLS patients on whom no medical direction has been given do not require a Base Hospital Form. The number and disposition of the BLS patients may be documented in the Comments Section of the Base Hospital Form on an ALS patient.

d.   EMS Agency approved MCI Base Hospital Forms may be utilized in incidents involving three (3) or more patients.

II.   Modification of the EMS Report Form

A.   Modifying the EMS Report Form (additions, deletions or changes) after the form has been completed or disseminated:

1.   Make corrections by drawing a single line through the incorrect item or narrative (the writing underneath the single line must remain readable).

2.   Make the changes on the original, noting the date and time the changes were made, with the signature of the individual making the changes adjacent to the correction. Ideally, changes should be made by the individual who initially completed the form. Under no circumstances should changes to either patient assessment or patient treatment documentation be made by an individual who did not participate in the response.

B.   Making substantive changes (documentation of additional medications, defibrillation attempts, pertinent comments, complaints, etc.) to the EMS Report Form:

1.   Photocopy the EMS Report Form with the changes and send the copy, along with a cover letter, to all entities that received the original form (EMS Agency, receiving facility, base hospital). The cover letter should explain the modifications and request that the modified copy be attached to the original copy.

2.   Do not re-write the incident on a new EMS Report Form because this would result in a mismatch in Sequence Number. If the form requiring corrections has been mutilated or soiled and cannot be photocopied, then a new form may be used to re-write the incident provided the Sequence Number of the new form has been replaced with the Sequence Number from the original form.

CROSS REFERENCES:

Prehospital Care Policy Manual:
Ref. No. 608, **Disposition of Copies of the EMS Report Form**
Ref. No. 519, **Management of Multiple Casualty Incidents**

SUBJECT: **EMERGENCY MEDICAL TECHNICIAN (EMT)**
SCOPE OF PRACTICE

REFERENCE NO. 802

PURPOSE: To define the scope of practice for an Emergency Medical Technician (EMT) in Los Angeles County.

AUTHORITY: California Code of Regulations, Title 22, Section 100063

DEFINITIONS:

California EMT Scope of Practice: Skills, procedures, and administration of medications allowed by California regulations.

Local EMT Scope of Practice: Skills, procedures or administration of medications approved for EMTs by the Los Angeles County EMS Agency Medical Director.

Most Accessible Receiving (MAR) Facility: The nearest licensed health facility that maintains and operates a basic emergency department.

Most Appropriate Receiving Facility: The nearest licensed health facility that is staffed, equipped, and prepared to administer emergency and/or definitive care appropriate for the needs of the patient.

PRINCIPLES:

1. EMT personnel certified in California shall be trained and tested in the EMT scope of practice in accordance with California regulations.

2. EMT personnel working in Los Angeles County shall be trained and tested in the Local EMT Scope of Practice approved by the EMS Agency Medical Director.

3. When EMT personnel arrive prior to an advanced life support (ALS) unit, they shall assess the patient and make appropriate care and transport decisions as per Reference No.808 – Base Hospital Contact and Transport Criteria and Reference No. 502 – Patient Destination.

4. When EMTs assist patients with a physician prescribed medication, an ALS unit must be enroute or the patient must be transported immediately to the most accessible receiving facility that meets the needs of the patient, if the ALS unit's estimated time of arrival (ETA) exceeds the ETA to the MAR.

5. If EMT personnel encounter a life-threatening situation, they should exercise their clinical judgment as to whether it is in the patient's best interest to transport the patient prior to the arrival of an ALS unit if their estimated time of arrival (ETA) exceeds the ETA to the MAR. The rationale for the decision to transport shall be documented on an EMS report form.

EFFECTIVE: 3-1-86
REVISED: 2-1-11
SUPERSEDES: 8-15-05

APPROVED: _____
Director, EMS Agency

_____
Medical Director, EMS Agency

PAGE 1 OF 5

UCLA Skills Guide Page 256

6. EMT personnel may honor a patient request for transport to a facility other than the MAR if the patient is deemed stable and only requires basic life support (BLS) as long as the ambulance is not unreasonably removed from the primary area of response.

7. EMTs may transfer care of a patient to another EMT team if necessary.

POLICY:

I. California EMT Scope of Practice

During training, while at the scene of an emergency, during transport of the sick or injured, or during interfacility transfer, a certified EMT or a supervised EMT student or certified EMT is authorized to do any of the following:

A. Evaluate the ill or injured patient

B. Render basic life support, rescue and emergency medical care to patients

C. Obtain diagnostic signs to include, but not limited to, the assessment of temperature, blood pressure, pulse and respiration rates, level of consciousness, and pupil status

D. Perform cardiopulmonary resuscitation (CPR), including the use of mechanical adjuncts to basic cardiopulmonary resuscitation

E. Use the following adjunctive airway breathing aids:

    1. oropharyngeal airway

    2. nasopharyngeal airway

    3. suction devices

    4. basic oxygen delivery devices

    5. manual and mechanical ventilating devices designed for prehospital use

F. Use various types of stretchers and body immobilization devices

G. Provide initial prehospital emergency care of trauma patients

H. Administer oral glucose or sugar solutions

I. Extricate entrapped persons

J. Perform field triage

K. Transport patients

L. Set up for ALS procedures, under the direction of an Advanced Emergency Medical Technician (AEMT) or paramedic.

M. Perform automated external defibrillation when authorized by an AED service provider.

N. Assist patients with the administration of physician prescribed emergency medications and devices, including but not limited to:

    1. patient operated medication pumps

    2. sublingual nitroglycerin

    3. epinephrine devices

II. Local EMT Scope of Practice

A certified EMT or a supervised EMT student in Los Angeles County shall perform the activities listed in the California Scope of Practice and may perform the following additional activities in the prehospital setting and/or during interfacility transport:

A. Airway management:

    1. Ventilate advanced airway adjuncts:

        a. endotracheal tube

        b. esophageal-tracheal airway device

        c. perilaryngeal airway device (King LTS-D)

        d. tracheostomy tube or stoma

    2. Suction a tracheostomy tube or stoma

B. Transport a patient deemed appropriate for transfer by the transferring physician, who may have one or more of the following

    1. nasogastric (NG) tube

    2. gastrostomy tube (GT)

    3. saline/heparin lock

    4. foley catheter

    5. tracheostomy tube

    6. ventricular assist device (VAD)

    7. surgical drain(s)

8. medication patches

NOTE: Excluded are thoracostomy (chest) tubes

C. Assist patients with the administration of physician prescribed self-administered emergency medications if indications are met and no contraindications are present. These medications include but are not limited to:

1. Sublingual nitroglycerin up to maximum of 3 doses (includes patient self administration) if systolic blood pressure is ≥ 100mm/Hg

2. Bronchodilator inhaler or nebulizer, if the patient is alert enough to use an inhaler or nebulizer

3. Epinephrine device (autoinjector) for signs/symptoms of severe allergic reaction and asthma

D. Monitor and maintain preset rate of intravenous (IV) infusions:

1. Glucose solutions

2. Isotonic salt solutions (Normal Saline)

3. Ringer's Lactate

E. Monitor and maintain preset rate of IV lines:

1. Pre-existing vascular access device (indwelling vascular access line)

2. Peripherally inserted central catheter (PICC) line

NOTE: Excluded are central venous catheter (CVP) monitoring devices, arterial lines and Swan Ganz Catheters

F. Monitor IV infusions with additives adjusted to a keep open (TKO) rate:

1. Folic acid – maximum – 1mg/1000mL

1. Multi-vitamins (MVI) – maximum 1 vial/1000mL

2. Magnesium Sulfate – maximum 2 grams/1000mL <u>only</u> in conjunction with multi-vitamins

3. Thiamine – maximum 100mg/1000mL

G. Monitor IV lines with additives at pre-set rate via infusion pump:

1. KCl 20mEq/1000mL

2. Total parenteral nutrition (TPN)

H. Transport patients with specialized infusion pumps:

1. Any prescribed medication with an automated or patient operated medication pump.

2. Any prescribed pain medication via a patient controlled analgesia (PCA) pump.

CROSS REFERENCES:

Prehospital Care Policy Manual:

Ref. No. 412, **Automated External Defibrillator (AED) EMT Service Provider Program Requirements**
Ref. No. 502, **Patient Destination**
Ref. No. 506, **Trauma Triage**
Ref. No. 510, **Pediatric Patient Destination**
Ref. No. 511, **Perinatal Patient Destination**
Ref. No. 512, **Burn Patient Destination**
Ref. No. 808, **Base Hospital Contact and Transport Criteria**

SUBJECT: EMT SCOPE OF PRACTICE   REFERENCE NO. 802.1

CALIFORNIA EMT SCOPE OF PRACTICE	LOS ANGELES COUNTY EMT SCOPE OF PRACTICE

ALL INDIVIDUALS CERTIFIED IN CALIFORNIA MUST BE TRAINED AND TESTED IN THE FOLLOWING SCOPE OF PRACTICE:

In addition to the California EMT Scope of Practice, the Medical Director of Los Angeles County has established the EMT Scope of Practice to include the following treatment and transport protocols.

ALL EMTs WORKING IN LOS ANGELES COUNTY MUST BE TRAINED AND TESTED IN THE FOLLOWING SCOPE OF PRACTICE:

1. Evaluate the ill or injured patient.
2. Render basic life support, rescue and emergency medical care to patients.
3. Obtain diagnostic signs to include, but not limited to the assessment of temperature, blood pressure, pulse and respiration rates, level of consciousness, and pupil status.
4. Perform cardiopulmonary resuscitation, including the use of mechanical adjuncts to basic cardiopulmonary resuscitation.
5. Use the following adjunctive airway breathing aids:
   a. oropharyngeal airway;
   b. nasopharyngeal airway;
   c. suction devices;
   d. basic oxygen delivery devices; and
   e. manual and mechanical ventilating devices designed for prehospital use.
6. Use various types of stretchers and body immobilization devices.
7. Provide initial prehospital emergency care of trauma.
8. Administer oral glucose or sugar solutions.
9. Extricate entrapped persons.
10. Perform field triage.
11. Transport patients.
12. Set up for ALS procedures under the direction of an AEMT or paramedic.
13. Perform automated-external defibrillation when authorized by an EMT AED Service Provider.
14. Assist patients with the administration of physician prescribed devices, including but not limited to, patient operated medication pumps, sublingual nitroglycerin, and self-administered emergency medications, including epinephrine devices.

AIRWAY MANAGEMENT

1. Ventilate advanced airway adjuncts: endotracheal tube, esophageal-tracheal airway device, perilaryngeal airway device (King LTS-D)., tracheostomy tube or stoma
2. Suction tracheostomy tube or stoma

TRANSPORT PATIENT WHO MAY HAVE MEDICAL DEVICES AND/OR MEDICATION PATCHES

1. Nasogastric tube
2. Gastrostomy tube
3. Saline/Heparin lock
4. Foley catheter
5. Tracheostomy tube
6. Ventricular Assist Device (VAD)
7. Surgical drains
8. Medication patches

Excluded are thoracostomy (Chest) tubes

ASSIST PATIENTS WITH ADMINISTRATION OF ANY PHYSICIAN PRESCRIBED SELF-ADMINISTERED EMERGENCY MEDICATIONS INCLUDING BUT NOT LIMITED TO:

1. Sublingual nitroglycerin up to maximum of 3 doses if blood pressure is maintained at 100mmHg (includes patient self administration)
2. Bronchodilator inhaler or nebulizer as prescribed if alert enough to use inhaler
3. Epinephrine device (autoinjector) as prescribed for S/S of severe allergic reactions or asthma

If medication assistance is rendered, an ALS unit must be enroute or the patient must be transported immediately to the most appropriate receiving facility per Ref. No. 502, Patient Destination.

LOCAL SCOPE OF PRACTICE

The medical director of the local EMS agency may establish policies and procedures to allow a certified EMT or a supervised EMT student in the prehospital setting and/or during interfacility transport to:
1. Monitor intravenous lines delivering glucose solutions or isotonic balanced salt solutions including Ringer's lactate for volume replacement;
2. Monitor, maintain, and adjust, if necessary in order to maintain, a preset rate of flow and turn off the flow of intravenous fluid; and
3. Transfer a patient, who is deemed appropriate for transfer by the transferring physician, and who has nasogastric (NG) tubes, gastrostomy tubes, heparin locks, foley catheters, tracheostomy tubes, and/or indwelling vascular access lines. Excluded shall be central venous pressure monitoring devices and arterial lines including Swan Ganz catheters.
4. Monitor preexisting vascular access devices and intravenous lines delivering fluids with additional medications pre-approved by the Director of the EMS Authority.

MONITOR AND MAINTAIN PRESET RATE INTRAVENOUS SOLUTIONS

1. Glucose solutions
2. Isotonic salt solutions (Normal Saline)
3. Ringer's lactate

MONITOR AND MAINTAIN PRESET RATE OF INTRAVENOUS LINES

1. Pre-existing Vascular Access Device
2. Peripheral Inserted Central Catheter (PICC) lines

Excluded are central venous catheter (CVP) monitoring devices, arterial lines and Swan Ganz catheters

MONITOR INTRAVENOUS INFUSIONS WITH ADDITIVES ADJUSTED TO A TKO RATE

1. Folic acid – maximum 1mg/1000mL
2. Multi-vitamins (MVI) – maximum 1 vial/1000mL
3. Magnesium Sulfate – maximum 2 Grams/1000mL only in conjunction with MVI
4. Thiamine – maximum 100mg/1000mL

MONITOR INTRAVENOUS INFUSIONS WITH ADDITIVES AT A PRE-SET RATE VIA AN INFUSION PUMP

1. KCl – maximum 20mEq/1000mL
2. Total Parenteral Nutrition (TPN)

AUTHORITY

California Code of Regulations, Title 22, Section 100063

TRANSPORT PATIENTS WITH SPECIALIZED INFUSION PUMPS

1. Any prescribed medication with an automated or patient operated pump
2. Any prescribed pain medication via a patient controlled analgesia (PCA) pump

SUBJECT:	**LOS ANGELES COUNTY PARAMEDIC**	(PARAMEDIC)
	SCOPE OF PRACTICE	REFERENCE NO. 803

PURPOSE: To define the scope of practice of a paramedic accredited in Los Angeles County.

AUTHORITY: California Health and Safety Code, Division 2.5, Section 1797.172
California Code of Regulations, Title 22, Chapter 4, Section 100145.

PRINCIPLES:

1. A basic statewide scope of practice shall be used for the training and testing of paramedics.

2. Paramedics must be trained and tested to demonstrate competence in performing the optional scope of practice.

3. Procedures or medications may be added as part of the local optional scope of practice or through a trial study.

4. A paramedic may perform any activity identified in the scope of practice of an EMT-I in Los Angeles County.

5. Paramedics shall be licensed in the State, accredited by the County and sponsored by an approved paramedic service provider in order to perform the scope of practice approved for paramedics.

6. Advanced life support activities carried out by paramedics at the scene of a medical or trauma emergency or during transport shall be under the following conditions only:

   A. Online medical direction by a base hospital physician or MICN.

   B. Direct medical supervision as outlined in Reference No. 816, Physician at the Scene.

   C. Procedures Prior to Base Contact (Reference No. 806) followed by base hospital contact.

   D. Standing Field Treatment Protocols (Reference No. 813); may only be used by paramedics employed and trained by paramedic service providers that have been approved to utilize Standing Field Treatment Protocols (SFTPs).

EFFECTIVE: 3-01-86
REVISED: 07-01-09
SUPERSEDES: 10-01-08

PAGE 1 OF 4

APPROVED: _____

Director EMS Agency

_____

Medical Director, EMS Agency

POLICY:

I.   Basic Los Angeles County Scope of Practice

   A.   Perform defibrillation and synchronized cardioversion.

   B.   Visualize the airway by use of the laryngoscope and remove a foreign body with forceps.

   C.   Perform pulmonary ventilation by use of lower airway multi-lumen adjuncts, stomal intubation and adult oral endotracheal intubation.

   D.   Institute intravenous (IV) catheters, saline locks, needles, or other cannulae (IV lines), in peripheral veins and monitor and administer medications through various external venous pre-existing vascular access devices (PVAD).

   E.   Administer intravenous isotonic balanced salt solutions and monitor glucose and Ringer's lactate solutions.

   F.   Obtain venous or capillary blood samples.

   G.   Use an electronic glucose measuring device.

   H.   Utilize Valsalva maneuver.

   I.   Perform needle thoracostomy utilizing the 2nd intercostal space, mid-clavicular line.

   J.   Monitor thoracostomy tubes.

   K.   Administer approved medications by the following routes: intravenous, intramuscular, subcutaneous, inhalation, transcutaneous, rectal, sublingual, oral, intranasal or topical.

   L.   Administer the following medications (using prepackaged unit dose products when available):

      1.   25% and 50% dextrose (may dilute 50% dextrose to make 25% solution).

      2.   Adenosine.

      3.   Aerosolized/nebulized albuterol by hand held nebulizer or approved FDA delivery device.

      4.   Aspirin.

      5.   Atropine sulfate.

      6.   Calcium chloride.

7. Diazepam (disaster caches only).

8. Diphenhydramine hydrochloride.

9. Dopamine hydrochloride.

10. Epinephrine.

11. Glucagon.

12. Midazolam.

13. Morphine sulfate.

14. Naloxone hydrochloride.

15. Nitroglycerin (spray only).

16. Pralidoxime chloride (2-PAMCl).

17. Sodium bicarbonate.

II. Local Optional Scope of Practice

A. Administer medications, using prepackaged unit dose products when available:

1. Amyl nitrite (disaster caches).

2. Amiodarone.

B. Monitor and adjust IV solutions containing up to 40 mEq/L of potassium chloride.

III. Additional Local Optional Scope of Practice (requires an EMS Agency approved training and quality improvement program prior to implementation)

A. Perform adult and pediatric intraosseous insertion during cardiac arrest.

B. Perform transcutaneous pacing for symptomatic bradycardia.

C. Administer Continuous Positive Airway Pressure (CPAP).

IV. Trial Studies

Procedures or medications may be implemented on a trial basis when approved by the Medical Director of the EMS Agency and the Director of the EMS Authority through the Paramedic Trial Studies section of the paramedic regulations.

V. Statewide Scope of Practice Not Approved for Use in Los Angeles County

A. Needle cricothyroidotomy.

B.   Endotracheal medication administration.

C.   Activated Charcoal.

D.   Furosemide.

E.   Lidocaine hydrochloride.

CROSS REFERENCES:

Prehospital Care Policy Manual:
Ref. No. 802   EMT-I Scope of Practice
Ref. No. 803.1 Los Angeles County Paramedic Scope of Practice
Ref. No. 806   Procedures Prior to Base Contact
Ref. No. 813   Standing Field Treatment Protocols
Ref. No. 816   Physician at the Scene
Ref. No. 1006   Paramedic Accreditation, Continuous Accreditation and Reaccreditation

LOS ANGELES COUNTY PARAMEDIC SCOPE OF PRACTICE

CALIFORNIA PARAMEDIC REGULATION	LOS ANGELES COUNTY POLICIES
Basic Scope - all individuals licensed in California must be trained and tested in these practices:	SAME AS CALIFORNIA REGULATIONS EXCEPT:
(A) Perform defibrillation and synchronized cardioversion	
(B) Visualize the airway by use of the laryngoscope and remove foreign body(-ies) with forceps	
(C) Perform pulmonary ventilation by use of lower airway multi-lumen adjuncts, the esophageal airway, stomal intubation and adult oral endotracheal intubation	
(D) Institute intravenous (IV) catheters, saline locks, needles, or other cannulae (IV lines), in peripheral veins; and monitor and administer medications through pre-existing vascular access	(D) Pre-existing vascular access device – external venous device only
(E) Administer intravenous glucose solutions or isotonic balanced salt solutions including Ringer's lactate solution	(E) Initiate normal saline solution only, may monitor glucose and Ringer's lactate solutions
(F) Obtain venous blood samples	
(G) Use glucose measuring device	
(H) Utilize Valsalva maneuver	
(I) Perform needle cricothyroidotomy	(I) Not utilized in Los Angeles County
(J) Perform needle thoracostomy	(J) 2nd intercostal space, mid-clavicular line only
(K) Monitor thoracostomy tubes	
(L) Monitor and adjust IV solutions containing potassium, equal to or less than 20 mEq/L	(L) Up to 40mEq/L
(M) Administer approved medications by the following routes: intravenous, intramuscular, subcutaneous, inhalation, transcutaneous, rectal, sublingual, endotracheal, oral or topical	(M) Endotracheal route not utilized
(N) Administer, using prepackaged products when available, the following medications:	(N) Medications:
(1) 25% and 50% dextrose	(1) 25% dextrose may be diluted from 50% dextrose
(2) activated charcoal	(2) Not utilized in Los Angeles County
(3) adenosine	
(4) aerosolized or nebulized beta$_2$ specific bronchodilators	(4) Aerosolized albuterol administered by hand-held nebulizer or FDA approved delivery device
(5) aspirin	
(6) atropine sulfate	
(7) pralidoxime chloride (2-PAMCI) protopam	
(8) calcium chloride	
(9) diazepam	(9) Disaster caches only
(10) diphenhydramine hydrochloride	
(11) dopamine hydrochloride	
(12) epinephrine	
(13) furosemide	(13) Not utilized in Los Angeles County
(14) glucagon	
(15) midazolam	
(16) lidocaine hydrochloride	(16) Not utilized in Los Angeles County
(17) morphine sulfate	
(18) naloxone hydrochloride	
(19) nitroglycerin preparations, except intravenous, unless permitted under local optional scope of practice	(19) Nitroglycerin spray only
(20) sodium bicarbonate	

Based on California Code of Regulations, Title 22, Chapter 4, Emergency Medical Technician-Paramedic
 	
EMT-I Scope of Practice – a paramedic may perform any activity.
 	
Paramedics must be trained and tested to demonstrate competence in performing the optional scope of practice.
	Local Optional Scope
	
	<u>Medications:</u>
	  Amyl Nitrite – (disaster caches)
	  Amiodarone
	  Potassium Chloride – up to 40mEq/L
	
	<u>Procedures (Requires EMS Agency approval):</u>
	  Adult/Pediatric Intraosseous insertion in cardiac arrest
	  Transcutaneous Pacing for symptomatic bradycardia
	  Continuous Positive Airway Pressure (CPAP)

7/01/09

DEPARTMENT OF HEALTH SERVICES
COUNTY OF LOS ANGELES

| SUBJECT: | **BASE HOSPITAL CONTACT** | (EMT-I/PARAMEDIC/MICN) |
| | **AND TRANSPORT CRITERIA** | REFERENCE NO. 808 |

PURPOSE: To identify the signs, symptoms, chief complaints, or special circumstances of patients for whom base hospital contact is required for medical direction and/or patient destination. This policy delineates when transport to an appropriate and approved facility is indicated.

AUTHORITY: California Health and Safety Code, Division 2.5, Section 1798 et seq.,
California Code of Regulations, Title 22, Section 100175
California Welfare and Institution Code, Section 5008

PRINCIPLES:

1.   Paramedics should contact their assigned base hospital.

2.   In situations not described in this policy, paramedics and EMT-Is should exercise their clinical judgment as to whether ALS intervention, base hospital contact and/or transport is anticipated or indicated.

3.   Children ≤ 36 months of age require base hospital contact and/or transport in accordance with this policy.

4.   When base hospital contact and/or transport are not performed in accordance with this policy, appropriate explanation and documentation shall be recorded on the EMS Report Form. **This does not apply to patients ≤ 36 months of age.**

5.   Circumstances may dictate that transport be undertaken immediately with attempts to contact the base hospital enroute.

6.   In situations where EMT-Is arrive on scene prior to the paramedics, EMT-Is shall not cancel the paramedic response if a patient meets any criteria outlined in Section I of this policy. An ALS unit shall be requested if one has not been dispatched, unless Principle 7 applies.

7.   In life-threatening situations in which the estimated time of arrival (ETA) of the paramedics exceeds the ETA to the most accessible receiving facility (MAR), EMT-Is should exercise their clinical judgment as to whether it is in the patient's best interest to be transported prior to the arrival of paramedics. EMT-Is shall make every effort to notify the MAR via the Hospital Emergency Administrative Radio (HEAR), telephone, dispatch, or other appropriate means of communication when exercising this principle.

        NOTE: The MAR for pediatric patients is the most accessible EDAP.

EFFECTIVE: 7-13-77   PAGE 1 OF 4
REVISED: 11-15-09
SUPERSEDES: 09-15-06

APPROVED: _____   _____
          Director, EMS Agency   Medical Director, EMS Agency

8.   Paramedics shall contact their designated receiving trauma center on all injured patients meeting trauma triage criteria and/or guidelines or, if in the paramedics' judgment, it is in the patient's best interest to be transported to a trauma center. When the receiving trauma center is not a base hospital (only applies to Childrens Hospital Los Angeles), paramedics shall contact their assigned base hospital.

9.   A paramedic team may transfer care of a patient to an EMT-I team in cases where, in the paramedics' judgment, the patient does not require ALS level care. If the patient's condition meets base hospital contact criteria, the base hospital must approve the EMT-I transport.

POLICY:

I.   Paramedics shall make base hospital contact for medical direction and/or patient destination on all patients meeting one or more of the following criteria:

A.   Signs or symptoms of shock

B.   Cardiopulmonary arrest (excluding patients defined in Ref. Nos. 814 and 815)

C.   Chest pain or discomfort

D.   Shortness of breath and/or tachypnea

E.   Pediatric Medical Care (PMC) guidelines as defined in Ref. No. 510

F.   Situations involving five or more patients who require transport (Contacting the Medical Alert Center constitutes base hospital contact)

G.   Altered level of consciousness as defined in the Medical Control Guidelines

H.   Suspected ingestion of potentially poisonous substances

I.   Exposure to hazardous materials with a medical complaint

J.   Abdominal pain in a pregnant or in a suspected pregnant patient

K.   Childbirth or signs of labor

L.   Suspected fractures of the pelvis or femur

M.   Facial, neck, electrical, or extensive burns:

1.   20% or greater BSA in adults

2.   15% or greater BSA in children

3.   10% or greater BSA in infants

N.   Trauma Triage Criteria and Guidelines as defined in Ref. No. 506.

O. Traumatic Crush Syndrome

P. Syncope or loss of consciousness, or acute neurological symptoms (i.e., blurred vision, weak and dizzy, numbness, etc) prior to or upon EMS personnel arrival.

Q. A patient meeting any criteria in Section I who refuses transport against medical advice (AMA). Base contact is required prior to the patient leaving the scene.

II. EMT-I or paramedic personnel shall transport all patients meeting one or more of the following criteria:

A. Abdominal pain

B. Suspected isolated fractures of the spine, skull, or hip

C. Abnormal vaginal bleeding

D. Suspected allergic reaction

E. Asymptomatic exposure to hazardous material known to have delayed symptoms

F. Gastrointestinal bleeding

G. Near drowning

H. Patients who are gravely disabled or a danger to themselves or others.

III. Prehospital personnel shall manage pediatric patients ≤ 36 months of age as follows:

A. All children ≤ twelve (12) months of age shall be transported, regardless of chief complaint and/or mechanism of injury **unless** the child meets the criteria outlined in Reference No. 814, Determination/Pronouncement of Death in the Field, e.g., rigor mortis, post-mortem lividity, evisceration of the heart, lung or brain, etc.

B. All children thirteen (13) months to thirty-six (36) months of age require base hospital contact and/or transport, except in isolated minor extremity injury.

C. If a parent or legal guardian refuses transport (AMA), base contact is required prior to the patient leaving the scene.

IV. Paramedics utilizing Standing Field Treatment Protocols (SFTPs) shall make base hospital contact for medical direction and/or patient destination on all patients meeting one or more of the following criteria:

A. If indicated in the SFTPs

B. For any criteria listed in Section I of this policy that is not addressed by SFTPs

C. Anytime consultation with the base hospital is indicated

CROSS REFERENCES:

Prehospital Care Policy Manual:
Ref. No. 411,   **Provider Agency Medical Director**
Ref. No. 502, **Patient Destination**
Ref. No. 506, **Trauma Triage**
Ref. No. 510, **Pediatric Patient Destination**
Ref. No. 515, **Air Ambulance Trauma Transport**
Ref. No. 519, **Management of Multiple Casualty Incidents**
Ref. No. 606, **Documentation of Prehospital Care**
Ref. No. 802, **Emergency Medical Technician – I Scope of Practice**
Ref. No. 813, **Standing Field Treatment Protocols**
Ref. No. 814, **Determination/Pronouncement of Death in the Field**
Ref. No. 815, **Honoring Prehospital DNR Orders**
Ref. No. 816, **Physician at Scene**
Ref. No. 832, **Treatment/Transport of Minors**
Ref. No. 834, **Patient Refusal of Treatment or Transport**

Medical Control Guidelines

Los Angeles County EMS Agency

Ref. No. 808.1 - BASE HOSPITAL CONTACT AND TRANSPORT CRITERIA

Field Reference

PRINCIPLES:

❶ Contact assigned base whenever possible.

❷ Clinical judgment should be exercised in situations not described in this policy.

❸ Children under three years of age require base hospital contact and/or transport in accordance with this policy.

❹ Thorough documentation is essential, especially if contact/transport is not performed in accordance with this policy (* EXCEPTION, See SECTION III).

❺ Circumstances may dictate immediate transport with base contact enroute.

❻ EMT-Is shall not cancel a paramedic response if a patient meets any criteria in Section I; an ALS Unit shall be requested if one has not been dispatched.

❼ In life threatening situations, consider BLS transport if ALS arrival is longer than transport time.

❽ Contact shall be made with the area's trauma center, when it is also a base hospital, on all injured patients meeting Trauma Criteria and/or Guidelines.

SECTION I – BASE CONTACT REQUIRED

- Signs or symptoms of shock
- Cardiopulmonary arrest (excluding those meeting Ref. No. 814, 815 & 821)
- Chest pain or discomfort
- Shortness of breath/ tachypnea
- PMC/PTC Criteria/Guidelines (Ref. No. 510)
- 5 or more patients requiring transport (contacting MAC constitutes base contact)
- Altered level of consciousness as defined in the Medical Control Guidelines
- Suspected ingestion of poisonous substance
- Exposure to hazardous materials with a medical complaint

- Abdominal pain pregnancy or suspected pregnancy
- Childbirth or signs of labor
- Suspected fractures of pelvis or femur
- Facial, neck, electrical, or extensive burns:
  20% or > in adults
  15% or > in children
  10% or > in infants
- Trauma Criteria/Guidelines (Ref. No. 506)
- Traumatic crush syndrome
- Syncope, loss of consciousness, acute neurological symptoms
- Refusal of transport (AMA), if meeting any criteria in Section I

SECTION II – TRANSPORT REQUIRED

- Abdominal pain
- Suspected isolated fractures of spine, skull or hip
- Abnormal vaginal bleeding
- Suspected allergic reaction
- Asymptomatic exposure to haz-mat (If known to have delayed symptoms)
- GI bleeding
- Near drowning
- Patients who are gravely disabled or a danger to themselves or others

SECTION III – PEDIATRIC PATIENTS

- Infants ≤ 12 months of age shall be transported, regardless of chief complaint and/or mechanism of injury

  EXCEPTION: Infants ≤ 12 months of age who meet Ref. No. 814, Determination/Pronouncement of Death in the Field, Section I.

- Children 13-36 months of age require base hospital contact and/or transport except isolated minor extremity injury

- If a parent or legal guardian refuses transport (AMA), base contact is required prior to leaving the scene

  EXCEPTION: Ref. No. 808, Principle 4 does not apply to patients ≤ 36 months of age.

SECTION IV – REQUIRED BASE CONTACT CRITERIA FOR SFTPs

- If indicated in the SFTPs
- For any criteria listed in Section I which is not addressed by SFTPs
- Whenever consultation with the base hospital is Indicated

SUBJECT: **DETERMINATION/PRONOUNCEMENT**
         OF DEATH IN THE FIELD

(EMT-I/PARAMEDIC/MICN)
REFERENCE NO. 814

PURPOSE: This policy is intended to provide prehospital personnel with parameters to determine whether or not to withhold resuscitative efforts and to provide guidelines for base hospital physicians to discontinue resuscitative efforts and pronounce death.

AUTHORITY: California Health and Safety Code, Division 2.5
               California Probate Code, Division 4.7
               California Family Code, Section 297-297.5

DEFINITIONS:

Agent: An individual, eighteen years of age or older, designated in a power of attorney for health care to make health care decisions for the patient, also known as "attorney-in-fact".

Immediate Family: The spouse, domestic partner, adult child(ren) or adult sibling(s) of the patient.

Conservator: Court appointed-authority to make health care decisions for a patient.

Advanced Health Care Directive (AHCD): A written document that allows an individual to provide health care instructions or designate an agent to make health care decisions for that person. AHCD is the current legal format for a living will or Durable Power-of-Attorney for Health Care (DPAHC).

PRINCIPLES:

1.   Resuscitative efforts are of no benefit to patients whose physical condition precludes any possibility of successful resuscitation.

2.   EMT-Is and paramedics **may determine** death based on specific criteria set forth in this policy.

3.   Base hospital physicians may **pronounce** death based on information provided by the paramedics in the field and guidelines set forth in this policy.

4.   If there is any objection or disagreement by family members or prehospital personnel regarding terminating or withholding resuscitation, basic life support (BLS) resuscitation, including defibrillation, should continue or begin immediately and paramedics should contact the base hospital for further directions.

EFFECTIVE: 10-10-80
REVISED: 2-1-07
SUPERSEDES: 7-1-03

APPROVED:

Director, EMS Agency

Medical Director, EMS Agency

PAGE 1 OF 5

UCLA Skills Guide Page 272

POLICY:

I.   Determination of death, base hospital contact not required:

    A.   A patient may be determined dead if, in addition to the absence of respiration, cardiac activity, and neurologic reflexes, one or more of the following physical or circumstantial conditions exist:

        1.   Decapitation

        2.   Massive crush injury

        3.   Penetrating or blunt injury with evisceration of the heart, lung or brain

        4.   Decomposition

        5.   Incineration

        6.   Pulseless, non-breathing victims with extrication time greater than fifteen minutes, where no resuscitative measures can be performed prior to extrication.

        7.   Blunt trauma patients who, based on paramedic's thorough patient assessment, are found apneic, pulseless, and without organized EKG activity* upon the arrival of EMS at the scene.

            Organized EKG activity is defined as narrow complex supraventricular.

        8.   Pulseless, non-breathing victims of a multiple victim incident where insufficient medical resources preclude initiating resuscitative measures.

        9.   Drowning victims, when it is reasonably determined that submersion has been greater than one hour

        10.   Rigor Mortis (Requires assessment as described in Section I. B.)

        11.   Post-Mortem Lividity (Requires assessment as described in Section I. B.)

    B.   If the initial assessment reveals rigor mortis and/or post-mortem lividity only, EMT-Is and/or paramedics shall perform the following assessments to confirm the absence of respiratory, cardiac, and neurologic function for determination of death in the field:

    NOTE: Assessment steps may be performed concurrently.

        1.   Assessment of respiratory status:

            a.   Assure that the patient has an open airway.

            b.   Look, listen and feel for respirations. Auscultate the lungs for a minimum of 30 seconds to confirm apnea.

2.   Assessment of cardiac status:

    a.   Auscultate the apical pulse for a minimum of 60 seconds to confirm absence of heart sounds.

    b.   Adults and children: Palpate the carotid pulse for a minimum of 60 seconds to confirm absence of pulse.

    c.   Infants: Palpate the brachial pulse for a minimum of 60 seconds to confirm absence of pulse.

3.   Assessment of neurological reflexes:

    a.   Check for pupil response with a penlight or flashlight to determine if pupils are fixed and dilated.

    b.   Check and confirm unresponsive to pain stimuli.

C.   Patients in atraumatic cardiopulmonary arrest, who do not meet the conditions described in Section I. A., require immediate BLS measures to be initiated while assessing for one or more of the following:

1.   A valid Do Not Resuscitate (DNR)

2.   A valid AHCD with one of the following present at scene:

    a.   An AHCD with written DNR instructions.

    b.   The agent identified in the AHCD requesting no resuscitation.

3.   Immediate family member present at scene:

    a.   With a Living Will or DPAHC on scene requesting no resuscitation.

    b.   Without said documents at scene, with full agreement of others if present, requesting no resuscitation.

4.   Parent or legal guardian is required and must be present at scene to withhold or terminate resuscitation for patients under 18 years of age.

5.   Patient in asystole without CPR <u>and</u> the estimated time from collapse to bystander CPR or EMS initiating BLS measures is greater than 10 minutes.

    NOTE: If one or more of the conditions in Section I. C. is met, BLS measures may be discontinued and the patient is determined to be dead.

II.   Patients in cardiopulmonary arrest requiring base hospital contact.

A.   Pediatric patients (equal to or less than 14 years of age) who do not meet Section I. A., of this policy should receive immediate BLS measures while establishing base contact.

B.   Base contact shall be established for all patients who do not meet the conditions described in Section I. of this policy. The following are general guidelines:

1.   Continuing resuscitation on scene is appropriate for patients in medical cardiopulmonary arrest until there is a return of spontaneous circulation (ROSC).

2.   Transporting patients without ROSC is discouraged.

C.   Base hospital physician pronouncement of death:

The base hospital physician may pronounce death when it is determined that further resuscitative efforts are futile. Patients without ROSC after 20 minutes of resuscitative efforts by EMS personnel should be considered candidates for termination of resuscitation. Exceptions may include hypothermia or patients who remain in, or whose rhythm changes to V-fibrillation or Pulseless V-tachycardia.

III.   Crime scene responsibility, including presumed accidental deaths and suspected suicides:

A.   Responsibility for medical management rests with the most medically qualified person on scene.

B.   Authority for crime scene management shall be vested in law enforcement. To access the patient(s), it may be necessary to ask law enforcement officers for assistance to create a "safe path" that minimizes scene contamination.

C.   If law enforcement is not on scene, prehospital care personnel should attempt to create a "safe path" and secure the scene until law enforcement arrives on scene.

IV.   Procedures following pronouncement of death:

A.   The deceased should not be moved without the Coroner's authorization, any invasive equipment (i.e., intravenous line, endotracheal tube) used on the patient should be left in place.

NOTE: If it is necessary to move the deceased in the event, the scene is unsafe or the deceased is creating a hazard, prehospital personnel may relocate the deceased to a safer location or transport to the most accessible receiving facility.

B   If the patient is confirmed by law enforcement or the Coroner not to be a coroner's case and the personal physician is going to sign the death certificate, any invasive equipment used during the resuscitation may be removed.

C.   Prehospital personnel should remain on scene until law enforcement arrives, during this time when appropriate, the provider should provide grief support to family member(s).

D.   Consider Critical Incident Stress Debriefing for all involved prehospital personnel for unusual cases or upon request.

V.   Documentation shall include:

A.   For patients determined to be dead, document the criteria utilized for death determination, condition, location, and position of the patient and any care provided.

B.   If the deceased was moved, the location and the reason why. If the Coroner authorized movement of the deceased, document the coroner's case number (if available) and the coroner's representative who authorized the movement.

C.   For patients on whom base hospital contact is initiated, time of pronouncement and name of the pronouncing physician must be documented. Paramedics should provide a complete description of the circumstances, findings, medical history, and estimated duration of full arrest.

D.   The name of the agent identified in the AHCD or immediate family member who made the decision to withhold or withdraw resuscitative measures shall be documented along with their signature on the EMS report form.

E.   If the patient was determined not be coroner's case and the patient's personal physician is going to sign the death certificate, document the name of the coroner's representative who authorized release of the patient and patient's personal physician signing the death certificate, and any invasive equipment removed.

CROSS REFERENCE:

Prehospital Care Policy Manual:
        Ref. No. 518, **Decompression Emergencies/Patient Destination**
        Ref. No. 519, **Management of Multiple Casualty Incidents**
        Ref. No. 606, **Documentation of Prehospital Care**
        Ref. No. 806, **Procedures Prior to Base Contact**
        Ref. No. 808, **Base Hospital Contact and Transport Criteria**
        Ref. No. 815, **Honoring Prehospital Do-Not-Resuscitate (DNR) Orders**
        Ref. No. 818, **Honoring Advanced Health Care Directives (AHCD)**
        Ref. No. 819, **Organ Donor Identification**

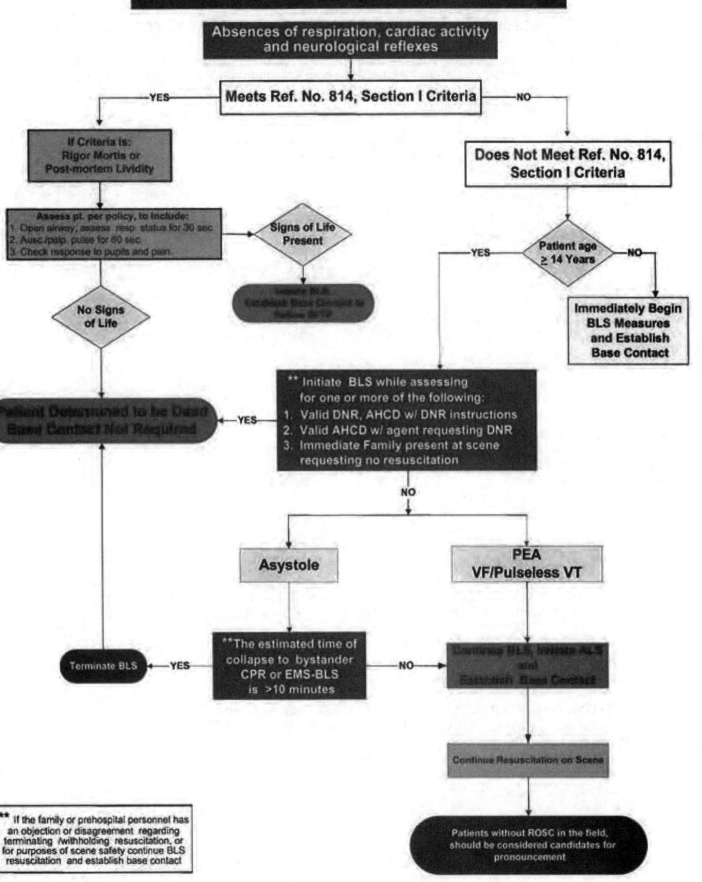

LA County Prehospital Care Policy Ref. No. 814, Determination/Pronouncement of Death in the Field

Absences of respiration, cardiac activity and neurological reflexes

Meets Ref. No. 814, Section I Criteria

YES — **If Criteria is:** Rigor Mortis or Post-mortem Lividity

NO — **Does Not Meet Ref. No. 814, Section I Criteria**

Assess pt. per policy, to include:
1. Open airway, assess resp. status for 30 sec.
2. Ausc./palp. pulse for 60 sec.
3. Check response to pupils and pain.

Signs of Life Present

Initiate BLS, Establish Base Contact to Refine DLTP

No Signs of Life

Patient age ≥ 14 Years

YES

NO — **Immediately Begin BLS Measures and Establish Base Contact**

Patient Determined to be Dead Base Contact Not Required

YES — ** Initiate BLS while assessing for one or more of the following:
1. Valid DNR, AHCD w/ DNR instructions
2. Valid AHCD w/ agent requesting DNR
3. Immediate Family present at scene requesting no resuscitation

NO

Asystole

PEA VF/Pulseless VT

Terminate BLS

YES — **The estimated time of collapse to bystander CPR or EMS-BLS is >10 minutes

NO — Continue BLS, Initiate ALS and Establish Base Contact

Continue Resuscitation on Scene

Patients without ROSC in the field, should be considered candidates for pronouncement

** if the family or prehospital personnel has an objection or disagreement regarding terminating /withholding resuscitation, or for purposes of scene safety continue BLS resuscitation and establish base contact

SC-1 12-06

DEPARTMENT OF HEALTH SERVICES
COUNTY OF LOS ANGELES

SUBJECT: **HONORING PREHOSPITAL DO-NOT-RESUSCITATE (DNR) ORDERS**

EMTI/PARAMEDIC/MICN)
REFERENCE NO. 815

PURPOSE: To allow prehospital personnel to honor valid Do-Not-Resuscitate (DNR) orders or Physician Orders for Life Sustaining Treatment (POLST) in the field and use supportive measures in accordance with the patient's wishes when death appears imminent.

AUTHORITY: California Health and Safety Code, Division 1, Part 1.8, Section 442 , Division 2.5. California Probate Code, Division 4.7, Section 4670 (Health Care Decisions Law)

DEFINITIONS:

Basic Life Support (BLS) measures:
Assisted ventilation via a bag-valve-mask device
Chest compressions
Automated External Defibrillator (AED) – only if an EMT-I is on scene prior to the arrival of paramedics

Resuscitation: Interventions intended to restore cardiac activity and respirations, including cardiopulmonary resuscitation, defibrillation, drug therapy, and other life saving measures.

Supportive Measures: Medical interventions used to provide and promote patient comfort, safety, and dignity. Supportive measures may include but are not limited to:

Airway maneuvers, including removal of foreign body
Suctioning
Oxygen administration
Hemorrhage control
Hydration
Glucose administration
Pain control (i.e., morphine)

Valid DNR Order for Patients in a Licensed Health Care Facility: A written document in the patient's medical record with the patient's name and the statement "Do Not Resuscitate", "No Code", or "No CPR" which is signed and dated by a physician, or a verbal order to withhold resuscitation given by the patient's physician who is physically present at the scene and immediately confirms the DNR order in writing in the patient's medical record, or POLST.

Physician Orders for Life Sustaining Treatment: A standardized, signed, designated physician order form printed on brightly colored paper that addresses a patient's wishes about a specific set of medical issues related to end-of-life care.

Valid DNR Order for Patients at a Location Other Than a Licensed Facility:
State Emergency Medical Services Prehospital Do Not Resuscitate (DNR) Form (Ref. No. 815.1), fully executed (photocopies are acceptable) **or** a State Emergency Medical Services Authority approved DNR medallion (Ref. No. 815.2) **or** POLST.

EFFECTIVE: 6-1-92
REVISED: 1-1-09
SUPERSEDES: 10-15-0

PAGE 1 OF 2

APPROVED: _____   _____
Director   Medical Director

EMERGENCY MEDICAL SERVICES
PREHOSPITAL DO NOT RESUSCITATE (DNR) FORM

An Advance Request to Limit the Scope of Emergency Medical Care

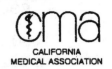

**CALIFORNIA
MEDICAL ASSOCIATION**

I, _____, request limited emergency care as herein described.

(print patient's name)

I understand DNR means that if my heart stops beating or if I stop breathing, no medical procedure to restart breathing or heart functioning will be instituted.

I understand this decision will **not** prevent me from obtaining other emergency medical care by prehospital emergency medical care personnel and/or medical care directed by a physician prior to my death.

I understand I may revoke this directive at any time by destroying this form and removing any "DNR" medallions.

I give permission for this information to be given to the prehospital emergency care personnel, doctors, nurses or other health personnel as necessary to implement this directive.

I hereby agree to the "Do Not Resuscitate" (DNR) order.

_____   _____
Patient/Surrogate Signature   Date

_____
Surrogate's Relationship to Patient

I affirm that this patient/surrogate is making an informed decision and that this directive is the expressed wish of the patient/surrogate. A copy of this form is in the patient's permanent medical record.

In the event of cardiac or respiratory arrest, no chest compressions, assisted ventilations, intubation, defibrillation, or cardiotonic medications are to be initiated.

_____   _____
Physician Signature   Date

_____   _____
Print Name   Telephone

_____
Address

THIS FORM WILL NOT BE ACCEPTED IF IT HAS BEEN AMENDED OR ALTERED IN ANY WAY

PREHOSPITAL DNR REQUEST FORM

White Copy: To be kept by patient
Goldenrod Copy: To be kept in patient's permanent medical record
Pink Copy: If authorized DNR medallion desired, submit this form with Medic Alert enrollment form to: Medic Alert Foundation, Turlock, CA 95381

DEPARTMENT OF HEALTH SERVICES
COUNTY OF LOS ANGELES

SUBJECT: **STATE EMS AUTHORITY APPROVED**
             DNR MEDALLION   REFERENCE NO. 815.2

1.   Medic Alert Foundation
       2323 Colorado Avenue
       Turlock, CA 95382
       Phone: 1-800-ID-ALERT (1-800-432-5378)
       FAX: 1-800-863-3429
       www.medicalert.org

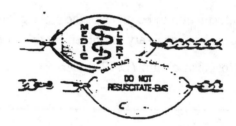

EFFECTIVE DATE: 8-1-93   PAGE 1 OF 1
REVISED: 2-12-07
SUPERSEDES: 8-1-93

APRPROVED: _____   _____
                Director, EMS Agency   Medical Director, EMS Agency

DEPARTMENT OF HEALTH SERVICES
COUNTY OF LOS ANGELES

SUBJECT: **PHYSICIAN AT THE SCENE**

PURPOSE: To establish guidelines for interaction between paramedics and a patient's personal physician, or physicians at the scene of a medical emergency who may not be the patient's personal physician.

NOTE: The guidelines set forth in this policy are intended for physicians at the scene who are <u>not</u> responding as a Provider Agency Medical Director.

AUTHORITY: California Health and Safety Code, Section 1798.6(a) provides that "authority for patient health care management in an emergency shall be vested in that licensed or certified health care professional . . . at the scene of an emergency who is most medically qualified specific to the provision of rendering emergency medical care."

DEFINITION:

Provider Agency Medical Director: A physician designated by an approved EMS Provider Agency to advise and coordinate the medical aspects of field care who meets the criteria outlined in Reference No. 411.

PRINCIPLES:

1. Although the law does not preclude a physician at the scene of a medical emergency from <u>rendering</u> patient care, it does prohibit them from <u>directing</u> paramedic personnel in advanced life support procedures. Such direction must come from the base hospital unless direct voice communication with the base hospital cannot be established or maintained. A Provider Agency Medical Director on scene may direct paramedics in advanced life support procedures per Reference No. 411.

2. Instructions by a private physician who is not on scene are subject to approval by the base hospital physician or Mobile Intensive Care Nurse (MICN) who is in direct voice contact with the paramedic.

3. A Provider Agency Medical Director may direct EMS personnel in lieu of base hospital contact.

POLICY:

I. Physician Identification

    A. Paramedics shall obtain proper identification, consisting of a California Physicians and Surgeons License, and note the physician's name, license number, and license expiration date on the EMS Report Form.

    B. When a physician on scene does not have identification or is in phone contact only, base hospital contact should be made to determine the extent of

EFFECTIVE: 1-1-81
REVISED: 1-01-07
SUPERSEDES: 5-15-94

APPROVED: _____   _____
           Director, EMS Agency   Medical Director, EMS Agency

permissible interaction between the paramedics and the physician.

II.   Patient Care

A.   Paramedics shall contact the base hospital and notify them of the presence of the physician on scene. If base hospital contact cannot be established immediately, it shall be made as soon as possible and a full report rendered.

B.   When communication cannot be established or maintained, paramedics may assist the physician and may provide advanced life support under the direction of the physician provided that their instructions are consistent with local EMS Agency policies and procedures.

C.   If either the paramedics or the base hospital physician perceive any problem(s) with the instructions of the patient's personal physician or physician on scene, the base hospital physician or MICN should speak directly with this physician to clarify or resolve the issue. If this direct contact is not possible, paramedics should follow the direction of the base hospital so that patient care is not delayed or compromised.

D.   When the physician on scene chooses to assume or retain responsibility for medical care, paramedics shall instruct the physician that they must take total responsibility for the care given. They must also accompany the patient until the patient arrives at a hospital and responsibility is assumed by the receiving physician unless relieved of the responsibility by the base hospital.

III.   Patient Destination

A.   Except when the physician on scene has accepted responsibility for patient care, patient destination shall be determined by the base hospital in accordance with EMS Agency policies.

B.   When the physician at the scene has accepted full responsibility for patient care, the patient may be transported to a general acute care hospital with a licensed basic emergency department chosen by the physician.

C.   If the paramedic provider agency determines that such transport would unreasonably remove the transport unit from the area, an alternate destination shall be agreed upon between the physician at the scene and the base hospital physician.

D.   If the patient's condition permits, alternate transportation may be arranged.

E.   If the patient's condition requires immediate transport, the decision of the base hospital physician or MICN shall be followed.

CROSS REFERENCE:

Prehospital Care Policy Manual
Ref. No. 411, **Provider Agency Medical Director**
Ref. No. 502, **Patient Destination**
Ref. No. 804, **Paramedic Scope of Practice**
Ref. No. 514, **Prehospital EMS Aircraft Operations Protocol**

DEPARTMENT OF HEALTH SERVICES
COUNTY OF LOS ANGELES

SUBJECT: **ORGAN DONOR IDENTIFICATION**   REFERENCE NO. 819

PURPOSE: To establish procedures for emergency medical personnel to comply with
statutory requirements to make a "reasonable search" for documentation which
identifies patients as organ/body part donors when death appears imminent.

AUTHORITY: California Health and Safety Code, Division 7, Chapter 3.5, Sections 7150, <u>et
seq</u>.

DEFINITIONS:

Imminent death: For the purposes of this policy, "imminent death" means any situation in which
illness or injuries in the adult patient are so severe that, in the opinion of
emergency medical personnel, death will occur before the patient arrives at the
hospital. For purposes of this policy, this definition does not include conscious
patients, regardless of the severity of illness/injury.

Reasonable search: A reasonable search consists of a brief, rapid attempt made by
emergency medical personnel to locate the patient's driver's license or other
documentation of anatomical gift intent. **IN NO EVENT SHOULD A SEARCH BE
CONDUCTED IF THAT EFFORT WILL DEPRIVE THE PATIENT OF LIFE-
SAVING CARE OR TRANSPORT.**

Document of gift: A document of gift is a card, a statement attached to or imprinted on a motor
vehicle operator's license, a will, or other writing used to make an anatomical gift.

PRINCIPLES:

1.   Individuals 18 years and older may make anatomical gifts and identify themselves as
donors either by documentation provided by the California Department of Motor Vehicles
attached to the motor vehicle operator's or chauffeur's licenses or by other document of
gift satisfying the law.

2.   The requirement to make a "reasonable search" for documentation either that a patient is
an organ donor or that they have refused to make an anatomical gift applies to
emergency medical personnel (EMT-1, Paramedics) who are treating a patient in whom
death appears imminent.

PROCEDURES:

1.   When emergency medical personnel are treating or transporting a patient whose death
appears imminent, they shall make a reasonable search for the organ donor
documentation.

EFFECTIVE: 1-1-93   PAGE 1 OF 2
REVISED: 4-15-09
SUPERSEDES: 4-11-06

APPROVED: _____   _____
                   Director, EMS Agency   Medical Director, EMS Agency

2. If the documentation is located, emergency medical personnel shall report this information verbally to the following, as indicated:

    a. The MICN, if base contact is made.

    b. The attending physician in the emergency department.

    c. Law enforcement officer or coroner's personnel at the scene if the patient has died on scene and will not be transported to the hospital.

DOCUMENTATION:

1. In addition to the verbal reports described above, paramedics shall enter brief remarks in the "Comments" section of the EMS Report Form, e.g., "organ donor per driver's license, base hospital (or coroner, or law enforcement, etc.) advised verbally".

2. If so advised, MICNs shall make a brief note to this effect on the Base Hospital Form.

DEPARTMENT OF HEALTH SERVICES
COUNTY OF LOS ANGELES

SUBJECT: **PHYSICIAN ORDERS FOR LIFE**   (EMT-1, PARAMEDIC, MICN)
             SUSTAINING TREATMENT (POLST)   REFERENCE NO. 821

PURPOSE: To allow prehospital personnel to honor valid POLST forms and provide end-of-life care in accordance with the patient's wishes.

AUTHORITY: California Health and Safety Code, Division 1, Part 1.8, Section 442,
H&S Code, Division 2.5
California Probate Code, Division 4.7, Section 4670 (Health Care Decisions Law)

DEFINITIONS:

Valid Physician Orders for Life Sustaining Treatment (POLST): A signed, designated physician order form that addresses a patient's wishes about a specific set of medical issues related to end-of-life care.

Advanced Health Care Directive: A document that allows patients who are unable to speak for themselves to provide health care instructions and/or appoint a "Power-of-Attorney for Health Care".

PRINCIPLES:

1. California law supports a patient's fundamental right to control decisions relating to their own health care, including the decision to have life-sustaining treatment.

2. Use of the original POLST form is strongly encouraged. Photocopies and faxes of signed POLST forms are legal and valid. The document must be signed by the patient or conservator and physician.

3. The POLST form is designed to supplement, not replace, an existing Advance Health Care Directive. If the POLST form conflicts with the Advance Health Care Directive, the most recent order or instruction of the patient's wishes governs.

POLICY:

I. Confirm that the patient is the person named in the POLST. This will normally require either the presence of a witness who can reliably identify the patient or the presence of an identification band/tag.

II. Basic Life Support (BLS) measures should be initiated pending verification of the valid POLST form.

III. If treatment contrary to the POLST directive(s) has been started, base hospital contact is required prior to discontinuing care.

EFFECTIVE: 1-30-09   PAGE 1 OF 2
REVISED:
SUPERSEDES:

APPROVED: _____   _____
           Director, EMS Agency   Medical Director, EMS Agency

IV.   Medical interventions should be initiated, consistent with the provider scope of practice, based upon the instructions on the POLST form.

V.   If the patient is transported, the POLST should be transported with the patient.

VI.   EMS Report Form Documentation

       A.   Describe the care given.
       B.   Print the base hospital physician's name, if consulted, and the date of the POLST.
       C.   Attach, when possible, a copy of the POLST to the provider agency's copy of the EMS Report Form.

CROSS REFERENCES:

Prehospital Care Policy Manual:
Ref. No. 502,   **Patient Destination**
Ref. No. 606,   **Documentation of Prehospital Care**
Ref. No. 802,   **Emergency Medical Technician-I Scope of Practice**
Ref. No. 803,   **Paramedic Scope of Practice**
Ref. No. 808,   **Base Hospital Contact and Transport Criteria**
Ref. No. 814,   **Determination/Pronouncement of Death in the Field**
Ref. No. 815,   **Honoring Prehospital Do-Not-Resuscitate (DNR) Orders**
Ref. No. 815.1, **State of California, Emergency Medical Services Prehospital Do-Not-Resuscitate (DNR) Form**
Ref. No. 815.2, **State Emergency Medical Services Authority Approved DNR Medallion**
Ref. No. 821.1, **Physician Orders for Life Sustaining Treatment**

HIPAA PERMITS DISCLOSURE OF POLST TO OTHER HEALTH CARE PROFESSIONALS AS NECESSARY

Physician Orders for Life-Sustaining Treatment (POLST)

First follow these orders, then contact physician. This is a Physician Order Sheet based on the person's current medical condition and wishes. Any section not completed implies full treatment for that section. Everyone shall be treated with dignity and respect.

EMSA #111 B
(Effective 1/1/2009)

Last Name
First /Middle Name

Date of Birth	Date Form Prepared

A Check One	**CARDIOPULMONARY RESUSCITATION (CPR):** *Person has no pulse and is not breathing.*

☐ **Attempt Resuscitation/CPR** ☐ **Do Not Attempt Resuscitation/DNR** (**A**llow **N**atural **D**eath)
(Section B: Full Treatment required)

When not in cardiopulmonary arrest, follow orders in **B** and **C**.

B Check One	**MEDICAL INTERVENTIONS:** *Person has pulse and/or is breathing.*

☐ **Comfort Measures Only** Use medication by any route, positioning, wound care and other measures to relieve pain and suffering. Use oxygen, suction and manual treatment of airway obstruction as needed for comfort. Antibiotics only to promote comfort. *Transfer if comfort needs cannot be met in current location.*

☐ **Limited Additional Interventions** Includes care described above. Use medical treatment, antibiotics, and IV fluids as indicated. Do not intubate. May use non-invasive positive airway pressure. Generally avoid intensive care.

☐ *Do Not Transfer to hospital for medical interventions. Transfer if comfort needs cannot be met in current location.*

☐ **Full Treatment** Includes care described above. Use intubation, advanced airway interventions, mechanical ventilation, and defibrillation/cardioversion as indicated. *Transfer to hospital if indicated. Includes intensive care.*

Additional Orders: _____

_____

C Check One	**ARTIFICIALLY ADMINISTERED NUTRITION:** *Offer food by mouth if feasible and desired.*

☐ No artificial nutrition by tube. ☐ Defined trial period of artificial nutrition by tube.
☐ Long-term artificial nutrition by tube.

Additional Orders: _____

D	**SIGNATURES AND SUMMARY OF MEDICAL CONDITION:**

Discussed with:
☐ Patient ☐ Health Care Decisionmaker ☐ Parent of Minor ☐ Court Appointed Conservator ☐ Other:

Signature of Physician
My signature below indicates to the best of my knowledge that these orders are consistent with the person's medical condition and preferences.

Print Physician Name	Physician Phone Number	Date
Physician Signature (required)	Physician License #	

Signature of Patient, Decisionmaker, Parent of Minor or Conservator
By signing this form, the legally recognized decisionmaker acknowledges that this request regarding resuscitative measures is consistent with the known desires of, and with the best interest of, the individual who is the subject of the form.

Signature (required)	Name (print)	Relationship (write self if patient)
Summary of Medical Condition		Office Use Only

SEND FORM WITH PERSON WHENEVER TRANSFERRED OR DISCHARGED

Patient Name (last, first, middle)		Date of Birth	Gender: M F
Patient Address			

Contact Information

Health Care Decisionmaker	Address		Phone Number
Health Care Professional Preparing Form	Preparer Title	Phone Number	Date Prepared

Directions for Health Care Professional

Completing POLST

- Must be completed by health care professional based on patient preferences and medical indications.
- POLST must be signed by a physician and the patient/decisionmaker to be valid. Verbal orders are acceptable with follow-up signature by physician in accordance with facility/community policy.
- Certain medical conditions or medical treatments may prohibit a person from residing in a residential care facility for the elderly.
- Use of original form is strongly encouraged. Photocopies and FAXes of signed POLST forms are legal and valid.

Using POLST

- Any incomplete section of POLST implies full treatment for that section.

Section A:

- No defibrillator (including automated external defibrillators) should be used on a person who has chosen "Do Not Attempt Resuscitation."

Section B:

- When comfort cannot be achieved in the current setting, the person, including someone with "Comfort Measures Only," should be transferred to a setting able to provide comfort (e.g., treatment of a hip fracture).
- IV medication to enhance comfort may be appropriate for a person who has chosen "Comfort Measures Only."
- Non-invasive positive airway pressure includes continuous positive airway pressure (CPAP), bi-level positive airway pressure (BiPAP), and bag valve mask (BVM) assisted respirations.
- Treatment of dehydration prolongs life. A person who desires IV fluids should indicate "Limited Interventions" or "Full Treatment."

Reviewing POLST

It is recommended that POLST be reviewed periodically. Review is recommended when:

- The person is transferred from one care setting or care level to another, or
- There is a substantial change in the person's health status, or
- The person's treatment preferences change.

Modifying and Voiding POLST

- A person with capacity can, at any time, void the POLST form or change his/her mind about his/her treatment preferences by executing a verbal or written advance directive or a new POLST form.
- To void POLST, draw a line through Sections A through D and write "VOID" in large letters. Sign and date this line.
- A health care decisionmaker may request to modify the orders based on the known desires of the individual or, if unknown, the individual's best interests.

California Coalition for Compassionate Care

The Coalition is the lead agency for implementation of POLST in California. This form is approved by the Emergency Medical Services Authority in cooperation with the California Coalition for Compassionate Care and the statewide POLST Task Force.

For more information or a copy of the form, visit **www.finalchoices.org**.

SEND FORM WITH PERSON WHENEVER TRANSFERRED OR DISCHARGED

SUBJECT: **SUSPECTED CHILD ABUSE/NEGLECT**　　　　(EMT-I,PARAMEDIC,MICN)
REPORTING GUIDELINES　　　　　　　　　REFERENCE NO. 822

PURPOSE: To provide guidelines for the identification of suspected child abuse and the reporting procedure for prehospital care personnel.

AUTHORITY: California Penal Code, Chapter 916, Sections 11164 - 11174.3.

DEFINITIONS:

Agencies authorized to accept mandated reports: Any police department or sheriff's department and the Department of Children and Family Services (DCFS). School District Police and security departments are not included.

Child: Any person under the age of eighteen.

Mandated reporter: Any healthcare practitioner, child care custodian, or an employee of a child protective agency. This includes EMTs and paramedics.

Neglect: The negligent failure of a parent or caretaker to provide adequate food, clothing, shelter, medical/dental care, or supervision.

Physical abuse: A physical injury, including death, to a child that appears to have been inflicted by other than accidental means.

Sexual abuse: Sexual assault on, or the exploitation of, a minor. Sexual assault includes rape; rape in concert (aiding or abetting or acting in concert with another person in the commission of a rape) incest; sodomy; oral copulation; penetration of genital or anal opening by a foreign object; and child molestation. It also includes lewd or lascivious conduct with a child < age 14 years, which may apply to any lewd touching if done with the intent of arousing or gratifying the sexual desires of either the person involved or the child. Sexual exploitation includes conduct or activities related to pornography depicting minors and promoting prostitution by minors.

PRINCIPLES:

1.　　The purpose of reporting suspected child abuse/neglect is to protect the child, prevent further abuse of the child and other children in the home, and begin treatment of the entire family. The infliction of injury, rather than the degree of that injury, is the determinant for intervention by DCFS and law enforcement.

2.　　California Penal Code, Sections 11166 and 11168, require mandated reporters to promptly report all suspected non-accidental injuries, sexual abuse, or neglect of children to local law enforcement and/or to DCFS. In Los Angeles County, it is recommended that a prompt verbal report be made to **both** the DCFS and local law enforcement.

EFFECTIVE: 6-1-83
REVISED: 4-1-09
SUPERSEDES: 3-1-06

APPROVED: _____　　　_____
　　　　　Director, EMS Agency　　　　　　Medical Director, EMS Agency

PAGE 1 OF 4

3. It is not necessary for the mandated reporter to determine child abuse but only to suspect that it may have occurred. Law enforcement, DCFS and the Courts determine whether child abuse/neglect has, in fact, occurred. **Children under the age of four, especially less than six months, are at highest risk.**

4. Current law mandates all healthcare professionals to report suspected child abuse/neglect that they know of or observe in their professional capacity. They are required to sign a statement acknowledging their understanding of this (See Ref. No. 822.1 for a sample form). Any person who fails to report as required may be punished by six months in jail and/or a $1,000 fine.

5. When a mandated reporter knows of or has observed child abuse/neglect, that individual is **required** to report by telephone to local law enforcement and/or to DCFS immediately, or as soon as practically possible, and complete the suspected child abuse report form **within 36 hours.**

6. The primary purpose of the Department of Justice (DOJ) Suspected Child Abuse Report Form (SS 8572) is to make all agencies aware of possible abuse/neglect. This will lead to a thorough investigation and protection of the child.

7. When two or more mandated reporters are present at scene and jointly know or suspect an instance of child abuse/neglect, a selected member of the reporting team can make the telephone report, and fill out and sign a single written report. Any member who knows that the designated reporter failed to uphold their agreement shall thereafter make the report. If paramedics are not selected as the designated reporters, they shall document the name and agency of the appointed team member on the EMS Report Form to indicate that the reporting obligation has been met.

8. Those persons legally required to report suspected child abuse are immune from criminal or civil liability for reporting as required.

POLICY:

I. Reporting Procedure

    A. Notify local law enforcement **immediately** if a child is suspected to be in imminent danger.

    B. Call the 24-hour Child Abuse Hotline at (800) 540-4000 as soon as possible to make the verbal report to DCFS. It is recommended that the Child Abuse Report Form be completed prior to verbal notification. Prehospital care providers should be aware of their local law enforcement reporting procedures and telephone numbers for notification.

    C. Complete the suspected child abuse/neglect form according to the instructions on the back of the form (Ref. No. 822.2 and 822.2a). **Within 36 hours,** send the completed report to local law enforcement and DCFS (3075 Wilshire Blvd., 5th Floor, Los Angeles, California, 90010).

    D. Document the following on the EMS Report Form

        1. The name of the DCFS social worker and/or name, department and badge number of the law enforcement officer.

2.   Time of notification.

3.   Disposition of child if not transported.

II.   Form SS 8572 Reporting Instructions

A.   Complete the SS 8572 for all reported suspected cases of child abuse/neglect.

Note: SS 8572 may be obtained by calling (800) 540-4000.

B.   Fill out the report as completely and clearly as possible using lay terminology.

1.   Section A - Case Identification is to be completed by the investigating agency authorized to receive the report.

2.   Section B - Reporting Party is to be completed by the person who initiated the report. Include name/title, address, phone number (include area code), date of report and signature.

3.   Section C - Report Sent To

a.   Check the appropriate box that identifies the designated agency authorized to receive the report.

b.   Enter the name and address of the agency to which this report is being sent.

c.   Enter the name, phone number and the date/time of the official contacted at the designated agency authorized to receive the report.

d.   The date and time are extremely important as they provide legal proof of verbal report.

4.   Section D - Involved Parties

a.   Victim: Enter the name, address, physical data, present location and phone number where the victim is located (attach additional sheets if multiple victims). If the birth date is not known, enter the approximate age.

b.   Siblings: Enter the name and physical data of siblings living in the same household as the victim. It is important to indicate when there are other children in the home even if no definitive information is available.

c.   Parents: Enter the names, physical data, addresses and phone numbers of father/stepfather and mother/stepmother. If the information is unavailable, then document "information not available".

5.   Section E - Incident Information

a.   Enter the date, time and place where the incident occurred or was observed and check the appropriate boxes.

b.   Check the type of abuse (there may be more than one type of abuse).

c. Write objectively; carefully describe all injuries and evidence of sexual assault, if applicable.

d. When obtaining information from the individual who is witness to the alleged abuse/neglect, attempt to use direct quotes when describing the incident.

e. If the parent, guardian or person accompanying the child changes their description of the occurrence, document both versions (use extra paper if needed).

f. If known, document prior incidents involving the victim.

g. When documenting neglect situations, stress the endangerment of the child. Endangerment is a key factor in the timely investigation of these cases.

h. Indicate circumstances which may contribute to an abusive/ neglectful situation (e.g., handicapped child or parent, substance abuse, spousal abuse, lack of resources, etc.).

III. SS 8572 Distribution

A. Retain the yellow copy for your records.

B. Submit the top three copies (white, blue and green) to the applicable child protective agency.

CROSS REFERENCES:

Prehospital Care Policy Manual:
Ref. No. 822.1,   **Sample Employee Acknowledgment as a Mandated Reporter**
Ref. No. 822.2,   **Suspected Child Abuse Report Form SS 8572**
Ref. No. 822.2a, **Definitions and General Instructions for Completion of Form SS 8572**

SUSPECTED CHILD ABUSE REPORT

To Be Completed by Reporting Party
Pursuant to Penal Code Section 11166

A. CASE IDENTIFICATION

TO BE COMPLETED BY INVESTIGATING CPA

VICTIM NAME: _____

REPORT NO./CASE NAME: _____

DATE OF REPORT: _____

B. REPORTING PARTY

NAME/TITLE

ADDRESS

PHONE ( )   DATE OF REPORT   SIGNATURE

C. REPORT SENT TO

☐ POLICE DEPARTMENT   ☐ SHERIFF'S OFFICE   ☐ COUNTY WELFARE   ☐ COUNTY PROBATION

AGENCY   ADDRESS

OFFICIAL CONTACTED   PHONE ( )   DATE/TIME

D. INVOLVED PARTIES

VICTIM

NAME (LAST, FIRST, MIDDLE)   ADDRESS   BIRTHDATE   SEX   RACE

PRESENT LOCATION OF CHILD   PHONE ( )

SIBLINGS

	NAME	BIRTHDATE	SEX	RACE		NAME	BIRTHDATE	SEX	RACE
1.					4.				
2.					5.				
3.					6.				

PARENTS

NAME (LAST, FIRST, MIDDLE)   BIRTHDATE   SEX   RACE   NAME (LAST, FIRST, MIDDLE)   BIRTHDATE   SEX   RACE

ADDRESS   ADDRESS

HOME PHONE ( )   BUSINESS PHONE ( )   HOME PHONE ( )   BUSINESS PHONE ( )

E. INCIDENT INFORMATION

IF NECESSARY, ATTACH EXTRA SHEET OR OTHER FORM AND CHECK THIS BOX. ☐

1. DATE/TIME OF INCIDENT   PLACE OF INCIDENT   (CHECK ONE)   ☐ OCCURRED   ☐ OBSERVED

IF CHILD WAS IN OUT-OF-HOME CARE AT TIME OF INCIDENT, CHECK TYPE OF CARE:

☐ FAMILY DAY CARE   ☐ CHILD CARE CENTER   ☐ FOSTER FAMILY HOME   ☐ SMALL FAMILY HOME   ☐ GROUP HOME OR INSTITUTION

2. TYPE OF ABUSE: (CHECK ONE OR MORE)   ☐ PHYSICAL   ☐ MENTAL   ☐ SEXUAL ASSAULT   ☐ NEGLECT   ☐ OTHER

3. NARRATIVE DESCRIPTION:

4. SUMMARIZE WHAT THE ABUSED CHILD OR PERSON ACCOMPANYING THE CHILD SAID HAPPENED:

5. EXPLAIN KNOWN HISTORY OF SIMILAR INCIDENT(S) FOR THIS CHILD:

SS 8572 (Rev. 1/93)

INSTRUCTIONS AND DISTRIBUTION ON REVERSE

DO NOT submit a copy of this form to the Department of Justice (DOJ). A CPA is required under Penal Code Section 11169 to submit to DOJ a Child Abuse Investigation Report Form SS-8583 if (1) an active investigation has been conducted and (2) the incident is **not** unfounded.

Police or Sheriff-WHITE Copy; County Welfare or Probation-BLUE Copy; District Attorney-GREEN Copy; Reporting Party-YELLOW Copy

SUBJECT: **ELDER ABUSE AND DEPENDENT**   (EMT-I, PARAMEDIC, MICN)
          ADULT ABUSE REPORTING GUIDELINES   REFERENCE NO. 823

PURPOSE: To define the required reporting procedures for prehospital care personnel regarding known or suspected elder or dependent adult abuse.

AUTHORITY: Welfare and Institutions Code Sections 15600, <u>et seq.</u>
California Code of Regulations, Title 22, 100160 and 100075

DEFINITIONS:

Abandonment: The desertion or willful forsaking of an elder or dependent adult by anyone having care or custody of that person under circumstances in which a reasonable person would continue to provide care or custody.

Abuse of an elder or a dependent adult: Physical abuse (including sexual abuse), neglect, financial abuse, abandonment, isolation, abduction, or other treatment with resulting physical harm or mental suffering, or the deprivation by a care custodian of goods or services that are necessary to avoid physical harm or mental suffering.

Dependent Adult: Any person between the ages of 18 and 64 years, who has physical or mental limitations that restrict their ability to carry out normal activities or to protect their rights. This includes, but is not limited to, persons who have physical or developmental disabilities. It also includes individuals whose physical or mental abilities have diminished because of age, as well as any 18 to 64 year-old who is admitted as an inpatient to a 24-hour health facility.

Elder: Any person who is 65 years of age or older.

Mandated Reporter: Any person who has assumed full or intermittent responsibility for care or custody of an elder or dependent adult, whether or not that person receives compensation, including administrators, supervisors, and any licensed staff of a public or private facility that provides care or services for elder or dependent adults, or any elder or dependent adult care custodian, health practitioner, or employee of a county adult protective services agency or a local law enforcement agency is a mandated reporter.

Neglect: The negligent failure of any person having care or custody of an elder or dependent adult to exercise that degree of care that a reasonable person in a like position would exercise.

Physical abuse: Assault, battery, unreasonable physical constraint, prolonged or continual deprivation of food or water, sexual assault or battery or rape (including spousal rape, incest, sodomy, oral copulation, or penetration by a foreign object).

Reasonable suspicion: An objectively reasonable suspicion of abuse that a person should entertain, based upon the facts, and drawing upon the person's training and experience.

EFFECTIVE: 10-10-80
REVISED: 1-15-09
SUPERSEDES: 10-15-06

APPROVED: _____   _____
         Director, EMS Agency   Medical Director, EMS Agency

PAGE 1 OF 4

Self-neglect: Failure of the elder or dependent adult to exercise a reasonable degree of care in providing for their own needs in such areas as personal hygiene, food, clothing, shelter,

PRINCIPLES:

1.   Elder and dependent adults may be subjected to abuse, neglect or abandonment.

2.   Health care providers are mandated to report known or suspected abuse, neglect or self-neglect of elder or dependent adults to protect and ensure the safety of these individuals.

3.   When two or more mandated reporters are present at the scene and jointly have knowledge of a known or reasonably suspected instance of elder or dependent adult abuse, the telephone report can be made by a selected member of the reporting team. Any member who has knowledge that the designated reporter failed to uphold their agreement shall thereafter make the report. Transfer of care to the hospital does not meet the reporting obligation.

4.   Reports made under this law are confidential. The identity of persons making reports of elder or dependent adult abuse is also confidential. This information is shared between the investigating and licensing agencies. This information will be shared with the district attorney in a criminal prosecution resulting from the report, by court order, or when the reporter waives confidentiality.

5.   Reporting is the individual responsibility of the mandated reporter. No supervisor or administrator may prohibit the filing of the required report.

POLICY:

I.   EMT-Is, Paramedics, and MICNs are mandated reporters and shall file a telephone and written report whenever, in their professional capacity or within the scope of their employment, the following occurs:

A.   The reporter has observed or has knowledge of an incident or injury that reasonably appears to be the result of abuse, neglect or self-neglect; or

B.   The reporter is told by an elder or a dependent adult that he or she has experienced behavior constituting abuse, neglect or self-neglect; or

C.   The reporter reasonably suspects abuse, neglect or self-neglect.

II.   Mandated reporters have immunity from civil and criminal liability for making a good faith report of a known or suspected elder or dependent adult abuse. This immunity includes taking photographs of the victim to submit with the report.

III.   Failure to report abuse, neglect or self-neglect of an elder or dependent adult is a misdemeanor, punishable by not more than six months in the county jail or by a fine of $1,000 or both. A mandated reporter who willfully fails to report abuse, neglect or self-abuse of an elder or dependent adult, where that abuse results in death or great bodily injury, is punishable by not more than one year in the county jail or by a fine of not more than $5,000 or both.

IV.   REPORTING PROCEDURES:

   A.   VERBAL REPORTS:

      1.   Reports of abuse, neglect or self-neglect shall be made immediately by telephone to the appropriate agency as defined in Reporting Procedure II

      2.   Reports are to include the following information, if available:

         a.   The name, address, telephone number, and occupation of the person making the report.

         b.   The name, address, and age of the elder or dependent adult.

         c.   Date, time, and place of the incident.

         d.   Other details, including the reporter's observations and beliefs concerning the incident.

         e.   Any statement relating to the incident made by the victim.

         f.   The name(s) of any individual(s) believed to have knowledge of the incident, and

         g.   The name(s) of the individual(s) believed to be responsible for the incident and their relationship to the victim.

   B.   WRITTEN REPORTS:

      1.   The Report of Suspected Dependent Adult/Elder Abuse form SOC 341 (Reference No. 823.1) must be completed and submitted to the agency initially contacted **within two business (working) days of the verbal report**. To request a supply of SOC 341 report forms, send a letter or facsimile to:

               California Department of Social Services Warehouse
               P.O. Box 980788
               West Sacramento, CA 95798-078
               Facsimile: (916) 371-3518

      2.   Reports shall be filed according to the following:

         a.   When the suspected/known abuse occurred in a long-term care facility, state mental health hospital, or state development center, report to either:

            i.   Local law enforcement agency, or

ii.   Long Term Care Ombudsman
        1527 Fourth Street, Suite 250
        Santa Monica, CA 90401
        Telephone: (800) 334-WISE (800-334-9473)
        After Hours: (800) 231-4024 (State Crisis Line)
        Facsimile: (310) 395-4090

3.   When the suspected/known abuse occurred in the community, report to either:

   a.   Local law enforcement agency

   b.   Adult Protective Services
          Centralized Intake Unit
          3333 Wilshire Boulevard, Suite 400
          Los Angeles, CA 90010

          Telephone: (888) 202-4248
          After hours: (877) 4-SENIORS (877-477-3646)
          Facsimile: (213) 738-6485

VI.   EMS REPORT FORM DOCUMENTATION:

Prehospital care personnel should document on the narrative section of the EMS Report Form the name of the responding agency (i.e. EMS Provider, Law Enforcement) designated to meet the reporting obligation.

CROSS REFERENCES:

Prehospital Care Policy Manual:

Ref. No. 823.1, **Report of Suspected Dependent Adult/Elder Abuse Form (SOC 341)**
Ref. No. 823.1a, **Report of Suspected Dependent Adult/Elder Abuse Form Instructions**

"Elder and Dependent Adult Abuse Reporting -- A Guide for the Mandated Reporter," June 2001, Los Angeles County Community and Senior Services

PURPOSE: To describe the guidelines for treatment and/or transport of a patient under the age of eighteen.

AUTHORITY: California Family Code 6922, 6926, 6927, 6929(4)b, 7002(a)(b)(c), 7122

DEFINITIONS:

Minor: A person less than eighteen years of age.

Minor not requiring parental consent is a person who:

Has an emergency medical condition and parent is not available
Is married or previously married
Is on active duty in the military
Is 15 years or older, living separate and apart from his/her parents and managing his/her own financial affairs
Is 12 years or older and in need of care for rape
Is 12 years or older and in need of care for contagious reportable disease or condition, or for substance abuse
Is an emancipated minor (decreed by court, identification card by DMV)
Is pregnant and requires care related to the pregnancy
Is in need of care for sexual assault

Legal Representative: A person who is granted custody or conservatorship of another person by a court of law.

Emergency: Condition or situation in which an individual has a need for immediate medical attention or where the potential for need is perceived by EMS personnel or a public safety agency.

PRINCIPLES:

1.   Consent

    A.   **Voluntary Consent:** Treatment or transport of a minor child shall be with the verbal or written consent of the parents or legal representative.

    B.   **Involuntary Consent:** In the absence of a parent or legal representative, emergency treatment and/or transport of a minor may be initiated without consent.

EFFECTIVE: 11-8-93
REVISED: 12-10-08
SUPERSEDES: 5-1-05

APPROVED:

Director, EMS Agency

Medical Director, EMS Agency

PAGE 1 OF 2

UCLA Skills Guide Page 298

PROCEDURES:

I.   Treatment/Transport of Minors

    A.   In the absence of a parent or legal representative, minors with an emergency condition shall be treated and transported to the health facility most appropriate to the needs of the patient (e.g. EDAP, PTC, PMC, Trauma Center, etc.)

    B.   Hospital or provider agency personnel shall make every effort to inform a parent or legal representative where their child has been transported.

    C.   If prehospital care personnel believe a parent or other legal representative of a minor is making a decision which appears to be endangering the health and welfare of the minor by refusing indicated immediate care or transport, law enforcement authorities should be involved.

II. Minors **Not** Requiring Transport

    A.   A minor child (excluding children ≤ twelve (12) months of age) who is evaluated by EMS personnel and determined not to be injured, to have sustained only minor injuries, or to have illnesses or injuries not requiring immediate treatment or transportation, may be released to:

        1.   Self (consideration should be given to age, maturity, environment and other factors that may be pertinent to the situation)

        2.   Parent or legal representative

        3.   A responsible adult at the scene.

        4.   Designated care giver

        5.   Law enforcement

    B.   Children ≤ 36 months of age require base hospital contact and/or transport in accordance with Reference No. 808.

    C   Prehospital care personnel shall document on the EMS Report Form to whom the patient was released.

CROSS REFERENCE:

Prehospital Care Policy Manual
Ref. No. 808, **Base Contact and Transport Criteria**
Ref. No. 822, **Suspected Child Abuse Reporting Guidelines**
Ref. No. 834, **Patient Refusal of Treatment or Transport**

California Association of Hospitals and Health Systems Consent Manual

DEPARTMENT OF HEALTH SERVICES
COUNTY OF LOS ANGELES

SUBJECT: **PATIENT REFUSAL OF TREATMENT
OR TRANSPORT**

(EMT-I/PARAMEDIC/MICN)
REFERENCE NO. 834

PURPOSE: To provide procedures for EMS personnel to follow when patients, parents, or legal representatives refuse medical treatment and/or ambulance transportation.

AUTHORITY: California Health and Safety Code, Division 2.5, Sections 1797.220, 1798, (a). California Welfare and Institution Code, Sections 305, 625, 5150, and 5170. Title 22, California Code of Regulations, Section 100169.

DEFINITIONS:

Adult: A person at least eighteen years of age.

Minor: A person less than eighteen years of age.

Minor Not Requiring Parental Consent is a person who:

- Is 12 years or older and in need of care for a reportable medical condition or substance abuse
- Is pregnant and requires care related to the pregnancy
- Is in immediate danger of suspected physical or sexual abuse
- Is an emancipated minor

Emancipated Minor: A person under the age of 18 years is an emancipated minor if any of the following conditions are met:

- Married or previously married
- On active military duty
- The person has received a declaration of emancipation pursuant to Section 7122 of the California Family Code, which includes all of the following: at least fourteen (14) years of age, living separate and apart from their parents and managing their own financial affairs (may be verified by DMV Identification Card)

Competent: A patient who is alert, oriented, has the capacity to understand the circumstances surrounding their illness or impairment, and the possible risks associated with refusing treatment and/or transport.

NOTE: Mental illness, drugs, alcohol intoxication, or physical/mental impairment may significantly impair a patient's competence. Patients who have attempted suicide, verbalized suicidal intent, or if other factors lead prehospital care personnel to suspect suicidal intent, should not be regarded as competent.

EFFECTIVE: 11-8-93
REVISED: 10-31-09
SUPERSEDES: 12-29-06

PAGE 1 OF 4

APPROVED: _____
Director, EMS Agency

_____
Medical Director, EMS Agency

UCLA Skills Guide Page 300

Emergency: A condition or situation in which an individual has an immediate need for medical attention, whether actual or perceived.

Implied Consent: This is a type of consent involving the presumption that an unconscious or incompetent person would consent to lifesaving care. This shall include minors with an emergency condition and a parent or legal representative is not available.

"Patient Not Requiring Transport" or "Release at Scene": A patient who, after a complete assessment by EMS personnel, does not meet any criteria listed in Ref. No. 808 and does not appear to require immediate treatment and/or transportation.

Refusing Care Against Medical Advice (AMA): A competent patient or a legal representative of a patient who refuses treatment and/or transport of the patient who meets any criteria listed in Ref. No. 808, or appears to require immediate treatment and/or transportation.

5150 Hold: A patient who is held against their will for evaluation under the authority of Welfare and Institutions Code, Section 5150, because the patient is a danger to themself, a danger to others, and/or gravely disabled (i.e., unable to care for self). This is a written order placed by a law enforcement officer, County mental health worker, or a health worker certified by the County to place an individual on a 5150 hold.

PRINCIPLES:

1.   A competent adult or emancipated minor has the right to determine the course of their medical care including the refusal of care. These patients must be advised of the risks and consequences resulting from refusal of medical care.

2.   A patient less than eighteen (18) years of age, with the exception of minors not requiring parental consent, must have a parent or legal representative to refuse evaluation, treatment, and/or transport for an emergency condition.

3.   A patient determined by EMS personnel or the base hospital to be incompetent may not refuse care AMA or be released at scene. Mental illness, drugs, alcohol intoxication, or physical/mental impairment may significantly impair a patient's competence. Patients who have attempted suicide, verbalized suicidal intent, or if other factors lead EMS personnel to suspect suicidal intent, should not be regarded as competent.

4.   At no time are EMS personnel to put themselves in danger by attempting to treat and/or transport a patient who refuses care.

POLICY:

I.   Refusal of Care AMA by a Competent Adult or Minor Not Requiring Parental Consent:

A.   EMS personnel shall advise the patient of the risks and consequences which may result from refusal of treatment and/or transport. The patient should be advised to seek immediate medical care.

B. If the patient's condition meets any criteria for base hospital contact and a BLS unit is alone on scene, an ALS unit should be requested.

C. When base hospital contact is made, contact should be made prior to the patient leaving the scene. Paramedics shall advise the base hospital of all the circumstances including care, transportation, reasons for refusal, and the patient's plans for follow-up care.

D. Paramedics shall have the patient or their legal representative, as appropriate, sign the release (AMA) section of the EMS Report Form. The signature shall be witnessed, preferably by a family member.

E. A patient's refusal to sign the AMA section should be documented on the EMS Report Form.

II. Refusal of Care AMA by an Incompetent Individual or a Minor Requiring Parental Consent:

A. The patient should be transported to an appropriate receiving facility under implied consent. A 5150 hold is not required.

B. If EMS personnel or the base hospital determines it is necessary to transport the patient against their will and the patient resists, or the EMS personnel believe the patient will resist, assistance from law enforcement should be requested in transporting the patient. Law enforcement may consider the placement of a 5150 hold on the patient but this is not required for transport.

C. Law enforcement should be involved whenever EMS personnel believe a parent or other legal representative of the patient is acting unreasonably in refusing immediate care and/or transport.

III. Patients Released at Scene:

A. EMS personnel shall advise the patient to seek follow-up treatment or immediate medical care, including re-contacting 9-1-1 if they develop symptoms at a later time. The advice given should be documented on the EMS Report Form.

B. EMS personnel should not require patients released at scene to sign the release (AMA) section of the EMS Report Form, as this implies that the patient is at significant risk by not utilizing the EMS system for treatment and/or transportation.

IV. Documentation:

An EMS Report Form must be completed for each incident of patient refusal of emergency medical evaluation, care and/or transportation. EMS personnel shall ensure that documentation includes, at a minimum, the following:

A. Patient history and assessment
B. Description of the patient which clearly indicates their decision-making capacity
C. What the patient is refusing (i.e., medical care, transport)

D.   Why the patient is refusing care
E.   Risk and consequences of refusing care
F.   Statement that the patient understands the risks and consequences of refusing care
G.   Signature of competent patient or legal representative refusing care
H.   Patient's plan for follow-up care

CROSS REFERENCE:

Prehospital Care Policy Manual

Ref. No. 808, **Base Hospital Contact and Transport Criteria**
Ref. No. 832, **Treatment/Transport of Minors**

DEPARTMENT OF HEALTH SERVICES
COUNTY OF LOS ANGELES

SUBJECT: **COMMUNICABLE DISEASE EXPOSURE AND**   (EMT-I, PARAMEDIC, MICN)
             TESTING   REFERENCE NO. 836

PURPOSE: To provide guidelines for prehospital care personnel exposed to blood or other potentially infectious material.

AUTHORITY: California Health and Safety Code, Division 105, Chapter 3.5, Sections 120260-120263
California Health and Safety Code, Sections 1797.188 -189, 120980, 121050-121070, 121140
U.S. Department of Labor-Occupational Safety and Health Administration Bloodborne Pathogens Standard 1910.1030 (2006)
California Occupational Safety and Health Standards
Exposure Control Plan for Bloodborne Pathogens (2001)
Ryan White HIV/AIDS Treatment Modernization Act of 2006
Code of Federal Regulations, Title 45, Section 164.512.b.4 (October 2007)
California Code of Regulations, Title 8, Section 5193 (Register 2007, No. 46)

DEFINITIONS:

Attending physician of the source patient: Any physician or surgeon who provides health care services to the source patient.

Available blood or patient sample: Blood, other tissue, or material legally obtained in the course of providing health care services and in the possession of the physician or other health care provider of the source patient **prior to the release of the source patient from the physician's or health care provider's facility.**

Body Substance Isolation (BSI): A method of infection control designed to approach <u>all</u> body fluids as being potentially infectious. It is the preferred infection control concept for EMS personnel.

Certifying physician: Any physician consulted by the exposed individual for the exposure incident.

Communicable disease: Any disease that is transferable through an exposure incident, as determined by the certifying physician.

Exposed individual: Any individual health care provider, first responder, or any other person, including, but not limited to, any employee, volunteer, or contracted agent of any health care provider, who is exposed, within the scope of their employment, to the blood or other potentially infectious materials of a source patient.

Exposure certification: A determination by the certifying physician on the exposure's significance.

EFFECTIVE: 1-1-95
REVISED: 2-1-09   PAGE 1 OF 5
SUPERSEDES: 6-1-08

APPROVED: _____   _____
             Director, EMS Agency   Medical Director, EMS Agency

Legal representative: For purposes of giving consent to communicable disease testing, whenever the word "source patient" is used herein, it shall also be deemed to mean the source patient's legal representative.

Personnel Protective Equipment (PPE): Specialized clothing or equipment worn by personnel for protection from exposure to blood or other potentially infectious material. See "universal precautions".

Significant exposure: Direct contact with blood or other potentially infectious materials of a patient in a manner that is capable of transmitting a communicable disease.

Source patient: Any person receiving health care services whose blood or other potentially infectious material is the source of a significant exposure to prehospital care personnel.

Universal Precautions: A method of infection control in which human blood and certain human body fluids are treated as if known to be infectious for blood borne pathogens.

PRINCIPLES:

1. Prehospital personnel must observe "body substance isolation" in situations where there is a potential for contact with blood, body fluids, or other potentially infectious material.

2. Prehospital care personnel are frequently exposed to blood and other potentially infectious materials of patients whose communicable disease infection status is unknown. Prehospital personnel who experience a significant exposure to these substances are permitted, under certain conditions, to learn the communicable disease infection status of the source patient.

3. Early knowledge of infection with a communicable disease is important to allow exposed persons to make informed health care decisions and take measures to reduce the transmission of the infection to others.

4. A health care provider shall not draw blood or patient sample for the sole purpose of communicable disease testing if the source patient refuses communicable disease testing. If the source patient's communicable disease status is unknown and the patient refuses communicable disease testing; only available blood or patient sample may be tested for any communicable disease.

5. California law prohibits an exposed individual from attempting to directly obtain informed consent to communicable disease testing from a source patient.

POLICY:

I. EVALUATION AND CERTIFICATION OF AN EXPOSURE

A. In the event of an exposure to blood or other potentially infectious material of a patient, exposed prehospital care personnel are to follow their provider agency's post-exposure protocol, including the completion of the Communicable Disease Exposure and Notification Form (Ref. No. 836.2) or the equivalent. The exposed individual shall make a written request for exposure certification within 72 hours of the exposure and a physician should promptly evaluate the exposure. No physician or other exposed individual shall certify their own exposure; however, an employing physician may certify the exposure of one of their employees.

Note: Prehospital care personnel with a significant exposure should seek medical evaluation and treatment immediately.

B.   The physician shall provide written certification of the exposure's significance within 72 hours of the request. The certification shall include the nature and extent of the exposure.

C.   The exposed individual shall be counseled regarding the likelihood of transmission, limitations of the tests performed, need for follow up testing, and the procedures that the exposed individual must follow regardless of the source patient's test results.

D.   Within 72 hours of certifying the exposure as significant, the certifying physician shall provide written certification to the source patient's attending physician. The certification shall: a) indicate that a significant exposure has occurred, b) request information regarding the communicable disease status of the source patient and the availability of blood or other patient samples. The source patient's attending physician shall respond to the request for information within three (3) working days.

Note: Many source patients are discharged from the emergency department; therefore, the exposure certification should be made immediately available to the emergency department where the source patient is being treated. This may allow the source patient to consent to communicable disease testing while still in the emergency department.

II.   COMMUNICABLE DISEASE STATUS OF SOURCE PATIENT

A.   KNOWN COMMUNICABLE DISEASE STATUS

1.   If the source patient's communicable disease status is known, the source patient's attending physician shall obtain consent to disclose the communicable disease status to the exposed individual.

2.   If the source patient cannot be contacted or refuses to consent to the disclosure, then the exposed individual may be informed of the communicable disease status by the attending physician as soon as possible after the exposure has been certified as significant.

B.   UNKNOWN COMMUNICABLE DISEASE STATUS

1.   If the communicable disease status of the source patient is unknown, and blood or other patient samples are available, and the exposed individual has tested negative on a baseline test for communicable diseases, the source patient shall be given an opportunity to give a voluntary, written, informed consent to test for communicable diseases.

2.   The source patient shall be provided with medically appropriate pretest counseling and referred to appropriate posttest counseling and follow-up if necessary. The source patient shall be offered medically appropriate counseling whether or not he or she consents to testing.

3.   Within 72 hours after receiving a written certification of significant exposure, the source patient's attending physician shall make a good faith effort to notify the source patient about the significant exposure. A good faith effort to notify includes, but is not limited to, a documented attempt to locate the source patient by telephone or by first-class mail with certificate of mailing. An attempt to locate the source patient and the results of that attempt shall be documented in the source patient's medical record.

4.   An inability to contact the source patient after a good faith effort or the inability of the source patient to provide informed consent **shall constitute a refusal of consent,** provided all the following conditions are met:

   a.   The source patient has no authorized legal representative,
   b.   The source patient is incapable of giving consent, and
   c.   In the opinion of the attending physician, the source patient will be unable to grant informed consent within the 72-hour period required to respond.

5.   **If the source patient refuses consent to test for communicable diseases, any available blood or patient sample of the source patient may be tested. The source patient shall be informed that the available blood or patient sample will be tested despite their refusal, and the exposed individual shall be informed of the results regarding communicable diseases.**

6.   If the source patient is deceased, consent to perform a test for any communicable disease on any blood or patient sample of the source patient legally obtained in the course of providing health care services at the time of the exposure shall be deemed granted.

7.   The source patient shall have the option not to be informed of the test result. If a patient refuses to provide informed consent to communicable disease testing and refuses to learn the results of testing, documentation of the refusal shall be signed. The source patient's refusal to sign shall be construed a refusal to be informed of the test results. Test results shall only be placed in the source patient's medical record when the patient has agreed in writing to be informed of the results. If the source patient refuses to be informed of the test results, the test results shall only be provided to the exposed individual in accordance with applicable Federal and State occupational health and safety standards.

III.   CONFIDENTIALITY AND LIABILITY

   A.   The exposed individual shall be informed that any identifying information about the communicable disease test results and medical information regarding the communicable disease status of the source patient shall be kept confidential and may not be further disclosed, except as authorized by law. The exposed individual shall be informed of the civil and criminal penalties for which they would be **personally** liable for violating Health and Safety Code Section 120980.

B. The costs for communicable disease testing and counseling of the exposed individual, and/or the source patient, shall be borne by the employer of the exposed individual.

C. The source patient's identity shall be encoded on the communicable disease test result record.

D. If the health care provider has acted in good faith in complying with Health and Safety Code Chapter 3.5, the health care provider shall not be subject to civil or criminal liability or professional disciplinary action for:

1. Performing communicable disease test on the available blood or patient sample of the source patient.

2. Disclosing the communicable disease status of a source patient to the source patient, the source patient's attending physician, the certifying physician, the exposed individual, or any attending physician of the exposed individual.

E. Any health care provider or first responder or any exposed individual who willfully performs or permits the performance of a test for communicable disease on a source patient that results in economic, bodily, or psychological harm to the source patient, without adhering to the procedure set forth in Health and Safety Code Chapter 3.5 is guilty of a misdemeanor, punishable by imprisonment in the county jail for a period not to exceed one year, or a fine not to exceed ten thousand dollars ($10,000), or both.

IV. CORONER'S CASES

If the source patient is pronounced dead in the field, the County Medical Examiner/Coroner may test for any communicable disease when an autopsy is performed. The certifying physician or the exposed prehospital care personnel's employer shall notify the County Medical Examiner/Coroner of the exposure. If the County Medical Examiner/Coroner confirms a diagnosis of any communicable disease in the source patient, they shall notify the County Health Officer, who in turn shall apprise the exposed individual of the source patient's communicable disease status. The County Medical Examiner/Coroner shall adhere to the procedure defined in Health and Safety Code 1797.189 in carrying out this process.

V. SOURCE PATIENT IN CUSTODY OR CHARGED WITH A CRIME

If the source patient is in custody or charged with a crime and refuses to voluntarily consent to communicable disease testing, Health and Safety Code 121060, 121060.1 and 121065 allows for the exposed health care provider to petition the court. The court will require the source patient to provide three specimens of blood to be tested for HIV, hepatitis B and hepatitis C by court order (Ref. No. 836.3).

CROSS REFERENCES:

Prehospital Care Policy Manual:
Ref. No. 836.1, **Communicable Disease Exposure and Testing Flow Chart**

Ref. No. 836.2, **Communicable Disease Exposure and Notification Report Form**
Ref. No. 836.3, **Court Petition for Order to Test Accused Blood**

PURPOSE: To provide guidelines on the use of restraints in the field or during transport for patients who are violent or potentially violent, or who may harm self or others.

AUTHORITY: California Code of Regulations, Title 22, Sections 100075 & 100160; Welfare and Institutions Code, 5150; California Administrative Code, Title 13, Section 1103.2; Health and Safety Code, Section 1798.

PRINCIPLES:

1. The safety of the patient, community, and responding personnel is of paramount concern when following this policy.

2. Restraints are to be used only when necessary in situations where the patient is potentially violent or is exhibiting behavior that is dangerous to self or others.

3. Prehospital personnel must consider that aggressive or violent behavior may be a symptom of medical conditions such as head trauma, alcohol, drug related problems, metabolic disorders, stress and psychiatric disorders. Base contact criteria shall be strictly adhered to for those conditions that require it.

4. The responsibility for patient health care management rests with the highest medical authority on scene. Therefore, medical intervention and patient destination shall be determined by EMS prehospital personnel in conjunction with the base hospital. Authority for scene management shall be vested in law enforcement.

5. The method of restraint used shall allow for adequate monitoring of vital signs and shall not restrict the ability to protect the patient's airway or compromise neurological or vascular status.

6. Restraints applied by law enforcement require the officer to remain available at the scene or during transport to remove or adjust the restraints for patient safety.

7. This policy is not intended to negate the need for law enforcement personnel to use appropriate restraint equipment that is approved by their respective agency to establish scene management control.

POLICY

I. Forms of Restraining Devices

A. Restraint devices applied by prehospital personnel must be either padded hard restraints or soft restraints (i.e., vest with ties, velcro or seatbelt type). Both methods must allow for quick release.

EFFECTIVE: 02-15-95
REVISED: 10-15-09
SUPERSEDES: 05-01-06
APPROVED: _____
Director, EMS Agency

_____
Medical Director, EMS Agency

PAGE 1 OF 3

UCLA Skills Guide Page 310

B.   The following forms of restraint shall NOT be applied by EMS prehospital care personnel:

    1.   Hard plastic ties or any restraint device requiring a key to remove.
       EXCEPTION: see Section IV: Interfacility Transport of Psychiatric Patients.

    2.   Restraining a patient's hands and feet behind the patient.

    3.   "Sandwich" restraints, using backboard, scoop-stretcher or flats.

    4.   Materials applied in a manner that could cause vascular, neurological or respiratory compromise (e.g., gauze bandage or tape).

II.   Application and Monitoring of Restraints by EMS Personnel

A.   Restraints shall be applied in such a manner that they do not cause vascular, neurological or respiratory compromise.

B.   Restrained extremities should be evaluated for pulse quality, capillary refill, color, temperature, nerve and motor function immediately following application and every 15 minutes thereafter. It is recognized that the evaluation of nerve and motor status requires patient cooperation, and thus may be difficult or impossible to monitor.

C.   Patients shall not be transported in a prone position. Prehospital personnel must ensure that the patient's position does not compromise the patient's respiratory/circulatory systems, and does not preclude any necessary medical intervention to protect or manage the airway should vomiting occur.

D.   Restraints may be attached to the frame of the gurney. Restraints shall not be attached to movable side rails of a gurney.

III.   Application of Restraints by Law Enforcement

A.   Restraint devices applied by law enforcement must provide sufficient slack in the restraint device to allow the patient to straighten the abdomen and chest and to take full tidal volume breaths.

B.   Patients shall not be transported in a prone position. Prehospital personnel must ensure that the patient's position does not compromise the patient's respiratory/circulatory systems, and does not preclude any necessary medical intervention to protect or manage the airway should vomiting occur.

C.   Restraint devices applied by law enforcement require the officer's continued presence to ensure patient and scene management safety. The officer shall accompany the patient in the ambulance. In the unusual event that this is not possible, the officer should follow by driving in tandem with the ambulance on a pre-determined route. A method to alert the officer of any problems that may develop during transport should be discussed prior to leaving the scene.

IV.   Interfacility Transport of Psychiatric Patients

    A.   A two-point, locking, padded cuff and belt restraint and/or two-point locking, padded ankle restraints may be used only in the interfacility transport of psychiatric patients.

    B.   Transport personnel must be provided with a written restraint order from the transferring physician or their designee as part of the transfer record.

    C.   Transport personnel must assess the restraint application and evaluate the circulation to the affected extremities prior to transport and every 15 minutes thereafter. Any abnormal findings require the restraints to be removed and reapplied or supporting documentation.

    D.   Transport personnel shall have immediate access to the restraint key at all times during the transport.

    E.   If an unrestrained patient becomes aggressive or violent enroute, refer to Policy, Section II, Application and Monitoring of Restraints by EMS Personnel.

V.   Required Documentation on the Patient Care/EMS Report Form

    A.   Reason restraints were applied.

    B.   Type of restraints applied.

    C.   Identity of agency/medical facility applying restraints.

    D.   Assessment of the circulatory and neurological status of the restrained extremities. Any abnormal findings require the restraints to be removed and reapplied or supporting documentation.

    E.   Assessment of the cardiac and respiratory status of the restrained patient.

CROSS REFERENCE:

Prehospital Care Policy Manual:
Ref. No. 502, **Patient Destination**
Ref. No. 702, **ALS Unit Inventory**
Ref. No. 808, **Base Hospital Contact and Transport Criteria**

COUNTY OF LOS ANGELES
DEPARTMENT OF HEALTH SERVICES

SUBJECT: **EMT-I CERTIFICATION**   REFERENCE NO. 1014

PURPOSE: To define the eligibility requirements and application procedures for EMT-I certification and recertification in Los Angeles County.

AUTHORITY: California Code of Regulations, Title 22, Section 100078-100083

DEFINITIONS:

EMT-I Certifying authority: an agency or person authorized to certify and recertify, as an Emergency Medical technician-I, an individual who has complied with the requirements of this policy as follows:

1.   The program director of an approved training program offered by a public safety agency may certify and recertify an individual who complies with the requirements of this policy.

2.   The medical director of the local EMS agency shall certify and recertify all other applicants for EMT-I certification who have complied with the requirements of this policy.

Local EMS Agency: the agency, department, or office having primary responsibility for administration of emergency medical services in a county. In Los Angeles County, the local EMS Agency is the Department of Health Services, Emergency Medical Services Agency.

Certifying Examination: an examination either developed by the EMS Authority or the EMT-I Certifying Authority and administered or approved by the EMT-I Certifying Authority, given to an individual applying for certification as an EMT-I. The examination shall include both written and skills testing portions designed to determine an individual's competence for certification as an EMT-I.

Emergency Medical Technician-I or EMT: a person who has successfully completed an EMT-I Basic course, has passed all required tests, and who has been certified by an EMT-I Certifying Authority.

POLICY:

I.   Certification

        A.   To be eligible for EMT-I certification, an individual shall meet the following requirements:

                1.   Have a course completion record or other documented proof of successful completion of an approved EMT-I Basic course.

                2.   Apply for certification within two (2) years of being issued a course completion record.

EFFECTIVE DATE: 12-1-87   PAGE 1 OF 5
REVISED: 9-15-08
SUPERSEDES: 4-30-98

APPROVED: _____   _____
                Director, EMS Agency   Medical Director, EMS Agency

3. Pass, by pre-established standards, a competency-based skills certifying examination administered by the approved EMT-I training program.

4. Pass a competency-based written certifying examination administered by the approved EMT-I certifying authority.

5. Be eighteen (18) years of age or older.

6. Meet all requirements set forth in Section 1798.200 of the Health and Safety Code. (Ref. No. 1014.1)

B. An individual currently licensed in California as a paramedic is deemed to be certified as an EMT-I.

C. An individual who meets one of the following criteria shall be eligible for EMT-I certification by successfully completing an approved EMT-I refresher course and completing the certification requirements in Section I, A, 2-6:

1. Possesses or has possessed in the last four (4) years a valid California EMT-I certification.

2. Possesses or has possessed in the last four (4) years a valid out-of-state or a National Registry EMT-Basic certification and has completed training equivalent to the United States Department of Transportation (DOT) Emergency Medical Technician National Standard Curriculum.

3. Has possessed a valid California EMT-II certification or paramedic certification or license.

4. Possesses or has possessed a valid out-of-state or National Registry EMT-Intermediate certification, or paramedic certification or license.

5. Has documentation of successful completion of an out-of-state EMT-I Basic course within the last two (2) years which meets the requirements of the United States Department of Transportation (DOT) Emergency Medical Technician National Standard Curriculum.

D. Certification procedures for candidates previously certified as EMT-Is, but whose certification has expired for more than four (4) years, are the same as an initial certification.

E. Certification as an EMT-I shall be for a maximum of two (2) years from the date of the EMT-I certifying authority examination, except that in the case of an individual currently licensed as a paramedic, who is deemed to be certified as an EMT-I pursuant to subsection B, the expiration date of the EMT-I certification shall be two (2) years from the expiration date of the current paramedic license.

NOTE: An individual who exercised the above option must complete certification requirements in Section III, A, 1-5 prior to expiration of the EMT-I certification. This includes a written and skills examination.

F.   The certification expiration date will be the final day of the final month of the two (2) year period.

II.   Certification by Challenge

A.   To be eligible for EMT-I certification by challenge, an individual shall:

1.   Meet one of the following requirements;

a.   Currently be licensed as a physician, registered nurse, physician assistant, vocational nurse, or as a paramedic licensed or certified out-of-state.

b.   Provide documented evidence of having successfully completed an emergency medical service training program of the Armed Forces, including the Coast Guard of the United States, within the preceding two(2) years which meets the Department of Transportation (DOT) EMT-Basic course guidelines.

c.   Provide documented evidence of active service in the last two (2) years in a prehospital emergency medical classification of the Armed Services, including the Coast Guard of the United States, which does not have formal recertification requirements.

2.   Successfully complete an EMT-I refresher course approved in Los Angeles County.

3.   Complete the certification requirements as defined in Section I, A, 2-6.

B.   Challenge candidates shall be permitted to take the EMT-I certifying skills and written examinations one time only. Unsuccessful challenge candidates will be required to take an EMT-I Basic course and meet all other eligibility requirements to be certified as an EMT-I.

III. Recertification

A.   To be eligible for EMT-I recertification, an individual shall:

1.   Possess a current California EMT-I certification.

2.   Possess documentation of successful completion of one of the following:

a.   An approved EMT-I refresher course.
b.   Twenty-four (24) hours of approved EMT-I continuing education (CE) obtained at any time throughout the current certification period.
c.   A letter from an approved paramedic training program indicating the candidate has completed a minimum of twenty-four (24) hours of approved EMT-I continuing education.

NOTE: All candidates recertifying by CE must show documentation of classroom and laboratory instruction in basic life support knowledge and skills to include airway management and

cardiopulmonary resuscitation as described in Section IV, A of this policy.

3.   Pass once every four (4) years a competency-based skills certifying examination administered by an approved EMT-I training program or BLS CE provider. A minimum of nine (9) skills must be tested including:

   a.   Patient Assessment
   b.   Ventilation via Bag-Valve-Mask Device
   c.   One Rescuer CPR: Adult
   d.   One Rescuer CPR: Infant
   e.   Assist with Administration of Physician Prescribed Medications (Expanded Scope of Practice)
   f.   Two optional skills from the Los Angeles County EMT-I Curriculum

4.   Pass once every four (4) years a competency-based certifying written examination administered by the certifying authority.

5.   Meet all requirements set forth in Section 1798.200 of the Health and Safety Code (Ref. No. 1014.1).

   NOTE: Certification is for two (2) years. EMT-Is who are not in a testing cycle will be required to test if the above requirements are not completed prior to the expiration date.

IV.   Recertification by Continuing Education

A.   EMT-Is recertifying with continuing education shall submit:

1.   Course completion certificates showing a minimum of twenty-four (24) hours of classroom and laboratory instruction. Not including recertification testing, in basic life support knowledge.

2.   Documentation of mandatory skills to include airway management and cardiopulmonary resuscitation (CPR). A current AHA Healthcare Provider card or American Red Cross Professional Rescuer card will meet airway management and CPR requirements.

B.   An individual who is currently licensed in California as a paramedic may be given credit for continuing education hours in basic life support earned as a paramedic to satisfy the continuing education requirements for EMT-I recertification.

V.   Application for Certification through the Los Angeles County EMS Agency

A.   Individuals eligible for EMT-I certification through the Los Angeles County EMS Agency may be certified by submitting an application packet consisting of:

1.   An EMT-I Certification Application form (Ref. No. 1014.1).

2.   A non-refundable fee.

3.   Two (2) passport size color photographs for EMT-I Certification card.

4.   Three (3) self-addressed, stamped, legal sized envelopes. Only one envelope if the EMT-I candidate is not in a testing cycle.

B.   Initial certification, out-of-county certification, or challenge certification candidates must complete a "BID-7" fingerprint card to be submitted by the EMS Agency to the California Department of Justice for a criminal background check.

Recertification, out-of-county certification, or challenge certification candidates must:

1.   Provide a recent certification card and/or other qualifying documents.

2.   Submit an EMT-I application packet every two (2) years prior to the EMT-Is certification expiration date.

3.   Pay the established fee.

4.   Complete a "BID-7" fingerprint to be submitted by the EMS Agency to the California Department of Justice for a criminal background check, if previous certification was out-of-county or prior to 1991.

C.   Application packets must be submitted to

County of Los Angeles EMS Agency
Office of Prehospital Certification
10100 Pioneer Boulevard, Suite 200
Santa Fe Springs, CA 90670

VI.   Training Program Responsibilities

To comply with the requirements of the certification/recertification application process, an approved EMT-I training program shall:

A.   Issue a course completion certificate to each person who has successfully completed the EMT-I Basic course or refresher course.

B.   Submit a course completion roster within 15 days to:

County of Los Angeles EMS Agency
Office of Prehospital Certification
10100 Pioneer Boulevard, Suite 200
Santa Fe Springs, CA 90670

CROSS REFERENCES:

Prehospital Care Policy Manual:
Ref. No. 906,   **Criteria for Approval of EMT-I Training Programs**

UCLA CENTER FOR PREHOSPITAL CARE

Pharmacology for Basic Life Support Providers

PHARMACOLOGY
FOR
BASIC LIFE SUPPORT
PROVIDERS

The pharmacology section for basic life support providers is designed to furnish relevant information regarding the medications that have been added to the EMT-Basic Scope of Practice in Los Angeles County. It incorporates all the medications that are in the 1994 EMT-Basic: National Standard Curriculum developed by the Department of Transportation (DOT). In addition, it contains information about established intravenous infusions that may be transported by EMT-Basic providers in Los Angeles County.

ALBUTEROL SULFATE (Proventil®, Ventolin®)

Classification: Bronchodilalor

Actions: Dilates bronchioles
Reduces airway resistance

Indications: Bronchospasm caused by:

- Acute asthma
- COPD
- Bronchitis
- Toxic gas inhalation

- Near drowning
- Drug overdose
- Pulmonary edema

Crush syndrome

- Suspected hyperkalemia
- Crush force > 4 hours

Contraindications: Maximum prescribed inhalation dose taken by patient
Inhaler not prescribed for patient

Adverse Effects:
Cardiovascular
tachycardia
hypertension

Respiratory
cough
wheezing

Neurological
tremors
nervousness
headache
dizziness

Gastrointestinal
nausea

Administration: EMT-Basic providers are not authorized to carry bronchodilators, but may assist patient with their own physician prescribed albuterol inhaler.
One spray inhaled by using either the metered dose inhaler with or without a spacer device. May repeat 1 spray in 35 minutes one time.

Pediatric: < 12 years   Not recommended for prehospital use
> 12 years   Same as adult

Onset: Within 5 minutes

Duration: 4-6 hours

2-1

ALBUTEROL SULFATE (Proventil®, Ventolin®)
(Continued)

Precautions: The albuterol inhaler is for EMERGENCY SUPPORTIVE THERAPY ONLY and is not a substitute for immediate medical care. An ALS unit must be enroute or the patient must be transported immediately to the nearest emergency department if ALS response is not available.

Hypoxic patients may experience dysrhythmias. Monitor pulse periodically for irregularity. Administer supplemental O_2 before and after treatment to decrease hypoxemia.

Note:

Directions for Using Metered Dose Inhaler Without a Spacer Device

1. Shake container vigorously several times.
2. Instruct patient to exhale deeply.
3. Instruct patient to place lips around mouthpiece.
4. Instruct patient to take a slow, deep breath and depress the medication canister while patient inhales.
5. Instruct patient to remove mouthpiece and hold breath for as long as possible.
6. Instruct patient to exhale slowly through pursed lips.
7. Replace patient 0, and reevaluate breath sounds.
8. Repeat procedure one time if needed.

Directions for Using Metered Dose Inhaler With a Spacer Device

1. Shake container vigorously several times.
2. Remove cap from spacer.
3. Attach spacer to inhaler.
4. Instruct patient to exhale deeply.
5. Instruct patient to place lips around mouthpiece.
6. Depress the medication canister to fill the spacer chamber.
7. Instruct patient to take several slow, deep breaths to inhale medication in spacer. (There may be a whistling sound if the patient inhales too rapidly.)
8. Instruct patient to remove mouthpiece and hold breath for as long as possible.
9. Instruct patient to exhale slowly through pursed lips.
10. Replace patient 02 and reevaluate breath sounds.
11. Repeat procedure one time if needed.   (1/00)

Included in Los Angeles County "Expanded" Scope of Practice

2-2

CHARCOAL (ACTIVATED)
(Acta-Char®, Actidose®, Charcoaid®, Insta-Char®, Liqui-Char®)

Classification: Chemical absorbent

Actions: Absorbs ingested drugs and chemicals

Indications: Suspected drug overdose or ingestion of poisons

Contraindications: Altered level of consciousness or risk of decreased consciousness in the field

Absent gag reflex

Adverse effects:

Gastrointestinal	*Respiratory*
vomiting	aspiration

Administration: *Use preparations without Sorbitol* 25-50g PO (*per os* or "by mouth") as tolerated

Pediatric:

0-2 years	Not recommended for, prehospital use.
> 2 years	Same as adult.

Onset: Immediate

Duration: 24 hours

Precautions: DO NOT ADMINISTER IF THERE IS A POTENTIAL FOR ALTERED LEVEL OF CONSCIOUSNESS. There is a risk of vomiting and aspiration if a decrease in consciousness occurs. Patient must be able to drink without assistance.

DO NOT ADMINISTER CHARCOAL WITH SORBITOL TO PATIENTS LESS THAN 2 YEARS OLD. Sorbitol acts as a potent cathartic and may cause fluid and electrolyte disturbances.

Note: Shake bottle vigorously prior to administration to ensure that charcoal is thoroughly suspended.

Charcoal is most effective if administered within 30 minutes of overdose or poison ingestion.

Charcoal does not absorb cyanide, ethanol, methanol, ferrous sulfate, caustic alkali or mineral acids. (1/00)

Not included in Los Angeles County Scope of Practice

2-3

DEXTROSE PREPARATIONS (ORAL)
DEXTROSE CARBONATE SOLUTION
and
GLUCOSE PASTE / GLUCOSE GEL

Classification: Hyperglycemic agent (carbohydrate)

Actions: Immediate source of glucose, needed for cellular metabolism

Indications: Conscious diabetic patient who has signs/symptoms of hypoglycemia

Contraindications: Unresponsive patients
Patients who are unable to swallow or have a diminished gag reflex
Patients complaining of nausea

Adverse Effects:

Gastrointestinal	*Respiratory*
vomiting	aspiration
	obstructed airway

Administration:

Solution	75-100g (10g/oz) PO, sipped slowly
Paste/Gel	1 tube of paste/gel swallowed or 1inch placed between cheek and gum.

Pediatric:

Solution	1g/kg PO, sipped slowly
Paste/Gel	Not recommended for prehospital use

Onset: Within 20 minutes

Duration: Depends on the degree and cause of hypoglycemia

Precautions: Administer solution only to patients who can hold the bottle and drink without assistance or administer paste/gel if the patient has the ability to swallow. There is a risk of airway obstruction, vomiting, and aspiration if the patient is unable to swallow or has a diminished gag reflex.

Note: The entire amount does not need to be administered if the patient's condition improves.

Signs/Symptoms of hypoglycemia: rapid onset, cool, moist skin, hunger, bizarre/combative behavior, anxiety, restlessness, weakness, appearance of intoxication or stroke such as slurred speech and staggering gait, and seizures. (1/00)

Included in Los Angeles County 'Expanded" Scope of Practice

2-6

DEXTROSE 5% IN WATER (D$_5$W) SOLUTION

Classification:	Isotonic/hypotonic solution (5g dextrose/100ml water)
Actions:	Provides some sugar for cellular metabolism Supplies body water
Indications:	Intravenous access for drug administration
Contraindications:	Not significant during interfacility transport
Adverse Effects:	Increases free water and may cause intracellular edema
Administration:	May transport with infusion adjusted to a TKO rate by hospital personnel.
Pediatric:	Must transport with a volume-control set and rate adjusted to a TKO rate by hospital personnel.
Onset:	Immediate
Duration:	20-40 minutes
Precautions:	Monitor infusion rates frequently; if signs of fluid overload, turn off IV drip. Infusion may result in fluid overload. Check IV site frequently and if infiltration is noted, turn off IV drip. IV may infiltrate during transport.
Note:	Signs of fluid overload: jugular vein distention (JVD), rapid respirations, shallow tidal volume, fine auscultatory crackles, dyspnea, and peripheral edema. Signs of infiltration: swelling and pain around IV site. (1/00)

2-7

EPINEPHRINE HYDROCHLORIDE (Adrenalin®)

EPIPEN AUTO-INJECTOR

Classification: Sympathomimetic agent (catecholamine)

Actions: Dilates bronchioles
Constricts blood vessels

Indications: Anaphylaxis (severe allergic reaction)

Contraindications: Not significant in above indication

Adverse effects:

Cardiovascular	*Neurological*
tachycardia	seizures
hypertension	cerebral hemorrhage
chest pain	headache
ventricular fibrillation	tremors
	dizziness
	anxiety

Gastrointestinal
nausea/vomiting

Administration: EMT-Basic providers are not authorized to carry the EpiPen Auto-injector, but may assist patients with their own physician prescribed device.

EpiPen Auto-injector (0.3mg) IM in the upper-outer thigh. No repeat.

Pediatric: EpiPen Jr. Auto-injector (0.15mg) IM in the upper-outer thigh. No repeat.

Onset: 5-10 minutes

Duration: 20 minutes

Precautions: The EpiPen is for EMERGENCY SUPPORTIVE THERAPY ONLY and is not a substitute for immediate medical care. An ALS unit must be enroute or the patient must be transported immediately to the nearest emergency department if ALS response is not available.

2-8

EPINEPHRINE HYDROCHLORIDE (Adrenalin®)

DO NOT INJECT INTO BUTTOCKS, HANDS, FEET, OR ADMINISTER INTRAVENOUSLY. Injection into buttocks, hands or feet may result in loss of blood flow to the affected area and result in delayed absorption and tissue necrosis. Intravenous injection may result in an acute myocardial infarction or cerebral hemorrhage.

Only administer if solution is clear and not expired. A solution that is discolored, contains particles, or if outdated may be chemically altered and may lose its potency or result in muscle damage.

Note:　　　The EpiPen contains 2ml (2mg) of epinephrine. The Auto-injector delivers 0.3ml (0.3mg); approximately 1.7ml remains in the pen after activation.

Insect stings may cause anaphylaxis or bites, foods, drugs, other allergens, exercise, or may be spontaneous.

Signs/symptoms of anaphylaxis: flushed skin, nervousness, syncope, tachycardia, thready or unobtainable pulse, hypotension, convulsions, vomiting, diarrhea, abdominal cramps, urinary incontinence, wheezing, stridor, difficulty breathing, itching, rash, hives, and generalized edema.

Directions for Using EpiPen Auto-injector

1.　　Pull off gray safety cap.
2.　　Cleanse injection site with alcohol swab. **
3.　　Place black tip on the upper-outer thigh, at right angle to the leg.
4.　　Press EpiPen hard into thigh until Auto-Injector activates and hold in place for several seconds.
5.　　Remove EpiPen and place in needle container.
6.　　Massage the injection site for 10 seconds with alcohol swab.

** Patient's may have been instructed that they can use EpiPen through clothing. This is not recommended for basic life support providers. (1/00)

Included in Los Angeles County "Expanded" Scope of Practice.

2-9

FOLIC ACID (Vitamin B₉) INFUSION

Classification: Nutritional supplement (water-soluble vitamin)

Action: Aids in the development of red and white blood cells and formation of platelets

Indication: Suspected malnutrition, especially in the presence of chronic alcohol abuse, poor diet, and impaired food absorption

Contraindications: Not significant during interfacility transport

Adverse Effects: Not significant during interfacility transport

Administration: May transport a maximum IV solution concentration of 1mg/l000ml IV solution. Hospital personnel must adjust infusion to a TKO rate.

Pediatric: Concentration same as adult. Infusion must be on a volume control set and adjusted to a TKO rate by hospital personnel.

Precautions: Check IV site frequently and if infiltration is noted, turn off IV drip. IV may infiltrate during transport.

Note: Folic acid may be administered in conjunction with multi-vitamin infusion.

(1/00)

Included in Los Angeles County "Expanded' Scope of Practice

2-10

INSULIN
via
PATIENT-CONTROLLED PUMP

Classification: Hypoglycemic agent

Action: Decreases blood sugar

Indication: Insulin dependent diabetes

Contraindications: Not significant during interfacility transport

Adverse Effects: Hypoglycemia

Administration: EMT-Basic providers may not activate or adjust Infusion pump.

May transport patients with either an internal or external administration pump. Medication infusion is programmed for the individual patient and may only be activated by patient or caregiver.

Pediatric: Same as adult

Precautions: Evaluate level of consciousness and behavior frequently. Patients may experience hypoglycemia; If mild signs/symptoms develop, administer oral hyperglycemic agent.

Note: Signs/symptoms of hypoglycemia: nervousness, trembling, irritability, combative behavior, weakness, uncoordination, confusion, weak and rapid pulse, cold and clammy skin, drowsiness, seizures, and altered level of consciousness.

(1/00)

Included in Los Angeles County "Expanded" Scope of Practice

LACTATED RINGER'S SOLUTION

Classification: Isotonic solution (crystalloid)

Action: Replaces fluid and electrolytes lost from the intravascular and intracellular spaces

Indications: Initial fluid replacement for hypovolemia and dehydration
IV access for drug administration

Contraindications: Not significant during interfacility transport

Adverse effects: Circulatory fluid volume overload

Administration: May transport with infusion adjusted to a TKO rate by hospital personnel.

Pediatrics: Must transport with a volume-control. Hospital personnel must adjust set and rate to a TKO rate.

Onset: Immediate

Duration: < 1 hour

Precautions: Monitor infusion rate frequently. Infusion may result in fluid overload.

Check IV site frequently and if infiltration is noted, turn off IV drip. IV may infiltrate during transport.

Note: Signs of fluid overload: jugular vein distention (JVD), rapid respirations, shallow tidal volume, fine auscultatory crackles, dyspnea, and peripheral edema.

Signs of infiltration: swelling and pain around IV site.

(1/00)

MEPERIDINE HYDROCHLORIDE (DEMEROL®)
via
PATIENT-CONTROLLED ANALGESIC PUMP

Classification: Narcotic analgesic

Actions: Alters pain perception and produces euphoria

Indications: Moderate to severe pain

Contraindications: Not significant during interfacility transport

Adverse effects:

Cardiovascular	*Neurological*
tachycardia	sedation
radycardia	dizziness
hypotension	headache
hypertension	confusion
	tremors
	seizures
	hallucinations

Respiratory	*Gastrointestinal*
depression	nausea/vomiting
arrest	

Administration: EMT-Basic providers may not activate or adjust Infusion pump.

May transport with locked settings. Medication infusion is programmed for individual patient and may only be activated by patient or caregiver.

Pediatric: Same as adult

Onset: 2-5 minutes

Duration: Individual per patient program

Precautions: Monitor pulse quality and blood pressure. Infusion may cause hypotension.

If hypotension persists, place patient in shock position.

2-13

MEPERIDINE HYDROCHLORIDE (DEMEROL®)
via
PATIENT-CONTROLLED ANALGESIC PUMP
(continued)

Monitor respiratory status frequently and ventilate with bag-valve mask device if necessary. Infusion may cause respiratory depression or arrest.

Note: There are different Patient-Controlled Analgesic pumps. Transferring personnel must provide the EMT-B provider with emergency shut off instructions regarding the specific pump used.

(1/00)

Included In Los Angeles County "Expanded" Scope of Practice

2-14

MORPHINE SULFATE
via
PATIENT-CONTROLLED ANALGESIC PUMP

Classification:	Narcotic analgesic
Actions:	Alters pain perception and produces euphoria
Indications:	Moderate to severe pain
Contraindications:	Not significant during interfacility transport

Adverse effects:

Cardiovascular	*Neurological*
tachycardia	sedation
bradycardia	dizziness
hypotension	headache
hypertension	confusion
	tremors
	seizures
	hallucinations

Respiratory	*Gastrointestinal*
depression	nausea/vomiting
arrest	

Administration: EMT-Basic providers may not activate or adjust Infusion pump.

May transport with locked settings. Medication infusion is programmed for individual patient and may only be activated by patient or caregiver.

Pediatric: Same as adult

Onset: 2-5 minutes

Duration: Individual per patient program

Precautions: Monitor pulse quality and blood pressure. Infusion may cause hypotension.

If hypotension persists, place patient in shock position.

Monitor respiratory status frequently and ventilate with bag-valve mask device if necessary. Infusion may cause respiratory depression or arrest.

2-15

MORPHINE SULFATE
via
PATIENT-CONTROLLED ANALGESIC PUMP
(continued)

Note: There are different types of Patient-Control Analgesic pumps. Transferring personnel must provide the EMT-B provider with emergency shut off instructions regarding the specific pump used.

(1/00)

Included in Los Angeles County "Expanded" Scope of Practice

2-16

MULTI-VITAMIN INFUSION

Action:	Vitamins are organic compounds needed for growth, resistance to infection, and normal metabolism
Indication:	Suspected malnutrition
Contraindications:	Not significant during interfacility transport
Adverse Effects:	Not significant during interfacility transport
Administration:	May transport a maximum concentration of 1vial/1000ml IV solution. Hospital/home health personnel must adjust infusion to a TKO rate.
Pediatrics:	Concentration same as adult. Infusion must be on a volume-control set and adjusted to a TKO rate by hospital/home health personnel.
Precautions:	Check IV site frequently, if infiltration is noted, turn off IV drip. IV may infiltrate during transport.
Note:	Multi-vitamins for infusion contain both water and fat-soluble vitamins.
	When added to an IV infusion, it gives a yellow color to the fluid.

ADDENDUM

Magnesium Sulfate may be given ONLY in conjunction with multivitamins. Maximum 2 grams/1000ml.

Classification: Nutritional supplement

(1/00)

Included in Los Angeles County "Expanded' of Practice

2-17

NITROGLYCERIN

TABLETS or LINGUAL AEROSOL (Nitrolingua

Classification:	Vasodilator
Actions:	Dilates blood vessels Dilates coronary arteries Dc the heart
Indications:	Chest pain
Contraindications:	Blood pressure below 100 systolic. Patient has taken three doses prior to the arrival of EMT-B providers Sildenafil or other erectile dysfunction drugs within last 36 hours
Effects:	Cardiovascular Neurological hypotension throbbing headache bradycardia dizziness/faintness reflex tachycardia confusion rebound hypertension blurred vision Gastrointestinal General nausea/vomiting flushed skin dry mouth sublingual burning
Administration:	EMT-Basic providers are not authorized to carry nitroglycerin tablets or aerosol, but may assist patients with their own physician prescribed medication.

Tablet 1 tablet (1/150gr or 0.4mg) SL Spray 1 spray (0.4mg) SL or TM (transmucosal)

Pediatric:	Not recommended for prehospital use
Onset:	1-3 minutes
Duration:	30-60 minutes

Nitroglycerin administration is for EMERGENCY SUPPORTIVE THERAPY ONLY and is not a substitute for immediate medical care.   An ALS unit must be enroute or the patient must be transported immediately to the nearest emergency department if ALS response is not available.

2-18

340

NITROGLYCERIN
TABLETS or LINGUAL AEROSOL (Nitrolingual® Spray)
(Continued)

DO NOT ADMINISTER IF BLOOD PRESSURE IS BELOW 100mmHg SYSTOLIC. May cause hypotension due to vasodilation. Always take blood pressure before and 5 minutes after administration of Nitroglycerin.

DO NOT SHAKE CONTAINER. One spray delivers 0.4mg of nitroglycerin. If the container is shaken it will alter the dose delivered.

INSTRUCT PATIENT NOT TO INHALE SPRAY. Inhaling spray affects absorption rate.

Note:

Directions for Administering Nitroglycerin Tablets

* 1.   DO NOT ADMINISTER IF B/P IS BELOW 100 SYSTOLIC. Take blood pressure before administration.
2.   Place tablet under tongue and instruct patient not to swallow, but to allow tablet to dissolve under tongue.
3.   Retake blood pressure and pulse after 5 minutes. If hypotension develops, place patient in shock position.

Directions for Administering Nitroglycerin Aerosol

* 1.   DO NOT ADMINISTER IF B/P IS BELOW 100 SYSTOLIC. Take blood pressure before administration.
2.   Instruct patient not to inhale spray and do not shake container.
3.   Administer spray on or under the tongue.
4.   Retake blood pressure and pulse after 5 minutes. If hypotension develops, place patient in shock position.

(1/00)

* Minimum systolic pressure is 100 in LA County, 90 for DOT

Included in Los Angeles County "Expanded" Scope of Practice

2-19

OXYGEN

Classification:	Gaseous element (21% of room air)
Actions:	Essential element for normal metabolic function (aerobic metabolism)
	Assists in the breakdown of glucose into a useable energy form
Indications:	Hypoxemia
	Increased oxygen demand
	Chest pain of myocardial origin
	Respiratory insufficiency
	Cardiopulmonary arrest
Contraindications:	Not significant in above indications
Adverse effects:	Not significant in above indications
Administration:	Oxygen percentage may vary slightly depending on technique and equipment.

Delivery Device	Flow Rate	Delivered
Nasal Cannula	2-6 L/min	23-44%
Face Mask	8-15 L/min	40-60%
Face Mask with O_2 Reservoir	6-10 L/min	60-95%
Bag-Valve-Mask with O_2 Reservoir	10-15 L/min	40-90%
ET -- Bag-Valve Device with O_2 Reservoir	10-15 L/min	100%
ET -- T-tube	10-15 L/min	60-70%
ETC (combitube) -- Bag-Valve Device with O_2 Reservoir	10-15 L/min	40-90%

Pediatric:	Same as adult except the ETC (combitube) is contraindicated in pediatric patients less than 4 feet tall.

2-20

OXYGEN
(Continued)

Onset: 1-2 minutes

Duration: Up to 30 minutes

Precautions: Observe the patient closely for changes in respiratory and mental status. Be prepared to assist ventilations if necessary. In some CO_2 retaining COPD patients, administration of oxygen may decrease their respiratory drive.

DO NOT ADMINISTER MORE THAN 6L/min VIA NASAL CANNULA. Oxygen is not humidified and may dry out or irritate mucus membranes.

DO NOT USE HIGH FLOW OXYGEN-POWERED-BREATHING-DEVICES IN PEDIATRIC PATIENTS LESS THAN 12 YEARS OF AGE OR IN CONJUNCTION WITH AN ET TUBE. These devices may result in gastric distention or pneumothorax due to high pressures.

Note: Oxygen should never be withheld from a patient in respiratory distress.

High flow oxygen-powered-breathing-devices are manually triggered, or demand valves, which have a flow rate of 100 liters/minute.

(1/00)

2-21

POTASSIUM CHLORIDE (KCI) INFUSION

Classification: Electrolyte

Actions: Regulates nerve conduction and muscle contraction

Indications: Potassium deficiency

Contraindications: Not significant during interfacility transport

Adverse effects:

Cardiovascular
dysrhythmias
arrest

Neurological
paresthesia
muscular paralysis
confusion

Respiratory
depression
arrest

General
hyperkalemia
venous thrombosis

Gastrointestinal
nausea/vomiting
abdominal pain

Administration: Infusion pump is required. Hospital personnel must adjust rate.

May transport a maximum IV solution concentration of 20mEq/1000ml IV solution.

Pediatric: Same as adult. Infusion must be on a volume-control set and adjusted to a TKO rate by hospital personnel.

Precautions: Monitor pulse periodically for irregularity; if change in regularity occurs, turn of IV drip. KCI may cause dysrhythmias.

Check IV site frequently for infiltration; if present, turn off IV drip. IV may infiltrate during transport, and cause tissue necrosis.

Note: If concentration is greater than 2OmEq/1 000ml of IV solution, patient must be transported by ALS unit and patient placed on an ECG monitor. (1/00)

Included in Los Angeles County "Expanded' Scope of Practice

2-22

SODIUM CHLORIDE 0.9% (Normal Saline) SOLUTION

Classification: Isotonic solution

Actions: Replaces fluid and sodium lost from the intravascular and intracellular spaces

Indications: Initial fluid replacement for hypovolemia, dehydration, and crush syndrome
Intravenous access for drug administration

Contraindications: Not significant during interfacility transport

Adverse effects: Circulatory fluid volume overload

Administration: May transport with infusion adjusted to a TKO rate by hospital personnel.

Pediatric: Must transport with a volume-control set and the rate adjusted - to a TKO rate by hospital personnel or field paramedic in a multiple casualty situation.

Onset: Immediate

Duration: < 1 hour

Precautions: Infusion may result in fluid overload. Monitor infusion rate frequently; if signs/symptoms of fluid overload, turn off IV drip

IV may infiltrate during transport. Check IV site frequently; if infiltration noted, turn off IV drip.

Note: Signs of fluid overload: jugular vein distension (JVD), rapid respirations, shallow tidal volume, fine auscultatory crackles, dyspnea, and peripheral edema.

Signs of infiltration: swelling and pain around IV site. (1/00)

2-23

THIAMINE (Vitamin B₁) INFUSION

Classification: Nutritional supplement (water-soluble vitamin)

Action: Aids in metabolizing carbohydrates, fats and amino acids and
                     detoxifying alcohol

Indication: Suspected malnutrition, especially in the presence of chronic
                     alcohol abuse

Contraindications: Not significant during interfacility transport

Adverse Effects: Not significant during interfacility transport

Administration: May transport a maximum IV solution concentration of
                     100mg/1000ml IV solution. Hospital/home health personnel must
                     adjust infusion to a TKO rate.

Pediatric: Concentration same as adult. Infusion must be on a volume-
                     control set and rate adjusted to a TKO rate by hospital/home health
                     personnel.

Precautions: Check IV site frequently; if infiltration noted, turn off IV drip. There
                     is a potential for IV to infiltrate during transport.

Note: Thiamin may be administered in conjunction with multi-vitamin
                     infusion.

(1/00)

Included in Los Angeles County "Expanded" Scope of Practice

2-24

TOTAL PARENTERAL NUTRITION (TPN)

Classification: Caloric agent

Actions: Provides total- nutritional needs to sustain life

Indications: Patients unable to take food orally or absorb adequate nutrition through the gastrointestinal tract

Contraindications: Not significant during interfacility transport

Adverse effects: Not significant during interfacility transport

Administration: Must transport with an infusion pump. The infusion is adjusted for the individual patient and hospital or home health personnel may only adjust the rate.

Pediatric: Same as adult

Precautions: Prevent separation of IV tubing. A break in the system may result in an air embolism, which may be fatal.

      Prevent disruption of infusion and insure that an adequate amount of TPN solution is available throughout transport. Interruption of TPN infusions may result in hypoglycemia.

(1/00)

Included in Los Angeles County "Expanded" Scope of Practice

2-25

DEPARTMENT OF HEALTH SERVICES
COUNTY OF LOS ANGELES

SUBJECT: **COMMUNICABLE DISEASE EXPOSURE AND TESTING** (EMT-I, PARAMEDIC, MICN)
REFERENCE NO. 836

PURPOSE: To provide guidelines for prehospital care personnel exposed to blood or other potentially infectious material.

AUTHORITY: California Health and Safety Code, Division 105, Chapter 3.5, Sections 120260-120263
California Health and Safety Code, Sections 1797.188 -189, 120980, 121050-121070, 121140
U.S. Department of Labor-Occupational Safety and Health Administration Bloodborne Pathogens Standard 1910.1030 (2006)
California Occupational Safety and Health Standards
Exposure Control Plan for Bloodborne Pathogens (2001)
Ryan White HIV/AIDS Treatment Modernization Act of 2006
Code of Federal Regulations, Title 45, Section 164.512.b.4 (October 2007)
California Code of Regulations, Title 8, Section 5193 (Register 2007, No. 46)

DEFINITIONS:

Attending physician of the source patient: Any physician or surgeon who provides health care services to the source patient.

Available blood or patient sample: Blood, other tissue, or material legally obtained in the course of providing health care services and in the possession of the physician or other health care provider of the source patient **prior to the release of the source patient from the physician's or health care provider's facility.**

Body Substance Isolation (BSI): A method of infection control designed to approach all body fluids as being potentially infectious. It is the preferred infection control concept for EMS personnel.

Certifying physician: Any physician consulted by the exposed individual for the exposure incident.

Communicable disease: Any disease that is transferable through an exposure incident, as determined by the certifying physician.

Exposed individual: Any individual health care provider, first responder, or any other person, including, but not limited to, any employee, volunteer, or contracted agent of any health care provider, who is exposed, within the scope of their employment, to the blood or other potentially infectious materials of a source patient.

Exposure certification: A determination by the certifying physician on the exposure's significance.

EFFECTIVE: 1-1-95
REVISED: 2-1-09
SUPERSEDES: 6-1-08

PAGE 1 OF 5

APPROVED: _____   _____
Director, EMS Agency   Medical Director, EMS Agency

UCLA CENTER FOR PREHOSPITAL CARE

Medical Terminology, Reference Materials and Acronyms

MEDTERMS – Root Words

ROOT WORDS	MEANING
Abdomino	pertaining to the abdomen
Acou	to hear
Acq	pertaining to water
Acro	end of a part
Aden	gland
Adip	fat
Alb	white
Alg	pain
All	other
Anc, ang, ank	bend or hollow
Andr	male
Angi	blood vessel
Aort	aorta
Arter	artery
Arth, artic	joint
Asphyxia	suffocate
Asthenia	weakness
Aud, aur, aus	hearing
Bio	life
Brachy	short
Branchi	arm
Bronch	pertaining to the bronchi
Bucc	cheek
Burs	sac
Caes, cis	to cut
Call	thick
Calx, calca	heel of foot
Can	malignant
Caput, capitis	head
Carc	cancer
Card	heart
Carotid	arteries in neck
Carpus	wrist
Caus, caut	burn
Cell	pertaining to abdominal cavity
Cestesis	puncture of a body cavity or organ
Ceph	head
Cerv	neck
Chol	bile or gall
Chond	cartilage
Chrom	color
Cil	hairlike

MEDTERMS

ROOT WORDS	MEANING
Cond	knuckle
Core	pupil
Cori	skin
Corp	the body
Cry	cold
Cubitus	elbow
Cyan	blue
Cyc	circle
Cyst	cyst or bladder
Dent	tooth
Derm	skin
Digit	finger
Duct	guide
Edem	swelling
Embryo	fetal
Enter	intestines
Eryth	red
Esth	sensation
Eti	cause
Febr	fever
Flex	to bend
Foramen	an opening
Fract	to break
Gangl	junction of nerves
Gast	stomach
Gen, gon	to make or generate
Glomerulus	a plexus of capillaries
Gnosis	to have knowledge
Gram	a written record
Graph	to write
Gyn	female
Hem	blood
Hepa, hepata	liver
Heter	different
Homo	same
Humerus	upper arm
Hydr	water
Hyster	uterus
Id	personal or one's own
Idio	distinct
Ingui	anterior near groin
Lact	milk

MEDTERMS

ROOT WORDS	MEANING
Lev	left
Ligament	connective tissue holding bones together
Ling	tongue
Lith	stone
Mal	bad
Meatus	outside opening
Mega	large
Melan, melen	black
Menin	pertaining to the covering of the brain
Morb	disease
Myel	bone marrow or spinal cord
Myo	muscle
Nephr	kidney
Noct	night
Oa, oss, ost	bone
Ocul	eye
Odon	tooth
Oa, ov	egg
Opthalm	eye
Orch	testicles
Ot	eat
Palpate	touch
Pari, part	to bear
Pariet	outside or wall
Path	disease
Ped	feet, child
Percuss	to hit
Phag	swallow, to eat
Photo	light
Pleur	surrounding the chest cavity or lungs
Pneum	to breath
Pty	spit
Pur, pus, py	pus
Pyel	pelvic or kidney
Pyr	fever
Quad, quar	four
Ren	kidney
Rhin	nose
Rub	red
Sang	blood
Sclera	hard
Sebum	fat

MEDTERMS

ROOT WORDS	MEANING
Sect, seg	to cut
Sepsis	infected
Sept	wall
Sinus	hollow cavity
Somat	pertaining to the body
Sphincter	muscle that closes a tube
Spir	coil
Stasis	to stand
Stature	height
Status	condition
Stern	pertaining to the chest
Stoma	opening or mouth
Tachy	fast
Tact	touching
Talus	heel of foot
Tarsus	bones of feet
Tel	distant
Temp	pertaining to time or the temple of the head
Tendon	connective tissue connecting muscle to bone
Tetra	four
Tom	to cut
Toxic	poisonous
Trachea	windpipe
Trich	hairlike
Ur, urin	pertaining to urine
Vagina	pertaining to vagina
Varic	dilated vein
Vertebra	bones of the spine
Vertex	top of the skull
Vertigo	dizziness
Viscera	internal organs
Viscous	sticky

MEDTERMS - Prefix

PREFIX	MEANING
A, an	without
Ab	to move away from
Acr	pertaining to an arm or leg
Ad	to move toward
Aden	pertaining to a gland
Algi	pain
Amph	around
Ana	again
Angio	blood vessel
Ante	before
Anti	against
Arthro	a joint
Auto	self
Bi	two
Blast	immature cell
Bleph	eye
Brachy	short
Brady	slow
Cardio	heart
Cephal	head
Cerebro	brain
Chole	bile or gall
Circum	around
Contra	against
Co, com, con	together
Cost	rib
Cyst	bladder
Derma	skin
Di	two
Dia	completely
Dys	difficult or painful
E, ex	out of
Em	in
Endo, en	inside
Enter	intestinal
Epi	on top, upon
Erythro	red
Eu	health, wellness
Ex, exo	outside of
Extra	additional
Fore	in front of
Gastr	pertaining to the stomach

MEDTERMS

PREFIX	MEANING
Glasso	pertaining to the tongue
Gynec	pertaining to females
Hem, hema	blood
Hemi	half of
Hydra, hydro	water
Hyper	over or above
Hypo	under
Hyster	uterus
Idio	relating to a particular individual
In	not
Infra	below
Inter	between
Intra	within
Iso	equal
Kinesi	movement
Laparo	relating to the abdomen
Laryng, laryngo	the larynx
Lateral	the side
Leuk, leuko	white
Macro	large
Med, medi	the middle
Mega, mego	very large
Mes, meso	middle
Meta	above. Beyond
Metra, metro	uterine
Micro	small
Mono	singular or one
Myel, myelo	bone marrow
Myo, mye	muscular
Neo	new
Nephr	kidney
Neuro	nerve
Non	not
Olig	little
Oophor	ovary
Opthal	eye
Ot	ear
Pan	entire, all
Para	next to
Patho	disease
Per	through
Peri	around

MEDTERMS

PREFIX	**MEANING**
Phago	to eat or swallow
Pneumo	air or lung
Poly	many
Post	after
Pre	before
Pro	before
Proto	initial or first
Proct	rectum
Pseudo	false
Psych	the mind
Pulmo	lung
Py	pus
Pyel	kidney
Retro	backwards
Rhin	nose
Salping	tube
Sarco	skin
Semi	half
Sclero	hard
Sub	below
Super, supra	above
Sym	together or with
Tachy	fast
Tele	distant
Trans	across
Tri	three
Uni	one
Vaso	vessel
Venter, ventro	abdominal
Xantho	yellow

MEDTERMS - Suffix

SUFFIX	MEANING
algia, algesia	pain
blast	immature cell
cele	hernia
centesis	puncturing of body part
cyte	cell
derm, derma	skin
ectomy	cut or remove
emia	blood
emesis	vomiting
esthesia	sensation
form	shape
gram	making or tracing
graphy	a record
itis	inflammation
kinesis	motion
logia, logy	study of
lysis	to take apart
meter	measure
oma	tumor
osis	condition of
ostomy	an opening
pathy	disease
penia	small
phagia	to eat or swallow
phasia	speech
phobia	fear of
phylaxis	protection
plasty	reconstruct
plegia	a stroke
ptosis	falling
rhythmia	rhythm
rrhagia	to burst
rrhaphy	repair
rrhea	flow
scope	an instrument, to see
scopy	to examine with an instrument
stomy, stomosis	to create an opening
taxia	movement
trophia	to nourish
uria	urine

MEDTERMS
GENERAL ABBREVIATIONS

ABBREVIATION   MEANING

a.c.	before meals
A&P	auscultation and percussion
AAA	American Ambulance Association
abd	abdomen
Ab	abortion
ACLS	advanced cardiac life support
ad lib.	As desired
AD	right ear
AED	automatic external defibrillator
AICD	automatic implantable cardioverter/defibrillator
AIDS	acquired immunodeficiency syndrome
ALS	advanced life support
amp	ampoule
AP	anteroposterior
aq.	Water
AHA	American Heart Association
ARC	American Red Cross
ARDS	acute respiratory distress syndrome
ARES	Amateur Radio Emergency Service
AS	left ear
ASA	aspirin
ASD	atrial septal defect
ASHD	arteriosclerotic heart disease
ATF	Alcohol, Tobacco, and Firearms
ATLS	advanced trauma life support
ausc.	auscultation
A-V	arteriovenous
BCLS	basic cardiac life support
b.i.d.	twice daily
BE	barium enema
BEC	basic emergency care
BLM	Bureau of Land Management
BLS	basic life support
BM	bowel movement
BP	blood pressure
Broncho	bronchoscopy
BSN	Bachelor of Science in Nursing
BTLS	basic trauma life support
BUN	blood urea nitrogen
BVM	bag valve mask
bx	biopsy

MEDTERMS
GENERAL ABBREVIATIONS

ABBREVIATION   **MEANING**

C-1...C-7	cervical vertebra
Ca	cancer
CA	California
CAD	coronary artery disease, computer aided dispatch
CAP	Civil Air Patrol
caps.	capsules
CAT	computerized axial tomography
CB	Citizen's Band radio
CBC	complete blood count
CC or C/c	chief complaint
cc	cubic centimeter
CCT	critical care transfer (transport)
CCU	cardiac care unit, coronary care unit
CDC	Center for Disease Control
CEU	continuing education units
CHF	congestive heart failure
CIS	critical incident stress
CISD	critical incident stress debriefing
cm	centimeter
CNS	central nervous system
CO	carbon monoxide
c/o	complaining of
CO_2	carbon dioxide
COPD	chronic obstructive pulmonary disease
CPC	Center for Prehospital Care
CPK	creatinine phosphokinase
CPR	cardiopulmonary resuscitation
C-section	cesarean section
CSF	cerebrospinal fluid
CT	computerized tomography
CVA	cerebrovascular accident
CYA	cover your ass
D&C	dilatation and curettage
D_5W	dextrose 5% in water
DAN	Diver's Alert Network
DC or D/C	discontinue
DEA	Drug Enforcement Agency
Derm.	Dermatology
DES	diethylstilbestrol
DFO	done fell out
DHS	Department of Health Services

MEDTERMS
GENERAL ABBREVIATIONS

ABBREVIATION   MEANING

Diff.	differential white blood count
DMAT	Disaster Medical Assistance Team
DNR	do not resuscitate
D.O.	Doctor of Osteopathic Medicine
DOA	dead on arrival
DOB	date of birth
DOE	dyspnea on exertion
DT	delirium tremens
DTR	deep tendon reflex
Dx	diagnosis
EBV	Epstein-Barr virus
ECC	external cardiac compressions
ECF	extended care facility
ECG	electrocardiogram
ECT	electroconvulsive shock therapy
ED	emergency department
ENA	Emergency Nurses Association
EEG	electroencephalogram
EKG	electrocardiogram
EMD	electromechanical dissociation of the heart, emergency medical dispatcher
EMS	emergency medical services
EMSA	Emergency Medical Services Authority
EMT	Emergency Medical Technician
EMT-D	Emergency Medical Technician/Automatic Defibrillator
EMT-A	Emergency Medical Technician/Ambulance
EMT-B	Emergency Medical Technician/Basic
EMT-P	Emergency Medical Technician/Ambulance/Paramedic
EMT-CT	Emergency Medical Technician/Cardiac Technician
EMT-2	Emergency Medical Technician/Calif. Intermediate
EMT-W	Emergency Medical Technician/ Wilderness
ENA	Emergency Nursing Association
ENT	ear, nose, throat
ER	emergency room
ESR	erythrocyte sedimentation rate
ET	endotracheal
ETA	estimated time of arrival
ETOH	ethanol (ethyl alcohol)
ETT	endotracheal tube, emergency trauma technician
exc	excision
F	Fahrenheit

MEDTERMS
GENERAL ABBREVIATIONS

ABBREVIATION   MEANING

FACP	Fellow of the American Academy of Physicians
FACS	Fellow of the American Academy of Surgeons
FAQ	frequently asked questions
FBS	fasting blood sugar
FD	fire department
FDA	Food and Drug Administration
Fe	iron
FEMA	Federal Emergency Management Agency
FHx	family history
FR	first response/first responder
FUO	fever of undetermined origin
Fx	fracture
GB	gallbladder
GC	gonorrhea
GI	gastrointestinal
Gm, gm	gram
GOA	gone on arrival
GPS	global positioning system
gr.	grain
GSW	gunshot wound
GTT	glucose tolerance test
gtt.	drops
gu	genitourinary
Gyn	gynecology
h. or hr.	hour
h.d.	at bedtime
h.p.f.	high powered fever
h.s.	at bedtime
H_2O	water
Hb, Hgb	hemoglobin
HCG	human chorionic gonadotropin
HCI	hydrochloric acid
HCO_3	bicarbonate
Hct	hematocrit
HDL	high density lipids
Hg	mercury
Hgb	hemoglobin
HIV	human immuno-deficiency virus
HVD	hypertensive vascular disease
Hx, hx	history
I	Iodine

MEDTERMS
GENERAL ABBREVIATIONS

ABBREVIATION   MEANING

IAFC	International Association of Fire Chiefs
IAFF	International Association of Fire Fighters
IC	intracardiac, incident commander
ICP	intracranial pressure
ICS	incident command system
ICU	intensive care unit
ID	identify / identification
IFT	interfacility transfer
IM	intramuscular
INH	Isoniazid
IO	interosseous
IPPB	intermittent positive pressure breathing
IUD	intrauterine device
IV,i.v.	intravenous
IVP	intravenous pyelogram
JAMA	Journal of the American Medical Association
JEMS	Journal of Emergency Medical Services
JOL	jaws of life
JVD	jugular venous distension
K or K+	potassium
KED	Kendrick Extrication Device
Kg	kilogram
KVO	keep veins open
L, l	left
l.p.f.	low powered field
L-1...L-5	lumbar vertebra
LA	left atria
Lat	lateral
lb.	Pound
LDL	low density lipids
LE	law enforcement, lower extremities, lupus erythematosus
LLQ	left lower quadrant of the abdomen
LMP	last menstrual period
LP	lumbar puncture
LPM	liters per minute
LPN	Licensed Practical Nurse
LR	Lactated Ringers
LSD	lysergic acid diethylamide
LUQ	left upper quadrant of the abdomen
LV	left ventricle
LVN	Licensed Vocational Nurse

MEDTERMS
GENERAL ABBREVIATIONS

ABBREVIATION   **MEANING**

lymphs	lymphocyte
LZ	landing zone
MAO	monoamine oxidase
MAST	military or medical anti-shock trousers
MCI	mass or multiple casualty incident
MCL	midclavicular line, modified chest lead
MD	Medical Doctor
mg	milligram
MHz	megahertz
MI	myocardical infarction
MICN	Mobile Intensive Care Nurse
MICP	Mobile Intensive Care Paramedic
MICU	mobile intensive care unit
ml	milliliter
mm	millimeter
mm Hg.	Millimeters of mercury
MOI	mechanism of injury
MRI	magnetic resonance imaging
MVA	motor vehicle accident
N.F.	National Formulary
Na	sodium
NaCl	sodium chloride
NASAR	National Association of Search and Rescue
NC	nasal cannula
NKA	no known allergies
neg.	negative
NG	naso-gastric
NIOSH	National Institute for Occupational Safety and Health
NP	Nurse Practitioner
NPO	nothing by mouth
NR	National Registry
NRB	non-rebreathing oxygen mask
NREMT	National Registry emergency medical technician's test
NREMT	Nationally Registered EMT
NRFM	non-rebreathing face mask
NS	normal saline
NSR	normal sinus rhythm
NTG	nitroglycerine
N/V	nausea and vomiting
O2	oxygen
OB	obstetrics

MEDTERMS
GENERAL ABBREVIATIONS

ABBREVIATION   MEANING

OBS	organic brain syndrome
OD	overdose, right eye
OEM	Office of Emergency Management
OEMS	Office of Emergency Medical Services
Opth	ophthalmology
OR	operating room
os	opening
OS	left eye
OSHA	Occupational Safety and Health Administration
Oto.	Otology
OU	each eye
Oz.	Ounce
P.A.	Physicians Assistant
p.c.	after meals
p.o.	orally (by mouth)
P&A	percussion and auscultation
PAC	premature atrial contractions
PaCO2	oxygen pressure
PALS	Pediatric Advanced Life Support
PASG	pneumatic anti-shock garment
PAT	paroxysmal atrial tachycardia
PCO2	carbon dioxide pressure
PD	police department
PDR	Physicians Desk Reference
PE	physical examination, pulmonary embolus
PEA	pulseless electrical activity
PEARL	pupils are equal and reactive to light
PEARLA	pupils are equal and reactive to light and accommodation
PET	positron emission tomography
pH.	Hydrogen ion concentration (acidity)
PHTLS	Pre-Hospital Trauma Life Support
PID	pelvic inflammatory disease
PND	paroxysmal nocturnal dyspnea
pos.	positive
POST	Peace Officer Standards of Training
POV	privately owned vehicle
PP	postprandial (after meals)
PPD	purified protein derivative (TB test)
PR	public relations
pre-op	preoperative (before operation)
PT	physical therapy

MEDTERMS
GENERAL ABBREVIATIONS

ABBREVIATION   **MEANING**

pt.	Patient
PTA	prior to admission
PVC	premature ventricular contractions
q.d.	every day
q.h.	every hour
q.i.d.	four times a day
q.n.	every night
QI	quality improvement
R/O	rule out
R,r,rt.	right
RA	rheumatoid arthritis, right atria
RACES	Radio Amateur Civil Emergency Services
RBC	red blood cell, red blood count
RDS	respiratory distress syndrome
RLQ	right lower quadrant of the abdomen
ROM	range of motion
RN	Registered Nurse
RP	reporting party
RSI	rapid sequence induction
RT	Respiratory Therapist
RV	right ventricle
Rx	therapy
S1...S5	sacral vertebra
SABA	supplied air breathing apparatus
SAED	semiautomatic external defibrillator
SAR	search and rescue
SCBA	self contained breathing apparatus
SC or SQ	subcutaneous
SCUBA	self contained underwater breathing apparatus
SFM	simple face mask
SIDS	sudden infant death syndrome
SOB	shortness of breath
SOP	standard operating procedure
SR	sedimentation rate
S/S	signs and symptoms
stat.	immediately
STD	sexually transmitted disease
STI	sexually transmitted infection
strep.	Streptococcus
subcu.	subcutaneous
Sub.Q.	subcutaneous

MEDTERMS
GENERAL ABBREVIATIONS

ABBREVIATION   MEANING

Sx.	symptoms
T	temperature
T&A	tonsillectomy and adenoidectomy
T1…T-12	thoracic vertebra
TA	traffic accident
tab.	tablet
TB	tuberculosis
TC	traffic collision
TIA	transient ischemic attack
TKO	to keep open
TNM	tumor, nodes, metastases
TPN	total parenteral nutrition
TPR	temperature, pulse, respirations
Tx.	treatment
U/A	urinalysis
ug	microgram
UHF	ultra high frequency
umb.	umbilicus
USFS	United States Forest Service
V-fib,VF	ventricular fibrillation
VA	Veteran's Administration, visual acuity
VD	venereal disease
VDRL	blood test for syphilis
VHF	very high frequency
WBC	white blood cell, white blood count
WEMT	wilderness emt
WWW	world wide web
y/o	years old

LADHS APPROVED ABBREVIATIONS – For Documentation
ABBREVIATION MEANING

a	before
Ab	abortion
abd	abdomen
adm	admission
AED	automatic external defibrillator
AIDS	acquired immune deficiency syndrome
AKA	above the knee amputation
ALC	altered level of consciousness
ALS	advanced life support
am	morning
AMA	against medical advice
amb	ambulation/ambulance
amt	amount
ant	anterior
a/o x3	alert, oriented times 3 parameters
approx	approximately
appt	appointment
ARDS	adult respiratory distress syndrome
ASA	aspirin
ASAP	as soon as possible
ASHD	atherosclerotic heart disease
BCP	birth control pills
BIB	brought in by
BKA	below the knee amputation
BLS	basic life support
BM	bowel movement
BOA	born out of asepsis
BOW	bag of waters
BP	blood pressure
BS	breath sounds
BSA	body surface area
c	with
C	centigrade
CA	cancer
CAD	coronary artery disease
cc	cubic centimeter
CC or c/c	chief complaint

LADHS APPROVED ABBREVIATIONS – For Documentation
ABBREVIATION MEANING

CHF	congestive heart failure
Cm	centimeter
C/O	complains of
CO_2	carbon dioxide
COA	condition on arrival
COPD	chronic obstructive pulmonary disease
CP	chest pain
CPR	cardiopulmonary resuscitation
CRF	chronic renal failure
CSF	cerebrospinal fluid
CSM	circulation, sensation, movement
CVA	cerebral vascular accident
CXR	chest x-ray
D&C	dilation and curettage
dc	discharge / discontinue
DM	diabetes mellitus
DNR	do not resuscitate
DOA	dead on arrival
DOB	date of birth
DOE	dyspnea on exertion
drg	dressing
DT's	delirium tremors
DVT	deep vein thrombosis
DX	diagnosis
EBL	estimated blood loss
ED/ER	emergency department / emergency room
EDAP	emergency dept. approved for pediatrics
EKG	electrocardiogram
EMS	emergency medical services
EMT	emergency medical technician
EMT-A	A emergency medical technician-advanced airway
EMT-D	emergency medical technician-defibrillation
EMT-P	emergency medical technician-paramedic
ET	endotracheal
ETA	estimated time of arrival
ETC	endotracheal combitube
ETOH	ethanol (alcohol)

LADHS APPROVED ABBREVIATIONS – For Documentation
ABBREVIATION MEANING

eval	evaluation
FB	foreign body
f/u	follow up
fx	fracture
G	gravida
GB	gallbladder
GI	gastrointestinal
gm	gram
GSW	gunshot wound
gtt	drop
GU	genitourinary
HMO	health maintenance organization
hosp	hospital
hr(s)	hour(s)
hs	at night
ht	height
HTN	hypertension
Hx	history
ICU	intensive care unit
Inc Ab	incomplete abortion
IUD	intrauterine device
IUP	intrauterine pregnancy
IV	intravenous
IVP	Intravenous push
JVD	jugular vein distention
KCL	potassium chloride
kg	kilogram
KO	knocked out (loss of consciousness)
KVO	keep vein open
L	liter
L	left
Lab	laboratory
lac	laceration
lb	pound
LLE	left lower extremity
LLL	left lower lobe (lung)
LLQ	left lower quadrant (abdomen)

LADHS APPROVED ABBREVIATIONS – For Documentation
ABBREVIATION MEANING

LMP	last menstrual period
LNMP	last normal menstrual period
LOC	level of consciousness/loss of consciousness
LUE	left upper extremity
LUL	left upper lobe (lung)
LUQ	left upper quadrant
MAR	most accessible receiving facility
max	maximum
MCL	mid clavicular line
MD/PMD	medical doctor / private medical doctor
mEq	milliequivalent
mg	milligram
MI	myocardial infarction
MICN	mobile intensive care nurse
min	minutes / minimum
ml	milliliter
mo	month
MS	multiple sclerosis / morphine sulfate
MVA	motor vehicle accident
NA	not applicable / not available
NAD	no apparent distress
narc	narcotic
NB	newborn
neg	negative
NKA	no known allergies
NP	nurse practitioner
npo	nothing per mouth
NSR	normal sinus rhythm
NTG	nitroglycerin
nv	nausea/vomiting
n/v/d	nausea / vomiting / diarrhea
O_2	oxygen
O_2 sat	oxygen saturation
OB/GYN	obstetrical / gynecological
OBS	organic brain syndrome
OD	overdose / right eye
OS	left eye

LADHS APPROVED ABBREVIATIONS – For Documentation
ABBREVIATION MEANING

OU	both eyes
p	after
P	para
PCCC	pediatric critical care center
PE	physical exam / pedal edema / pulmonary embolus
Peds	pediatric / pedestrian
perf	perforation
PERL	pupils equal, react to light
PIH	pregnancy induced hypertension
pm	evening
PMH	past medical history
PMS	pulse, motor, sensation
po	by mouth
post	posterior / after
PPD	purified protein derivative (TB skin test)
pr	per rectum
prn	as needed
PSI	passenger space intrusion
Psych	psychiatric
pt	patient
PTA	prior to arrival
pulm	pulmonary
PVC	premature ventricular contraction
q	every
R	right
rehab	rehabilitation
RLE	right lower extremity
RLL	right lower lob (lung)
RLQ	right middle quadrant (abdomen)
RML	right middle lobe (lung)
RN	registered nurse
r/o	rule out
RTS	revised trauma score
RUE	right upper extremity
RUL	right upper lobe (lung)
RUQ	right upper quadrant (abdomen)
Rx	prescription

LADHS APPROVED ABBREVIATIONS – For Documentation
ABBREVIATION MEANING

s	without
SC	specialty center
sec	second
SIDS	sudden infant death syndrome
SL	saline lock / sublingual
SOB	shortness of breath
sq	square
SQ	subcutaneous
SW	stab wound
TB	tuberculosis
TBC	total body check
Tbsp	tablespoon
TC	traffic collision
TIA	transient ischemic attack
TKO	to keep open (IV rate)
tsp	teaspoon
TV	tidal volume
unk	unknown
UTI	urinary tract infection
vag	vaginal
vol	volume
vs	versus
VS	vital signs
wk	weak
WNL	within normal limits
w/o	without
wt	weight
y/o	year old
yr	year
@	at
&	and
%	percent
2o	secondary to
=	equal
#	number
>	greater than

LADHS APPROVED ABBREVIATIONS – For Documentation
ABBREVIATION MEANING

<	less than
+	plus / positive
-	minus / negative

TEMPERATURE CONVERSIONS

Centigrade (C x9/5) +32 = F	Fahrenheit (F –32)x 5/9 = C
0	32
35.0	96.8
36.5	97.7
37.0	98.6
37.5	99.5
38.0	100.4
38.5	101.3
39.0	102.2
39.5	103.1
40.0	104
40.5	104.9
41.0	105.8
41.5	106.7

AIRWAY AND RESPIRATION

BVM

If administering with supplemental oxygen, give 400-600 ml. per ventilation or 6-7ml. / kg.

If administering without supplemental oxygen, give 700-1000 ml. per ventilation or 10ml. / kg

Device must have a 15/22 mm. fitting for face mask

Device must accept 30 L/min oxygen

Flow Restricted O2 Powered Ventilator

Must provide peak of 100% oxygen at up to 40L/min

Contra-Indicated in children, spinal or chest trauma

Must maintain cricoid pressure during use

Must have 60cm (H2O) pressure release valve

Suction Device   Suction no longer then 15 seconds at a time in an adult, 10 seconds in a child, and five seconds in an infant

Clean suction tubing with water if using over prolonged period

Must maintain vacuum of 300 ml when clamped.

Obtain correct depth by measuring from corner of patient's mouth to earlobe

Suction only in circular motions while withdrawing catheter

Use of rigid (Yankaur or tonsil tip) catheter is preferred in most adults and children

Use of a non-rigid (French or whistle tip) is preferred in stoma and incidents when a rigid catheter can cause complications

Oxygen Flow-Rates and Percents

Device	Oxygen Flow-Rate	Percent Oxygen
Nasal cannula	1-6 liters / min	24% - 44%
Simple face mask	8-15 liters / min	35% - 60%
Non-rebreather mask	10 – 15 liters / min	Up to 90% - 95%
Mouth to mask	15 liters / min	55%
BVM with reservoir	15 liters / min	Between 90 and 100%

BVM Bag Volumes

Infant	150 – 240 ml.
Pediatric	500 – 700 ml.
Adult	1200-1600 ml.

Normal Respiratory Ranges

Adults > 8 y	12 – 20
Children 1 – 8 y.	15 – 30
Infants 1-12 mo.	25 – 50
Neonates < 1 mo.	40 – 60

NEUROLOGICAL ASSESSMENTS

GLOSGOW COMA SCALE

Eye opening response
      Spontaneous (4)
      To voice (3)
      To pain (2) (includes tactile)
      None (1)

Best motor response
      Obeys commands (6)
      Localizes pain (5)
      Withdraws (4)
      Flexion (3)
      Extension (2)
      None (1)

Best verbal response
      Oriented (5)
      Confused (4)
      Inappropriate words (3) (e.g. patient often curses incomprehensibly)
      Sounds (2)
      None (1)

Prognostic indicator for head injury patients
Documented for all patients by paramedics in Los Angeles County

Initial Assessment (A.V.P.U.)
      Alert
      Verbal
      Painful
      Unresponsive

A.V.P.U. is utilized in the initial assessment

MINI- NEUROLOGICAL EXAM (DERM)

<u>D</u>epth of coma
- Eye opening (spontaneous, to voice, to pain, none)
- Verbal response (oriented, confused, inappropriate words, incomprehensible words, none)
- Specific orientation or note the patients response to stimulus applied

<u>E</u>yes (pupillary response)
- Size, equality, reaction to light

<u>R</u>espirations
- Rate, rhythm, tidal volume

<u>M</u>otor

- Motor response (obeys command, localizes, withdraws, flexion, extension, none)
- Assessment of distal circulation, motor and sensory functions in all extremities

Used to document neurological status in patients

ACRONYMS

Complete
Body
Check

Partial / Pertinent
Body
Check

Alcohol, arrhythmia, apena, anaphylaxis
Epilepsy, environment
Insulin
Overdose
Underdose, uremia
Trauma
Infection
Psychiatric, poisoning
Stroke, shock

Drug / dose
Indications / Integrity
Contra Indications / Clarity
Expiration

Level
Of
Consciousness

Depth of consciousness
Eyes
Respirations
Motor

Onset
Provocation / Palliation
Quality
Regional, Radiation, Recurrence
Severity
Time

Signs & Symptoms
Allergies
Meds
Past pertinent history
Last oral intake
Events prior

Body
Substance
Isolation

Shortness
Of
Breath

Alert
Verbal
Painful
Unresponsive

Airway
Breathing
Circulation
Deformity / **D**isability
Environment

C/C chief complaint

Mechanism
Of
Injury

UCLA CENTER FOR PREHOSPITAL CARE

Educational Enrichment for EMT's

TRANSPORTATION OF AMPUTATED BODY PARTS

Progress in surgical technique has made the potential for reattaching a severed part (reimplantation or replantation) a viable reality today. Some parts, like a severed ear, are relatively easy to attach as their revascularization and vitalization is the only concern. Replanting an arm or leg is much more difficult. Not only is reperfusing the limb a concern, but making the various ligaments, tendons and nerves functional is necessary if the reattached part is ever going to be more than prosthesis for improving body image. Even if the amputated part cannot be reattached, the skin may be used to cover the limb end.

In the prehospital setting, a paramedic or EMT should <u>NEVER</u> comment on whether a severed part can be replanted. It is impossible to determine the treatment possibilities in the field. This type of statement may turn out to be false and could set the patient up for having a poor relationship with the doctor or even result in a lawsuit for negligence if reimplantation is not attempted or is unsuccessful.

If there is any possibility that the amputated part can be reattached it must be properly cared for during transport. There has been conflicting information about how to transport and preserve amputated parts. Essentially measures should be taken to slow metabolism and decrease tissue death. Cold is a method of slowing metabolism and has been shown to protect non-perfusing tissues. However, cold can damage as well as preserve and it is impossible to provide the exact amount of cooling without doing damage in the prehospital setting. Protecting a part by soaking it in water (or balanced salt solution) can lead to maceration or edema, both affecting tissue survival.

Current recommendations for managing amputated body parts include "dry cooling and rapid transport". The amputated part should be put placed in a dry bag, sealed and the bag and placed in cool water. Ice cubes in the water is controversial, but may be valuable depending on the environmental temperature. AVOID DIRECT CONTACT BETWEEN ICE AND THE AMPUTATED PART.

USE OF CONSTRICTING BANDS IN THE TREATMENT OF SNAKEBITE

Bites by non-venomous snakes produce no more complications than would be caused by any other traumatic skin break. The bite of a poisonous snake involves the injection of a venom into the victim. Venom contains toxins and enzymes that paralyze the snake's prey and begin a digestive tissue destructive process. Many different methods for the treatment of snakebite have been proposed over the years. Most were aimed at attempting to remove the venom (cutting the bite and sucking out the fluids) or preventing its spread. (applying ice and/or constricting bands).

The medical literature is lacking on prospective randomized studies that document the best methods of dealing with snakebite. Most of the articles are published accounts of case studies and local guidelines or protocols. The main medical consensus seems to be that the use of anti-venom is the best method of dealing with the consequences of envenomation.

The following suggested treatments are either worthless or add too many of their own complications to be worthwhile:

1. Ice - applying ice to the skin causes frostbite. Its application to a snake bite injury has not been demonstrated to reduce the spread of injected venom and may cause further complications.

2. Cutting and sucking - again common sense might suggest that this is the best method of eliminating venom from a victims body, however, scientific data has not demonstrated that this is effective and can increase infection. The complication of creating an additional injury and route for infection are not worth the risks.

3. Constricting Band - it was also believed that if the problem in envenomation was the spread of the venom then containing it through the use of a constricting band must be of benefit. This is Not true. A study by Amaral CF et al in 1998 demonstrated that that the use of a "tourniquet" is "ineffective" in the treatment of snake bite injuries and anti-venom was the best treatment.

Many physicians in Los Angeles County, who are experts in this field, feel strongly that the best measure to take in prehospital care is to prevent the distribution of venom by immobilizing the extremity (splint or sling) and transporting to a hospital where anti-venom can be administered. They do not recommend constricting bands, but to keep the patient calm, the extremity at or below heart level, and immobilized.

Another LA County protocol is to NOT bring the actual snake to the hospital. There seems to be little benefit to doing this. First it exposes the rescuers and hospital personnel to harm by attempting to catch the snake. Even if the snake is dead it is still hazardous. ("Dead Rattle Snakes Can Bite" Mayo Clinic Health Letter 1999) Second it is generally well known by the health care workers what type of snakes are endemic in the geographical area and the exact type can be narrowed down (if necessary) by the description from the patient. If the snake was a pet, then the exact species should be readily identified by the owner.

SARS and Prehospital Responders; Questions that you might have; Answers that you need to know

By James Crabtree, Los Angeles County EMS Agency

What is SARS?

Severe acute respiratory syndrome (SARS) is a viral respiratory illness caused by a coronavirus, called SARS-associated coronavirus (SARS-CoV). SARS was first reported in Asia in February 2003 and was not known to exist as a disease before this date. Over the next few months, the illness spread to more than two dozen countries in North America, South America, Europe, and Asia. The SARS global outbreak of 2003 was eventually contained. This means that nobody is known to have SARS anywhere at this time. However, it is very possible that the disease could re-emerge. To find out the latest information about SARS, go to: www.cdc.gov/ncidod/sars/ and www.who.int/csr/sars/en/.

How many people had SARS?

According to the World Health Organization (WHO), during the SARS outbreak of 2003, a total of 8,098 people worldwide became sick with SARS; of these, 774 died. In the United States, there were 192 cases of SARS among people, all of whom got better. Most of the U.S. SARS cases were among travelers returning from other parts of the world with SARS. There were very few U.S. cases among close contacts of travelers, including health-care workers and family members. SARS did not spread more widely in the community in the United States.

How deadly is SARS?

As you can see, SARS was a factor in the deaths of about 10% of the people who developed it. This means that about 90% of the people who developed SARS later recovered. The greatest risk occurs in persons over the age of 60. In these cases there was an approximately 50% fatality rate.

What are the Symptoms of SARS?

In general, SARS begins with a high fever (temperature greater than 100.4°F [>38.0°C]). Other symptoms may include headache, an overall feeling of discomfort, and body aches. Some people also have mild respiratory symptoms at the outset. About 10 percent to 20 percent of patients have diarrhea. After 2 to 7 days, SARS patients may develop a dry cough. Most patients develop pneumonia.

How do you know if somebody has SARS?

During the 2003 outbreak, SARS was most easily identified by people who had high fevers (above 100.4°) and flu like symptoms, PLUS they had either recently traveled to a SARS area or they had close contact with somebody who had. Direct diagnosis of SARS is difficult to impossible. While there are laboratory tests to grow the virus and to determine the presence of SARS antibodies in the blood they are not always effective early on in the course of the disease. A SARS diagnosis is generally based on the patient's presenting symptoms and travel history and then by excluding all other causes of respiratory illnesses.

How does a person get SARS?

The main way that SARS seems to be spread is by close person-to-person contact. The virus that causes SARS is thought to be transmitted most readily by respiratory droplets (droplet spread) produced when an infected person coughs or sneezes. Droplet spread can happen when droplets from the cough or sneeze of an infected person are propelled a short distance (generally up to 3 feet) through the air and deposited on the mucous membranes of the mouth, nose, or eyes of persons who are nearby. The virus also can spread when a person touches a surface or object contaminated with infectious droplets and then touches his or her mouth, nose, or eye(s). In addition, it is possible that the SARS virus might spread through the air to greater distance than 3 feet (airborne spread) or by other ways that are not now known.

SARS seems to spread only when there is "close contact" what exactly does that mean?

In the context of SARS, close contact means having cared for or lived with someone who has SARS or having direct contact with respiratory secretions or body fluids of a patient with SARS. Examples of close contact include kissing or hugging, sharing eating or drinking utensils, talking to someone within 3 feet, and touching someone directly. Close contact does not include activities like walking by a person or sitting across a waiting room or office for a brief time.

Can I get SARS on my EMS related job?

As an emergency medical provider you might be called to care for somebody who has an undiagnosed flu like illness. The care you provide might expose you to droplet contamination while you are closer than 3 feet to the patient. (example: in the back of an ambulance) If the patient was contagious with SARS (or any other respiratory disease) it would be possible for you to catch it.

How do I protect myself?

Since we know how SARS is spread, we also know how to keep from getting it. The main method of transmission is inhaling or contacting droplets from when a SARS patient coughs or sneezes. These droplets can also be touched and then transfer the virus when somebody touches their eyes, nose or mouth. It is not known exactly how long the SARS virus lives in the environment, testing is ongoing but it looks like it may be several days.

Because SARS is spread by droplets, regular use of personnel protective equipment to stop these droplets is required. This includes gloves, gowns, eye protection and a filter type mask (N-95). It is important that you fully understand how to use the mask properly. Masks should be fit tested to ensure that they are sealed against your face and actually filter the inhaled air. Hand washing is also very important to prevent becoming sick and is too often forgotten after providing patient care.

How long are people contagious?
Up to 10 days after the fever has resolved. Experience suggests that SARS is not transmitted before the symptoms appear and most transmissions occurred late in the illness (when patients were already in the hospital)

Is there a disinfectant that kills the SARS virus?
Nothing is currently listed or approved as being able to kill the SARS virus on environmental surfaces. However similar viruses are known to be killed by using ammonia, bleach, alcohol and disinfectants that contain these chemicals.

Can I bring SARS home to my family?
People who had the SARS *disease* did transmit it to "close contacts" which included family members. However, transmission in casual 'community settings' occurred rarely and under specific situations that almost always included "close contact" with a SARS *patient*.
The best way to ensure that SARS is not spread to your family is to ensure that you don't catch the disease at all by strictly following the guidelines about protecting yourself. (see above)
It would be unlikely to bring the virus home on your clothing especially if you ensure that your work clothes are not contaminated with bodily fluids or droplets from suspected SARS patients.

Is there a vaccine against SARS? Is there a medicine to cure it?
No to both questions. SARS is still too new and not well enough understood to develop a vaccine against it. Because SARS is a virus there are no effective medications to fight it. Antibiotics are not effective. Antiviral medications have been tried but have not yet been shown to be effective. It is still not known if victims recover with immunity or are susceptible to reinfection.

If I believe that a patient has SARS who do I tell?
If during your assessment and evaluation you find symptoms and history that suggests SARS, tell the medical staff at the receiving hospital. At this time prehospital personnel are not required to formally report contagious diseases to the health department.

I heard that they quarantined EMS/Ambulance people in Toronto, could that happen here?
All persons who were suspected to have the *disease* SARS were ISOLATED. In hospitals they were not kept with any non-SARS patients, they wore masks to decrease droplet dispersion as well as other precautions to prevent them from giving the disease to others. These are the same type of precautions that you should take for a patient that had any contagious disease. Some EMS responders in Toronto did develop the disease SARS and they were kept in isolation.

Quarantine is when people who are not exhibiting the symptoms of a disease (people who are not sick) are asked to not move about in society or come in close contact with people such that they might unknowingly pass the disease to others. Essentially these people are asked to stay at home until it is certain that they do not have the disease. (10 days)

Some health care workers (including EMS) who were known to have been exposed to SARS patients but had not developed the disease SARS were asked to quarantine themselves. They either stayed completely at home (for 10 days) or they were put on a "work quarantine."

Work quarantine allowed some health care workers to continue to work at the hospital or health care setting where they were exposed to SARS as long as they remained well. Work quarantine was a necessary step to ensure that health care services could continue to be provided.

When at home people on work quarantine were asked to not leave their house and not have visitors into their home. Because they were working with and were known to have been exposed to SARS patients, they were asked to wear surgical type masks whenever they shared a room with their family, not share towels, drinking cups etc., wash their hands frequently and to sleep in a separate room. To determine very early if they were developing SARS, these health care workers were also asked to take their temperatures twice a day. The family members of people on work quarantine were not confined to their home unless they themselves began to develop the symptoms of SARS.

Remember that these work quarantine precautions were used to protect the community from health care workers were working regularly with known SARS patients. Health care workers who did not have regular known contact with SARS patients were not placed on work quarantine.

What measures did the Toronto fire department & ambulance people use to protect themselves on the job?

They instituted strict use of personal protective equipment including N-95 masks, gloves eye protection and gowns for all patient contacts during the SARS outbreak. The masks were reused for 12 hours as long as they were dry and undamaged. They were however, changed whenever a known SARS patient was encountered or when it was contaminated with blood or other body fluids. Frequent hand washing was reinforced.

Whenever possible they limited the number of people who had direct patient contact to just two. (Afterward it was reported that no responder developed SARS after having PROTECTED exposure to known SARS patients).

All patients were given surgical masks to wear unless they were receiving oxygen therapy by mask.

Other measures were instituted to insure that the virus did not spread among the close living conditions that exist in a fire department environment. Group training sessions of frontline staff from different locales was postponed. Field personnel who needed to enter the department headquarters and training buildings were medically screened before entering including measuring their temperature with a tympanic thermometer.

Items in the station house that had regular contact with the hands or facial area of many different users were wiped with a disinfectant at least daily. Such items included; telephones, door handles (especially washrooms), counter tops and tabletops, microphones for in-station announcements, computer keyboard and mouse, etc. Effort was made to ensure that all dishes and cutlery were thoroughly washed, and preferably air-dried.

References:
http://www.cdc.gov/ncidod/sars/factsheet.htm

Dementia in Emergency Situations

Dementia is one condition with many causes; the word means to be 'without a mind'. As a medical term dementia refers to the loss of the abilities to remember, process and apply information in a manner that makes a daily existence possible. Dementia is brain damage, damage that is caused by conditions that are irreversible, incurable and terminal. Many different types of dementias exist such as; Lewy Body, Frontotemporal, Vascular, Parkinson's, Creutzfeldt–Jakob disease and Normal Pressure Hydrocephalus. Other situations can also result in brain destruction leading to dementia such as chronic alcoholism and infections like encephalitis. Each source of damage shows itself with slightly different symptoms. Alzheimer's disease (AD) however is the most common type and the one that would sound familiar to most people, so it will be the main focus here.

In Alzheimer's disease unwanted proteins and chemicals (Beta Amyloid and Tau) accumulate inside brain tissue. These proteins interfere with nerve connections and destroy neurons resulting in the destruction of brain tissue. AD is a scary disease that people want to avoid. However unlike heart disease that can be avoided or lessened through diet and exercise, there is nothing that can stop Alzheimer's disease. In April of 2010 a National Institute of Health Expert Panel reviewed all available studies and concluded that the strongest risk factor for developing it is simply advancing age[1]. Diet, exercise, drugs or even doing puzzles cannot prevent it and currently there is no drug or treatment that can prevent or cure it.

The problem then becomes one of a disease that becomes more common with advancing age and can't be cured or stopped within a society that will see a huge growth in aged persons for the next 50 years. Medical science has lowered death rates from strokes, cancers, heart disease and even AIDS while the death rate from AD has increased 46%.[2] While the exact percentages of people who will develop AD or other dementia is not totally established, the number of Americans over age 65 is expected to double in the next 20 years eventually reaching 20% of the population. If just 10% of this group develops AD symptoms then the chances of dementia complicating an otherwise routine ambulance encounter are enormous. 21st century EMS responders need to be as comfortable in working with older dementia patients as they are working with children.

First it must be said that Alzheimer's disease is NOT a normal part of aging. It is a disease. During normal aging all human capabilities, physical and mental (including memory) will decline to some extent. Normal brain aging is not dementia. While AD is mainly a disease of people age 75 and up, it also occurs much earlier. The Alzheimer's Association estimates there are 500,000 Americans below age 65 with dementia, of all causes [2]. Medical literature records some people developing AD symptoms as early as their 30s.

The destructive changes of AD generally begin in the hippocampus of the brain where new memories are first formed. It then spreads through the brain areas that store; words and language, time and place, how to do daily routine tasks, recognition and naming normal objects and visual images, judgment and personality and the ability to solve problems. The symptoms of AD are not exactly the same for everyone who has it. The amount of loss or remaining capability that is seen in different persons with AD can be very inconsistent and surprising. There are AD people who are very capable of navigating and driving a car, but find it impossible to handle money or pay bills. Some dementia suffers will read the same page in a newspaper over and over again unable to remember what they had just seen, but can carry on a conversation such that you would never think there is anything wrong with them.

As the destruction progresses through each area of the brain the victim loses the abilities that are managed there. The forgetting starts with recent general memories, eventually AD erases the knowledge of who the sufferer is, which leads to changes in their personality. Performing complex, multipart tasks such as remembering the many steps it takes to make a sandwich will totally disappear. Later they forget how to perform all the skills of daily living such as dressing, eating, shaving and toileting, eventually even walking. Destruction in the frontal lobe leads to changes in moral behavior such as stealing and inappropriate sexual behavior. Loss of the cells that regulate self control means that uncontrolled anger, rage and violence in an otherwise passive person are not uncommon. Not being able to recognize images or place them into context, has some AD persons conversing with their own image in a mirror because they don't recognize their own face and instead interpret that image as being another person. As recent memories evaporate the dementia person regresses to having to base their daily existence on still older and older memories. This results in living life backwards. The AD person may not recognize their own children or spouse because the only memories they have left are from their life decades before their marriage. As the neuro connections are severed and their brain dies, they continually regress in knowledge and abilities.

Demonstrations of fear and paranoia related to everyday objects or behaviors (such as toileting & bathing) and hallucinations of all types are typical problems. Eventually the person forgets how to read and speak; their vocabulary may be just a few words. End stage Alzheimer's disease usually finds the person unable to walk and confined to bed with complications from the imposed inactivity. Death itself is usually related to malnourishment and pneumonia brought on by the inability to swallow and 'forgetting' to breathe. The slow relentless process from simple forgetting to death takes approximately 5-7 years but some people endure the decline for 20 or more years.

In this time span between the earliest symptoms and death, the person with AD needs increasing amounts of assistance to meet their daily needs. It quickly becomes impossible for somebody with dementia to live on their own. Generally a spouse or family member provides the care they need. These caretakers become affected by the disease almost as intensely as the original victim. It is said that there is never just one person suffering the effects of AD, there is always two. The bizarre behaviors of dementia require constant supervision. Insomnia and night time wandering by the AD person can prevent the caretaker from sleeping. The inability to leave an AD person alone for even short periods can make it difficult to even shop for daily supplies. 40% of caretakers suffer diagnosable depression [3]. Other symptoms caused by pure stress are so commonplace in caregivers as to be considered normal. It is incredibly difficult to care for someone who is slowly losing their mind. Dementia victims are living physically while dying intellectually.

How do these dementia symptoms affect prehospital and emergency care? Persons with AD or dementia cannot enter the normal world, so the responders must perform every task in a manner that fits the dementia frame of reference. Be prepared for strange behaviors such over dressing, inappropriate displays of anger and rage, even overt sexual advances. As the disease progresses AD persons cannot be oriented, learning becomes impossible, discipline and corrective measures have no effect on their behavior. It is natural to want a dementia patient to 'act normal' but they simply cannot. It becomes necessary for anyone working with them to accept their unnatural behavior as normal.

Paramedics and EMTs should treat dementia patients respectfully but be prepared to repeat, repeat and repeat everything you say. An early stage AD person called his daughter five times in one hour to ask what time they were getting together for dinner that night. Exasperated the daughter screamed "Dad, I have told you 5 times now!" Sensing the stress in her voice but unapologetic (because he only remembered asking just once) he then asked her "Ok, what part of Alzheimer's don't you understand?" In an emergency situation it is very likely they don't have any idea what happened to them or why you are there. They don't remember the car accident or falling down. They may not remember that they had chest pain or shortness of breath. Be prepared to explain things again and again. The hallucinations that AD can bring on can be as significant as with a psychotic patient. One caregiver describes her family member; "During the later stages she would think the blue veins on her hands and arms were blue worms and she would pick at herself to get them off. We finally had to put little gloves on her hands to keep her from damaging herself." An AD patient gets more confused when taken out of their environment, so keeping the area as calm and quiet as possible is to their advantage. Speak calmly and quietly to them when possible. They respond slower to questions than an average person so give them time to process the information before they can respond.

If an AD person doesn't remember why you are there, they also can't remember who or how many people are in the room. Always approach a dementia person from the front. Don't touch them without warning; they need time to process what is happening to them. AD persons commonly do not like to remove their clothing. You may have to perform an exam with much of their clothing in place. Upsetting them just to get them undressed can be a waste of both time and energy. If an AD person does become upset or combative, do not argue with them! The proper method of calming a dementia person is to distract and redirect them. Change the topic or ask another question or make small talk. They can quickly forget what was upsetting them.

Gathering information – AD people may talk and appear to be normal, mature people, but depending on the stage they are in, they may be 'children' and rescuers need to respond accordingly. They cannot always operate as adults. Speak in short simple sentences. They lose the first part of the sentence before they get to the end if it is too long. Break each question down to bare essentials. Talk to the pt, but verify the details with the family. You may need to gather actual details out of sight of patient. In one well handled prehospital encounter, the paramedics followed the patient's wife to the kitchen ostensibly 'to get the list of medications' but in reality it allowed the paramedic to talk to the patient's wife alone and understand what the actual problems were.

Because most dementia patients are elderly, you can expect them to have other medical problems beyond their initial chief complaint. This is also a population that will very likely will have paper work such as Durable Power of Attorney, (DPOA), Advanced Directives, DNRs etc. Before you rush into doing anything, talk about what treatments the patient and family actually wants you to perform.

Because the dementia brain does not work like a normal brain some medications may be totally inappropriate. When the caregiver says NOT to give a medication, believe it. Medication may have idiosyncratic reactions. Medications for anxiety and agitation such as midiazolam or Haldol may not help. It might make the behaviors worse or result in overly decreasing their LOC.

While it is more likely to become an issue after hospital arrival, NEVER leave AD person unattended. They very likely will wander. One Alzheimer's spouse described her trips to an ED. "On 3 of these trips, I went by other transport to the hospital, arriving after the ambulance and was delayed at the registration counter before joining him. He would usually be on the gurney in a curtained room--alone. Very shortly he'd be trying to climb off the gurney for one reason or another that made sense only to him. I would spend a lot of time distracting and diverting. TELL THE EMTs TO MAKE IT CLEAR TO THE EMERGENCY ROOM PERSONS--THE PATIENT CANNOT BE LEFT ALONE!" Do everything you can to keep the dementia person and the caregiver together.

As noted above, it is also very possible that the caregiver is the emergency patient. This creates an interesting situation because the AD person cannot be left alone. If the caregiver is ill or needs to be transported, then arrangements have to be made for a responsible person to look after the person with dementia, this may not be easy. The AD person may have to transported just out of convenience. An interesting situation arises if the caregiver is ill and responders on scene are not told or recognize that the other person has dementia. In at least one situation the husband with dementia wanted to follow the ambulance to the hospital despite the fact that he had lost his driving skills. Only because the wife was still able to tell the on scene personnel that he could not drive was a disaster averted.

References

1. http://www.nih.gov/news/health/apr2010/od-28.htm
2. Alzheimer's Association (2010) *2010 Alzheimer's Disease Facts and Figures*
3. Cohen et al, 1990, Gallagher, 1985, Schultz et al, 1995

USE OF PAINFUL STIMULI IN THE PREHOSPITAL SETTING

There is no readily available documentation concerning exactly what methods should be used to cause a painful stimuli. Some considerations based upon medical ethics include:

1. <u>The stimulation should not leave a permanent or temporary injury</u> (the first rule in medicine is to "do no harm").

   Some assessments and treatments do cause secondary complications, but the benefits must be outweighed by the risks. The information that is needed in the prehospital setting would <u>NEVER</u> indicate a need for the use of a painful stimulation that causes a permanent injury.

   Example of this type of stimulation that have occurred and caused considerable harm include: nipple pinching (sometimes by hemostat), cutting the skin, inserting objects under the finger nails, and inserting ammonia inhalants in each nostril (leading to hypoxia/toxic inhalation and severe burns of the mucus membranes).

2. <u>The use of painful stimulation should not be done punitively</u>.

   The continuous evaluation of patients in a hospital implies that their body is free from drugs or chemicals beyond those that are therapeutically prescribed. In the prehospital setting, patients routinely have their sensorium (level of consiousness) modified by recreational drugs and alcohol. Personal attitudes and biases on the part of the emergency responder can lead a rescuer to want to 'punish' a patient for their use of intoxicating chemicals. Anger at being woken up to respond to a non-emergency or an emergency of the patient's own making can lead a rescuer to intentionally cause pain not for assessment purposes, but rather to gain a personal satisfaction at "teaching somebody a lesson". Painful stimulation used for this reason represents torture and sadism.

   Example of this include repeated stimuli causing pain in drunks or drug addicts long after knowledge of their depth of coma has been obtained. The insertion of large bore IVs when their therapeutic use is not indicated is also a example.

3. <u>The level of pain applied, should be the minimal amount needed to elicit an assessable response</u>.

   There are limited treatments available to a prehospital care provider. The need to determine if there are responses to light pain versus deep pain is not appropriate in this setting. A complete diagnosis of specific areas of the brain that is involved can only be done in a hospital by an MD after reviewing other diagnostic materials such as CT scans, lab and specific neurological tests.

   Therefore, the question arises what type of painful stimuli should be applied in the field. EMT and paramedic textbooks advocate several methods for painful stimuli. Many of these are not appropriate and are *not to be used in Los Angeles County*.

   - <u>Pinching the patient's earlobe</u> - this does not cause enough reaction to warrant a true test unless fingernails are used, and this can result in tissue damage.

   - <u>Supraorbital pressure (pressure on the bone above the eye)</u> - this dose not cause enough reaction to warrant a true test. When no reaction is obtained, providers have attempted to apply direct pressure on the eyeball which is much more painful, but can result in injury to the eye.

- <u>Trapezius (muscle of the neck) pinch</u> - this can be very painful. Extremely painful stimuli is never appropriate.
- <u>Sternal rub</u> - this can be very painful, damage skin and underlying tissue and may be inaccurate if spinal trauma is present. Extremely painful stimuli is never appropriate.

Acceptable forms of painful stimuli that do not cause injury:
- Slight pressure on nailbed
- Interdigital pressure

*** If in doubt if the patient is truly unresponsive, assume the worst and treat accordingly.

LATEX ALLERGIES

An allergic reaction is a hyper stimulation of the immune system to a chemical or molecule that ordinary would not pose a threat to the body. It is not understood exactly how allergies develop or why some people have such a strong reaction to otherwise innocuous material, but the reactions are real and must be dealt with.

Latex is the natural rubber derived by harvesting the sap from the *Hevea brasiliensis* tree.

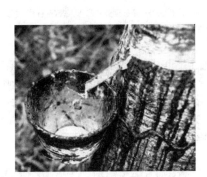

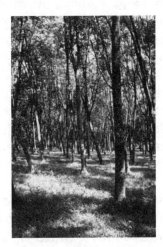

Well known for its durability, ease of processing and low cost it has been used in our society for a myriad of products. Beyond the gloves that people generally think of first, latex is used in condoms and even in road paving asphalt and roofing tar. Many of the proteins that cause latex allergy are also found in fruits--specifically, bananas, kiwis, and avocados, vegetables, nuts (especially chestnuts), and cereals.

Latex by definition is a water-based colloidal suspension of rubber particles. The rubber particles are not limited to natural rubber. There are two kinds of rubber particles in latex form: natural and synthetic rubber latex. The synthetic rubber products in latex form are just as common as natural rubber latex.

Allergy to this natural rubber protein has been misnamed "*latex allergy*". Gloves made from natural rubber latex have been called "*latex gloves*" for years. This term "*latex allergy*" implicates numerous other products which contain no natural rubber at all. Latex paint is the prime example of this paradox. Latex paint will not cause a natural rubber protein allergic reaction, but masking tape should be avoided by latex allergy sufferers because masking tape may be 100% natural rubber latex.

Essentially the issue is one of a reaction on the part of the patient and one on the part of the provider. A health care provider's main personal exposure is through gloves, patients are also exposed to gloves when healthcare providers wear them and may also receive very intense exposures from tape and IV equipment.

Protecting people from this antigen has legal implications. While not yet cited under workers compensation laws or the Americans with Disabilities Act, the employee and certainly the health care provider has some responsibility to keep natural rubber away from those that can be harmed by it. Identification of those at risk for a serious reaction and then providing an environment as latex free as possible is mandatory. Notations on charts, EMS Report forms, and wristbands will assist in providing this information to other healthcare providers.

An excellent resource for information about latex allergies exists at:
http://pw2.netcom.com/~nam1/latex_allergy.html

HYPERVENTILATION OF PATIENTS WITH HEAD INJURIES

For more than 20 years hyperventilation was considered the standard of care for the treatment of head injuries. Hyperventilation reduces raised intracranial pressure by causing cerebral vasoconstriction and reduction in cerebral blood flow by reducing the level of CO_2 in the blood. Therefore, it was thought that by constricting cerebral blood vessels and reducing the amount of blood in the brain would give the injured brain more room to "swell" which would reduce the overall intracranial pressure. Control of cerebral acidosis and reduction of elevated intracranial pressure were thought to be beneficial side effects. A rate of 24 or more breaths/minute for adults was advised.

Current research and technological capabilities have suggested that hyperventilation may do more harm than good. It has been shown that hyperventilation does indeed reduce cerebral blood flow, however, this reduced flow has now been shown to produce or exacerbate cerebral ischemia. Cerebral ischemia may harm otherwise viable neurons resulting in further brain damage.

In conclusion, head injured patients with reduced levels of consciousness should receive high levels of oxygen, but at a rate that would not result in hypocapnia (decreased level of CO_2 in the blood). Patients should only be hyperventilated if signs of cerebral herniation are present.

Hyperventilation may be defined as:

Adults ≥ 20 breaths /minute
Children ≥ 30 breaths /minute
Infants ≥ 35 breaths /minute

Signs of Increased intracranial pressure (ICP):

Level one of ICP (hyperventilation is indicated):

Blood pressure rises
Pulse rate slows
Abnormal respiratory pattern - Cheyne-Stokes
Localizes painful stimuli then progresses to only withdrawing from painful stimuli
Decorticate posturing (flexion of upper extremities and rigid lower extremities)

Level two of ICP (few patients recover with normal cerebral function):

Blood pressure continues to rise
Pulse continues to slow
Pupils may become fixed or react sluggishly
Abnormal respiratory pattern continues - central neurogenic hyperventilation
May exhibit decerebrate posturing (extension of the extremities)

Level three of ICP (last stage):

Blood pressure drops
Pulse become rapid and irregular
One or both pupils become dilated and fixed
Respirations may become ataxic (erratic)or absent
No response to painful stimuli and extremities become flaccid

***Any combination of these levels is possible

GLASGOW COMA SCALE

A patient would assume a comatose state due to trauma, metabolic, toxicological reasons such as inadequate oxygen and glucose to the brain or excessive carbon dioxide due to inadequate breathing, ingestion of poisons or drugs, etc. Evaluation of the depth of a coma can aid in the diagnosis and suggest treatments and prognosis. The most widely accepted method of evaluating a coma is the Glasgow Coma Scale. Originally published in 1974 by Teasedale and Jennett they suggested a scale for the assessment of coma and impaired consciousness. Originally promoted for use in hospitals by doctors, it has made its way to the prehospital setting and its use is taught to both paramedics and EMTs.

Essentially the GCS has the clinician give a <u>stimulus</u> to the patient and look for (and record) the <u>patient's response</u>. These stimulations range from nothing (spontaneous response) to the application of a painful stimuli. The less stimulation needed the less the depth of coma and presumably the better the patient outcome will be. The correlation of numbers to behaviors can be used to document and track a patient's progress (or lack of progress) and direct the therapeutic regimen.

GLASGOW COMA SCALE			LOS ANGELES COUNTY GLASGOW COMA SCALE		
Eye Opening			**Eye Opening**		
Spontaneous	4		Spontaneous	4	
To Voice	3		To Verbal Command	3	
To Pain	2		To Pain	2	
None	1		No Response	1	
Verbal Response			**Motor Response**		
Oriented	5		Obedient	6	
Confused	4		Purposeful	5	
Inappropriate Words	3		Withdraws	4	
Incomprehensible Words	2		Flexion	3	
None	1		Extension	2	
			No Response	1	
Motor Response			**Verbal Response**		
Obeys Command	6		Oriented	5	
Localizes Pain	5		Confused	4	
Withdraws (pain)	4		Inappropriate Words	3	
Flexion (pain)	3		Incomprehensible Sounds	2	
Extension (pain)	2		No Response	1	
None	1				

EYE INJURIES
PATCHING ONE EYE vs BOTH EYES

Eye injuries that are treatable in the field come in two varieties. Chemical burns and trauma (blunt & penetrating). In chemical burn situations the treatment is to throughly flush out the eye with water. This flushing process is generally done to both eyes and can take some time, so it is continued enroute and patching one or both eyes is not an issue. However, when it comes to trauma, the decision to patch one eye or both exists.

A traumatic force to the eye may result in a potential for many different types of injuries that range from corneal abrasions to detached retinas. Sometimes trauma can produce obvious injuries such as impalement, extrusion or enucleation, but in most cases only a detailed exam in a hospital, using specialized equipment, can evaluate the extent of the injury.

Use of an eye patch has been the treatment of choice for years. A patch covers any open wound and prevents further contamination or infection and if properly applied, it can prevent the expulsion of ocular humors through a global laceration by avoiding external pressure. *But should just the affected eye be patched or should both eyes be covered?*

A decrease in movement of the affected eye is seen as being beneficial. It has been argued that by covering both eyes you would prevent the spontaneous movement that occurs in the affected eye because of the mechanism that links both eyes for stereoscopic vision. While decreasing the movement of the injured eye can be beneficial, studies have shown that patching both eyes does not reduce spontaneous eye movement, but may increase the anxiety and fear of the patient.

Patching both the injured and uninjured eye in the field causes "immediate blindness". Anyone who suffers an eye injury immediately wonders and fears that it is going to cause blindness. The act of intentionally causing blindness as a routine part of the treatment reinforces the patient's greatest fear and can cause panic. Panicked patients cannot answer questions effectively and are slow or incapable at following instructions. This makes patient management much harder. Safe ambulation is impaired and any other treatment or procedure must be explained more completely before instituting them (IV attempts, or even oxygen administration) which takes more time. Therefore, it is recommend that unless there is an injury that affects both eyes that requires patching, the prehospital provider should patch only the affected eye.

COOLING MEASURES IN PEDIATRIC PATIENTS

Body temperature is monitored and regulated by the anterior hypothalamus which acts as a thermostat by altering the balance of heat production and heat loss via the sympathetic nervous system. Fever results when the thermoregulatory set point in the hypothalamus is shifted upward. Fever is initiated as part of the inflammatory response by interleukin-1 and prostaglandin E2.

Fevers are a natural physical reaction to infectious disease and bodily stress. It has been seen as both a symptom of infection and as a disease in and of itself. Theories for its control and eradication range from doing nothing (it helps fight the infection) to aggressive treatment to lower the temperature (high temperatures are the underlying cause of febrile seizures). It has not yet been conclusively shown in the scientific literature whether the benefits of antipyretic (temperature reduction) therapy outweigh the risks in the treatment of the underlying cause.

Fever can be reduced by peripheral cooling (convection and evaporation being shown to be better than conduction), but because of the underlying physiology, the preferred treatment is with antipyretic medication. The medications indicated are aspirin (carries a high risk of Reyes Syndrome in pediatric patients), acetaminophen and ibuprofen. Prior to the development of these medications, physical cooling measures both active and passive were the only available treatment.

Active cooling involves the bathing or sponging with tepid water (ice cold water or alcohol should never be used). Passive cooling is defined as exposing skin to ambient temperatures. These measures are low cost and readily available, thus they were readily incorporated into the common sense, lay public treatment for fever.

In the prehospital setting, the limitations and risks of the use of medications resulted in using active and passive cooling measures as the 'standard of care' for routine treatment of fever in children. However, active cooling measures may result in an increased discomfort level, hypothermia and shivering thus further compromising the condition of the pediatric patient. In addition, unless antipyretic medications are given in conjunction with active cooling measures, the temperature may return and rise rapidly possibly resulting in a febrile seizure. Therefore, due to the risks involved in using active cooling measure, these methods are discouraged in prehospital care and <u>*passive cooling*</u> *(exposing the skin to air without an evaporation medium), being the safest alterative, is encouraged.*

PREHOSPITAL TREATMENT OF THERMAL BURNS

A thermal burn is a traumatic injury that affects the largest organ of the body — the skin. This makes it the worst 'single mechanism' trauma that can affect the body. Burn victims rarely die immediately from their burn injuries (immediate death from a burn situation generally comes in the form of an inhalation injury).

Burn patients generally succumb much later from complications arising from an inability of the skin to perform its biological tasks (i.e. temperature regulation, fluid containment, and infection barrier) Death comes from conditions as diverse as sepsis to suicide due to altered body image. The time from injury to death can be years in some cases.

The best method for treating a burn injury is to perform an intervention that will preserve as much of the remaining skin tissues as possible. There are direct benefits in reducing the depth of a burn injury and preserving as much unburned healthy tissue as possible. Burn treatment is related to the depth and area of a burn injury.

Treatments are traditionally classified based on determining whether the burn is a first, second or third degree (superficial, partial or full thickness). Unfortunately burn injuries always transition near their periphery and except in cases of incineration, a third degree full thickness injury will be surrounded by a second degree partial thickness and a first degree superficial burn at the demarcation line between healthy tissue and the burn injury. This can complicate care as treatments are slightly different depending upon the injury.

In all cases of a thermal burn the burning process <u>MUST</u> be stopped. Flames must be extinguished and the burning process within the tissues stopped. This is best accomplished with cool water. In cases of either minor or major body surface area (BSA) involvement, cooling should be started immediately and submersion and the use of soaking wet dressings for transport should be avoided. Never use ice or ice cold water for cooling.

Pain is a significant problem in superficial and partial thickness burns. There is no reliable method of determining exactly when the underlying burning process has been stopped. Traditionally a decrease in pain has been the most significant indicator of a reduction in the burning process. Even though there is no direct evidence that cool moist dressings actually reduce pain, the cooling sensation is sometimes a psychological benefit to the patient. EMTs do not have pharmacological methods of analgesia available to them nor is the use of analgesia routinely utilized by paramedics. Therefore continued application of cool water/wet dressings was the method used, in prehospital care, to control pain.

Unfortunately the over zealous application of water in burn situations carries its own risks. The greater the depth of the burn, the greater the potential for complications.

1. <u>Hypothermia</u> - damaged skin cannot regulate temperature effectively. When coupled with the very effective method of evaporation (and conduction) that happens when cool water is applied, a burn patient is more susceptible to hypothermia. This is further complicated of the addition of significant amounts of intravenous infusions that are given as part of intra-hospital therapy. The infused fluids are generally not warmed, thus further complicating the problem which began in the prehospital setting and the patient may be severely compromised.

2. <u>Maceration of tissue cells</u> - when cells are exposed to or submerged in water for extended periods of time, there is a reduction in the tensile strength and the cells soften which can increase the tendency toward destruction and tearing. Burn damaged skin can be expected to react quicker and more severely. Therefore, the continuous application of water to a burn injury can increase the injury and complicate the healing process and should be avoided.

Initial cooling of a burn injury is recommended then transporting the patient with dry dressings should be done as soon as possible. Sterile dressings are appropriate to minimize the possibility of infection, however if field conditions are not conducive to maintenance of sterility, a clean dressing should be maintained.

Transportation of patients with severe burns to the nearest facility or trauma center is of the utmost importance for stabilization. In Los Angeles county, burn beds are limited and beds may not be available and often these centers may not be equipped to handle the other emergency situations that may accompany these injuries. Therefore, patients should not be initially transported to a burn center unless directed by the base hospital or the Medical Alert Center.

Bleeding Control

Blood loss is often associated with soft tissue injury and may be either subtle or dramatic. Damage to arteries, veins or capillaries or a combination of vessels can result in life-threatening hemorrhage. Arterial bleeding is usually described as bright red and spurting; venous bleeding is dark reddish-blue and steadily flowing; capillary bleeding is bright red and oozing and may subside spontaneously. Regardless of where the bleeding is coming from it should be controlled. Control of bleeding takes priority over initiating IV access. No matter how minor the bleeding may appear, loss of red blood cells may result in loss of oxygen carrying potential, shock and ultimately lead to death.

Recently the EMS Agency has received questions regarding the appropriate treatment of bleeding in prehospital care. Traditionally control has been performed by the following sequential steps.
- Apply direct pressure over the wound using a sterile dressing
- Elevate the extremity while continuing to apply direct pressure
- Apply a pressure dressing (adding additional dressings if needed)
- Compress appropriate pressure points
- Immobilize the bleeding extremity and use an air splint or pneumatic pressure device
- Apply a tourniquet as a last resort

Direct pressure remains the recommended initial step in bleeding control. Most bleeding is controlled in 4-6 minutes. Direct pressure may involve use of finger tips or may require hand pressure. Providing pressure to the area and directly compressing the vessels decreases the blood flow and allows for the formation of a clot. Pressure must still be held after a dressing has been applied. If the dressing becomes saturated, it <u>must not be removed</u> as this may cause dislodgement of a clot that has started to form and lead to further bleeding. Additional dressings should be applied over the original dressing as needed.

If direct pressure is not successful in controlling the bleeding, then the next step recommended is to raise the extremity above the level of the heart. Direct pressure must still be continued since elevation alone will not stop bleeding. Caution must be used if there is a suspected fracture as elevating the extremity may result in converting a closed fracture to an open fracture and increased bleeding. If direct pressure and elevation has not controlled the bleeding, a pressure dressing should be applied (using elastic wraps) over the original dressings.

If direct pressure and elevation have not controlled the bleeding, the next step suggested is compressing appropriate pressure points, splinting the extremity and applying pneumatic pressure devices. However, no research has been published to support the effectiveness of elevation or the use of pressure points in slowing the blood flow. Therefore, some advocates believe that elevation and providing manual pressure directly over pulse pressure points are not practical steps and tourniquets should be applied early if direct pressure and use of a pressure dressing have not been effective.

The use of tourniquets may be used if all the above measures have failed. Caution must be used in the application of tourniquets since their use may cause damage to nerves, muscle, blood vessels and soft tissue resulting in the potential for loss of the extremity. However, this does not preclude the use of a tourniquet earlier if bleeding is perfuse or the extremity is so severely injured that it is determined a tourniquet is needed. Application of tourniquets is safe when applied properly. A wide bandage must be used and secured tightly to prevent cutting into the skin and underlying tissue. Once a tourniquet is applied, it should not be loosened or removed in the field without approval of a physician. The goal is to save a life, even at the expense of potentially losing a limb.

UCLA CENTER FOR PREHOSPITAL CARE

EMT-B
Skills
Progression

UCLA EMT PROGRAM
PSYCHOMOTOR PROGRESSION

Psychomotor Skill	Demo	Supervised Practice	Unsupervised Practice	Independent Study / Practice	Competency
BLS/CPR SKILLS					
• ONE PERSON ADULT					
• TWO PERSON ADULT					
• CHILD					
• INFANT					
• FBOA – ADULT, CHILD, INFANT					
• AUTOMATED EXTERNAL DEFIBRILLATION (AED)					
AIRWAY / BREATHING SKILLS					
• AIRWAY ADJUNCTS / SUCTIONING:					
o AIRWAY OPENING – MEDICAL					
o AIRWAY OPENING – TRAUMA					

Psychomotor Skill	Demo	Supervised Practice	Unsupervised Practice	Independent Study / Practice	Competency
○ NASOPHARYNGEAL AIRWAY					
○ NASOPHARYNGEAL SUCTIONING					
○ OROPHARYNGEAL AIRWAY					
○ OROPHARYNGEAL SUCTIONING					
○ SUCTIONING - TRACHEOSTOMY TUBE					
• OXYGEN THERAPY:					
○ MASK					
○ NC					
○ BLOW-BY					
○ TANK					

Psychomotor Skill	Demo	Supervised Practice	Unsupervised Practice	Independent Study / Practice	Competency
• VENTILATION:					
o POCKET MASK					
o COMBITUBE OR ET TUBE WITH A BAG-VALVE-DEVICE					
o BAG-VALVE-MASK DEVICE					
o FLOW RESTRICTED OXYGEN POWERED VENTILATION DEVICE					
• BREATH SOUNDS:					
o AUSCULTATION					
o AUDITORY					
• PULSE OXIMETRY					

UCLA CPC / EMT